SEARCHING FOR DR. HARRIS

STUDIES IN SOCIAL MEDICINE

Allan M. Brandt, Larry R. Churchill, and Jonathan Oberlander, editors

This series publishes books at the intersection of medicine, health, and society that further our understanding of how medicine and society shape one another historically, politically, and ethically. The series is grounded in the convictions that medicine is a social science, that medicine is humanistic and cultural as well as biological, and that it should be studied as a social, political, ethical, and economic force.

A complete list of books published in Studies in Social Medicine is available at https://uncpress.org/series/studies-social-medicine.

SEARCHING FOR DR. HARRIS

The Life and Times of a Remarkable
African American Physician

MARGARET HUMPHREYS

THE UNIVERSITY OF NORTH CAROLINA PRESS
Chapel Hill

© 2024 Margaret Humphreys

The text of this book is licensed under a Creative Commons AttributionNonCommercial-NoDerivatives 4.0 International License: https://creativecommons.org/licenses/by-nc-nd/4.0/

Designed by Jamison Cockerham
Set in Arno, Irby, and Cutright
by codeMantra

Manufactured in the United States of America

Cover art: Howard's Grove Military Hospital,
courtesy of Chicago Historical Society.

Complete Library of Congress Cataloging-in-Publication Data for this title is available at https://lccn.loc.gov/2024020847.

ISBN 978-1-4696-8005-7 (cloth: alk. paper)
ISBN 978-1-4696-8006-4 (pbk.: alk. paper)
ISBN 978-1-4696-8007-1 (epub)
ISBN 978-1-4696-8234-1 (pdf)

Publication of this open monograph was the result of Duke University's participation in TOME (Toward an Open Monograph Ecosystem), a collaboration of the Association of American Universities, the Association of University Presses, and the Association of Research Libraries. TOME aims to expand the reach of long-form humanities and social science scholarship including digital scholarship. Additionally, the program looks to ensure the sustainability of university press monograph publishing by supporting the highest quality scholarship and promoting a new ecology of scholarly publishing in which authors' institutions bear the publication costs. Funding from Duke University Libraries made it possible to open this publication to the world.

FOR TED,

MY GENIAL COMPANION,

AS ALWAYS,

FOR EVERYTHING

CONTENTS

List of Illustrations ix

Acknowledgments xi

INTRODUCTION 1

1 The Formative Years 17

2 The Migration to Ohio 34

3 Poetry and Politics 45

4 Revolution in Cleveland, 1858–1859 71

5 The Anglo-African Empire 88

6 Colonizing the Caribbean 110

7 The Great Transition, 1862–1864 134

8 Family Ties in Reconstruction, 1864–1869 151

9 Medicine and Politics, 1864–1869 172

10 Finding a Professional Home 198

11 A Roaring Fire, a Fading Light 215

CONCLUSION 243

Notes 251

Bibliography 281

Index 295

ILLUSTRATIONS

FIGURES

Dr. J. D. Harris, 1868 *xvi*

Public market in Fayetteville,
North Carolina, ca. 1930 *59*

Artibonite River valley, Haiti *125*

US Marine Hospital, Cleveland, Ohio *138*

Howard's Grove Hospital, Richmond, Virginia *147*

Fredericksburg, Virginia, ca. 1863 *184*

Republican candidate card for the
1869 election in Virginia *191*

South Carolina Lunatic Asylum, Columbia *201*

Room in Poplar Ward, St. Elizabeths
Hospital, Washington, DC *221*

Black patients making up a work
crew at St. Elizabeths *224*

MAP

Haiti *126*

ACKNOWLEDGMENTS

During the twenty years of this book's research and construction, an abundance of institutions and individuals assisted in its creation and improved its final form. The Duke History Department is generous in its support of faculty, and I was no exception. Frequent sabbaticals, travel money, and congeries of helpful and interested colleagues did much to encourage the project's ultimate completion. My academic appointment spans arts and sciences and the Duke medical school; in the latter my intellectual home is in the Trent Center for Bioethics, Humanities, and History of Medicine. Jeremy Sugarman, Peter English, and I helped birth the Trent Center in the early 2000s. Now it has grown to include narrative medicine, poetry and medicine, and multiple other enriching approaches to the phenomenon of medical care. Having such colleagues has in turn broadened my appreciation of caring in all its aspects. Jeffrey Baker, the current head of the center, has been unstinting in his support and enthusiasm for this project. My academic chair (the Josiah Charles Trent Chair for the History of Medicine) "lives" in the Trent Center and has provided me with designated research time and, occasionally, financial support for research assistants. For all this help, and confidence, I am grateful.

Fellowships and sabbaticals brought relief from teaching responsibilities and offered me open time to continue this work. In particular, a Frederick Burkhardt Residential Fellowship (ACLS) at the National Humanities Center, 2004–5, allowed me the opportunity and the desktop microfilm reader to thoroughly review the United States Sanitary Commission papers produced by the New York Public Library. A National Library of Medicine publication grant gave me time off from teaching in order to complete my work on *Intensely Human: The Health of the Black Soldier in the American Civil War* (2008), which has a chapter on the Black doctors who served in the Civil War, including a short section on Dr. Harris. Grants from the Trent Center funded two postdoc assistants—Shauna Devine and Marie Hicks—who cheerfully performed manuscript tasks great and small.

This work in turn attracted the attention of Jill Newmark, who was mounting an exhibition on the history of African American doctors at the National Library of Medicine. Her exhibit (and subsequent book) enriched my knowledge of the ways the US Civil War created opportunities for Black physicians. Jill also found a reference to J. D. Harris's *Love and Law, South and West*, sent me a reproduced copy, and opened up a new chapter of J. D.'s life for me. And she recently published a book drawn from her exhibit research on the lives of Black Civil War surgeons. All told, she has been a wonderful partner in this path of discovery.

It is hard to imagine a more congenial group of colleagues than those of the Duke History Department. While I had trouble convincing some editors of the intrinsic value of this work, my History Department friends were often "rah-rah" in support. John Martin told me repeatedly, "You have to write this." Thomas Robisheaux led a microhistory group ("Microlab") that introduced me to the concept of creating a narrative out of multiple, disparate sources. John Hope Franklin held a Duke History Department appointment in his later years when I had the privilege of meeting him. His book *The Free Negro in North Carolina, 1790–1860* (1943) was pivotal in my own understanding of the town where Harris was born and of the times in which he lived.

The chairs of the History Department over the years that this book was in progress were important in facilitating my time off for research and writing. In particular, I appreciate the support of Sally Deutsch, John Martin, Simon Partner, and Sumathi Ramaswamy. One colleague who made a key intervention was Ed Balleisen, who now spends much of his time away from the department managing the Bass Fellowships out of the main administration building. But on one lucky day when the stars aligned, I happened to see him in the faculty lounge checking his mail. He posed interested questions about the Harris research and then asked me, "Are you using Ancestry.com to find these people?" This suggestion opened the world of nineteenth-century online genealogical research to me, which added great depth to my understanding of the Harris family history.

Other colleagues at Duke offered friendship, encouragement, and collegiality that built my sense of intellectual community. These wonderful people include Jean O'Barr, Priscilla Wald, Diane Nelson, Peter English, Alex Roland, Kristen Neuschel, Claudia Koonz, Sally Deutsch, Reeve Huston, Peter Wood, Elizabeth Fenn, John Thompson, and Jack Cell. More recently Thavolia Glymph, Laura Lieber, Helen Softerer, Dirk Bonker, Adriane Lentz-Smith, Nicole Barnes, Phil Stern, Reeve Huston, and James Chappell have offered friendship and intellectual richness to my academic life. I presented talks on this project at the Franklin Humanities Center and the History of Medicine Library and appreciated feedback and ideas from colleagues there.

Any historian owes an enormous debt to librarians, a term I use broadly here for all the workers who make historical sources more accessible to researchers. The projects that have scanned thousands of books, including many nineteenth-century sources useful herein, have greatly shortened research time. I remember the pivotal moment when I was walking out to my car to go yet again to the library to find an old book when I said to myself, "Duh! It is probably already online." And it was. The librarians at the New York Public Library who scanned the US Sanitary Commission Records and then made them available for purchase enabled my deep research into that topic. Other librarians at the National Archives launched a massive project to scan the papers of the Freedmen's Bureau, which in turn were available to me toward the end of this research.

Librarians at Duke have made it easier to find Dr. Harris and understand relevant background. Elizabeth Dunn came up to me after I gave a very preliminary talk on Dr. Harris at the medical school and said simply, "I know who his father was." She then referred me to Catherine Bishir's book *Crafting Lives* (2013), which includes information about Jacob Harris. Carson Holloway and Kelly Lawton were able, cheerful, and patient in facilitating my use of Lilly Library. Rachel Ingold, the Duke History of Medicine Librarian, was always ready to help with specific questions or refer me to other staff in Perkins Library as need be. And the librarian in Perkins (whose name I did not record, alas) who forgave me and my new puppy for the damage he did to an old book will always be dear to my heart.

Special thanks are due to those who granted permission to use the illustrations in this book. The Harris family has been one key source of photographs. Greg Harris (great-grandson via Thoro Harris) assembled a scrapbook of family images, including the photograph of J. D. Harris. This, in turn, came from his relative William Rippey of Portland, Oregon, who is a great-grandson of Worthie Harris. Greg's information was useful in guiding the biographical information about J. D.'s family members.

The community of medical historians and editors beyond Duke has been an important source of support since I returned to academia in 1993. Judy Leavitt and Morris Vogel urged me to publish my first book on yellow fever and helped me over the barriers that seemed to block its path. Jackie Wehmueller at Johns Hopkins was a steady hand that guided my Civil War books into press, while Lucas Church at the University of North Carolina Press has been pivotal in seeing this book to production. The recent book exhibit at the American Association for the History of Medicine in Ann Arbor (2023) reminded me of the crucial role that academic presses play in building our field and binding us together.

That same meeting reinforced the strength of academic bonding among my peers. The list is long—so many conversations, invitations, and words of encouragement. It took the COVID shutdown to make me realize how isolated I would be without my AAHM friends and colleagues. I owe particular thanks to Jacalyn Duffin, Susan Lederer, Janet Golden, Susan Reverby, Nancy Tomes, Susan Lawrence, Gerry Oppenheimer, Joel Howell, John Harley Warner, Jim Downs, Richard Meckel, Wendy Kline, Marty Pernick, Ken Ludmerer, and Michael McVaugh. That recent meeting also brought home to me how many ghosts walked the halls with us, our mentors who are there in memory—and the many anecdotes stored in our memories. (Do you remember the time when Bob Joy . . . ?) Wendy Kline still has *that* drawing and holds it in readiness.

Ann Carmichael deserves special mention. She has been my companion in navigating the strange world of genomics and disease history and shares my new passion for the history of food. Duke professor Charles Nunn and the evolutionary medicine group have likewise kept my academic interests alive and growing in new directions.

My family had a deep impact on this project, more than I can adequately describe here. It all began with my mother (of course!). Mary Humphreys fought the racism of our small southern town without fear or timidity. She had worked with Howard Baker in college at the University of Tennessee (back when Republicans were liberals compared with the Southern Dixiecrats) and brought that sense of public duty to her newly married home in Paris, Henry County, Tennessee. She became part of the 1960 census process in Henry County and outed the local customs of both "voting the graveyard" and limiting the Black vote. She volunteered to teach English at the local Black high school. (Schools there were not integrated until the mid-1960s.) She found Black high school students who couldn't read and brought in elementary school reading books to teach them rather than just "pass the students on." Both my brother, Brooks, and I heard taunts of "N——lover" in our childhood. And we both grew up committed to civil rights. This book is a direct outcome of that childhood family value.

My son, William, is, if anything, even more attuned to structural racism and especially to the ways it emerges in historical texts. He copyedited parts of this manuscript and explained to me why I couldn't use this or that language (even though it had been the norm in prior decades). My husband and I funded the best education we could here in Durham, North Carolina—and he has responded by schooling us in the greater sensitivities needed in the modern age. He has taught me so much—about life, about motherhood, about myself. Thanks, Will.

But now I come to the hardest paragraph to write, because words are so inadequate. My husband, Ted Kerin, could not have been more supportive of my historical work over the years. He has been my technological consultant in too many ways to count. He managed to overcome my innate Luddism over and over in both my teaching (videos in class!) and at my writer's desk. His skills in visual arts perfected the beautiful images included in this book. But most importantly he is the calm harbor from all my emotional storms. He talks me down off the ledge. He is the perfect anodyne to my anxieties and blues. He shares my quirky, irreverent sense of humor (much needed to read the news of modern day). And he brought home two very silly goldendoodles, whose antics are a reliable cure for writer's block. This is undeniably his book. Thanks.

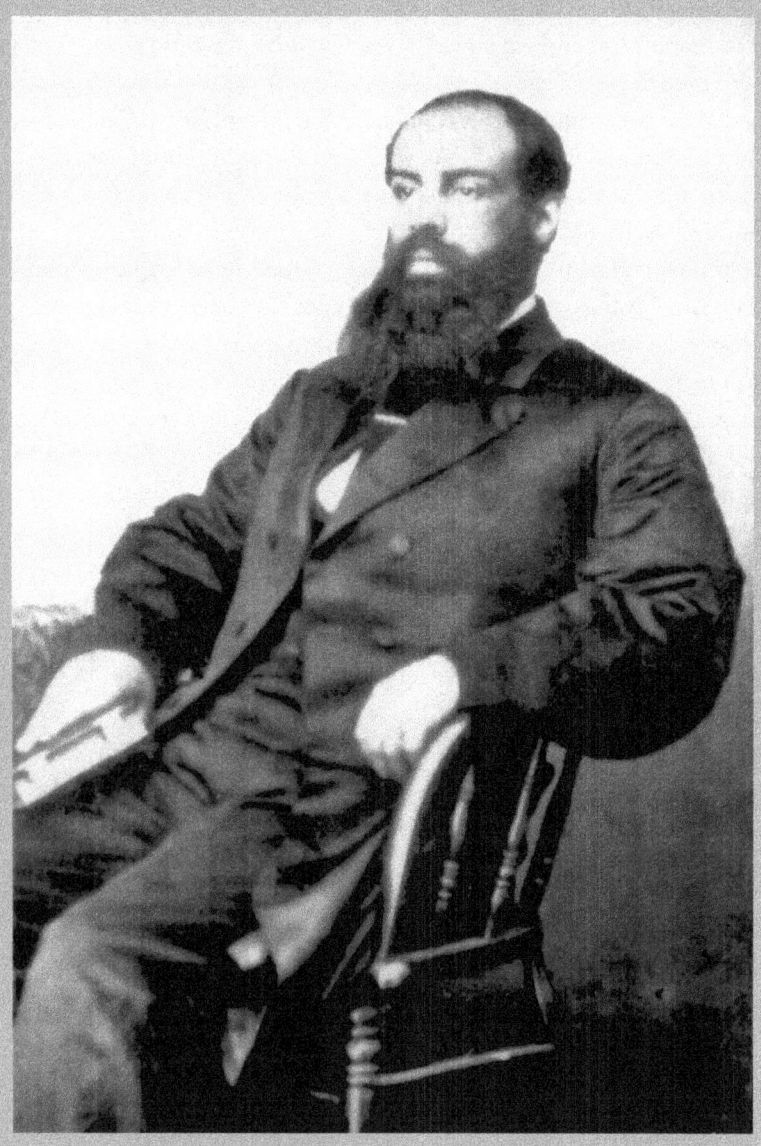

Dr. J. D. Harris, 1868.
Courtesy of William Rippey, MD.

SEARCHING FOR DR. HARRIS

Introduction

It was a chilly fall day in 2004 when I first met Dr. Harris. He was waiting for me in the faded microfilm images of an 1865 handwritten report by Dr. Ira Russell. Russell, a former US Army surgeon, had been asked by the US Sanitary Commission to survey the conditions of freedmen's hospitals in the former Confederate states. Russell himself had managed exemplary hospital wards for sick and injured Black Union troops during the war, so he was a natural choice to investigate how those men as well as the freed slaves were faring in the months following Appomattox.[1] As he walked through the shady trees toward the largest building of Howard's Grove Hospital in Richmond, Virginia, Russell must have wondered about the coming encounter. Was such a thing really possible in the suburbs of Richmond, conquered or no—a Black doctor working in the heart of the old Confederacy? Dr. Russell indeed found Dr. Harris at the hospital for freedmen in the early fall of 1865. The hospital, Russell observed, was "neat, orderly and well located." Its managing surgeon was one "Dr. Harris, a very intelligent colored gentleman from Cleveland Ohio." Russell noted that Harris had seen "a good deal of service, [was] familiar with the peculiarities of his race, and deeply interested in its elevation and welfare."[2]

Dr. Harris was unknown not only to me at that point but to the larger field of medical historians. He was not included on the short list of known Black physicians in the war enumerated by historians around 2005.[3] I was immediately curious about this man, but Russell never even mentioned his first name. How could I track down a person with such an infuriatingly common last name? The game was afoot! It was a thrill discovering that his initials were J. D., and later that these stood for Joseph Dennis. Even learning his life span dates (ca. 1833–84) was an illumination. At every step of the way, historians, librarians, archivists, and curators aided this quest. At one early lecture I gave on Dr. Harris, a librarian told me, "I know who his father was." At another, two graduate students came forward to say that they had read his records at St. Elizabeths Hospital for the mentally ill. Jill Newmark, then a curator at the National Library of Medicine creating an exhibit on Black doctors in the war, not only found the Harris photograph used as the frontispiece of this book but also ferreted out his published poem that underlies the story arc in chapter 3.[4] This volume represents the outcome of that long search, drawn from myriad archival and textual sources. It indeed took a village to raise this child.

My journey is entrenched in the methods and ideals of the social history of medicine. From the 1980s, the young firebrands studying the history of medicine and public health in American graduate programs dedicated themselves to foregrounding everyone *but* the "great white men" who had dominated the historical narrative to date. One seminal work that described the ambitions of this "turn" was an essay by Susan Reverby and David Rosner titled "Beyond 'the Great Doctors,'" published in the 1979 edited volume *Health Care in America: Essays in Social History*. They described a "new social history" that went beyond the "great man studies" written in the past. "This [new] history explicitly examines the growth and transformation of society's structures, institutions, and culture. Its current formulation has been shaped in part by contemporary political struggles," they explained. "The Civil Rights, Anti-War, and Women's movements all focused the historian's attentions on class and familial relations and the different historical experiences of minorities, women, and the working class."[5] They went on to admit the many challenges of such research. "In the absence of an abundance of the usual written sources to explore this history, social historians have turned to social science methodology, computer technology, and new sources of data such as manuscript censuses, city directories, and tax lists."[6]

There are many ways to perform "the social history of medicine," which remains the dominant paradigm in the academic history of medicine field. In 2018 I participated in a Society for Social Medicine conference in Liverpool where the conjoiner asked various scholars to define their view of the social history of medicine. While other panelists talked about studying institutions, actions of the state, and so on, I said that what distinguished social history is *whom* we study and *who* we think are worthy of historical attention.[7] Social historians ask different questions, value different events, and focus on different subjects than the more traditional "great man" history of medicine or traditional political history. In this case, by this book, I declare that the life of J. D. Harris was important. Even though he did not discover penicillin or lead the troops at Fort Wagner, there is glory in his story just the same.

Why is this life story worth telling? He overcame daunting structural racism that sought to block his ambitions at every turn, and he succeeded beyond any expectation that could have been formulated for this Black boy born free in rural North Carolina. This story both reveals these triumphs and illuminates why such success became possible in his time and place. It also shows the barriers that continued to limit the access to medical training and practice for Black men (and women) in nineteenth-century America. And, as I said at the Liverpool conference, "He is inspirational for medical students of colour, who should know that such heroes existed, even at the time of slavery."[8]

This book is a concrete proclamation that "Black lives matter." Yes, this phrase is the rallying cry of a modern movement that laments the large number of Black people killed by police in the United States and demands police reform. But I use it here as a reinvocation of the historiography that emerged in the mid-twentieth-century historical writings of John Hope Franklin and others. Each new generation of students needs to hear it again, to understand the lives of Black people of mid-nineteenth-century America, free and enslaved, and how such history continues to shape our modern polity.

This volume extends my prior work on the social history of race and disease in America. My first two books, *Yellow Fever and the South* (1992) and *Malaria: Poverty, Race and Public Health in the United States* (2001), explored the intersections of epidemic disease, poverty, and race within the political structures of the American South as well as the growing influence of federal public health measures in resolving them. Poverty was especially relevant to malaria and the misery of frontier and sharecropper lives, white and Black.

In my third and fourth books I drew on the voluminous records of the American Civil War in the US National Archives and elsewhere to illuminate the experiences of patients during that conflict. In 1990 Maris A. Vinovskis had published the provocative essay "Have Social Historians Lost the Civil War? Some Preliminary Demographic Speculations." Within military history the parallel of "great doctors" research is a focus on generals and battles and strategy. As with the Reverby and Rosner essay, the emergence of the social history of war was already well underway by the time that Vinovskis called for more of it. I answered that summons. In the first of these volumes, *Intensely Human: The Health of the Black Soldier in the American Civil War* (2008), I searched for information on the medical experiences of Black troops during the war. They were mostly served by white surgeons, although there were a few Black surgeons who cared for them. There is a short section on Dr. Harris in this volume.

The common paths of social history carry through into my more general history of Civil War medicine, *Marrow of Tragedy: The Health Crisis of the American Civil War* (2013). Here again the focus is not on great men or great battles but on the social determinants of medical care and medical outcomes, north and south. Chapters on the US Sanitary Commission, an exercise in applying the principles of public health to wartime conditions, continued another theme of social history of medicine. And the prominence of women in the care of sick troops is emphasized, especially in northern hospitals.

My research led me to Jill Newmark, a National Library of Medicine curator and historian who asked me to participate in an exhibit on the Black doctors who served in the Civil War. She has extended that work in her recently published book that chronicles what can be discovered about the Black surgeons who served the US Colored Troops during the war.[9] She could find only 14 Black surgeons (including Dr. Harris) out of the 10,000-plus surgeons in the Union army. Her research has extended and deepened my project in multiple ways.

As I have wrestled with the central themes of my biography of Dr. Harris, I have arrived at two organizing structures. The first describes how he conquered the many barriers of structural racism that hindered his professional development. The second looks at him not just as an accomplished professional but as an intelligent Black observer of the tumultuous world of mid-nineteenth-century America. So I suppose this leads us to an old-fashioned "life and times" structure but one that yields, I think, interesting results.

This volume builds on an older literature about the rise of "medical professionalism" in the early to mid-nineteenth-century United States. Doctors had been advocating for societal recognition of the special knowledge that made their occupation a "profession." From the 1840s they fought for medical licenses limited to those who had a "regular" medical training, and they created organizations such as the American Medical Association to mark this distinction through its membership. These special indicators recognized those with such a license as "official healers" that to some degree limited the rights of others to practice. This fight goes back at least to medieval Paris, when the "learned physicians" who had a university degree and could discourse in Latin sought a license from the Paris authorities to prevent those without such training from practicing medicine. They particularly disliked female practitioners, most notably a particular woman named Jacqueline who repeatedly ignored the law, delivering babies and distributing herbal remedies.[10] By the eighteenth century some professional order had been achieved in European cities, where physicians (Latin-educated college men), surgeons (technical men who had trained in English and often learned their trade in Scottish schools and the military), apothecaries (who made and sold remedies, including those ordered by physicians), and midwives (who cared for women and children) had been sorted. But this order was disrupted in the American colonies, where regularly trained medical men were scarce. Formal medical schools appeared in the American colonies only in the last half of the eighteenth century (at King's College in 1768 and Harvard in 1783), which left the colonies and nascent country wide open for a variety of practitioners.

Various medical labels emerged from styles of therapies. Those who emphasized herbal remedies might call themselves herbalists, Thomsonians, or later Eclectics. Herbal remedies (overlapping with "quack" potions) were widely available in fields and shops without prescription. Followers of homeopathy, based on the works of Samuel Hahnemann, could be found practicing in East Coast American cities, where they were popular with affluent women who might prefer their gentle remedies, especially for dosing babies. This cacophony pushed those physicians trained in formal medicine, tracing their roots back to Hippocrates, Galen, and the great medical professors of England and France, to take a stand as "regular" physicians and to demand that the state license them as such. Licenses per se may not have had all that much impact, especially in the frontier areas, but they became crucial during the Civil War. Those 10,000 men who acted as official government surgeons during the war had to demonstrate attendance at a "regular" medical school, training in a "regular" hospital, and allegiance to the "regular" medical formulary. The US and Confederate armies imposed a blanket new standard for orthodoxy.

Medical school admission became a major hurdle for Black people and women seeking entrance into the regular medical profession. Those sympathetic to women students responded by creating their own medical training sites, such as the New England Hospital for female physicians in Boston.[11] Eclectic medical colleges, which promoted the use of herbal remedies, were also likely to sell admission tickets to women. One such was Dr. Mary Walker, who even received a brief appointment with Union troops stationed in East

Tennessee toward the end of the Civil War.[12] Black activist Martin Delany challenged Harvard Medical School to admit him in 1850, and its professors did, along with two other African American students bound for Africa and supported by the American Colonization Society. To their shame, Harvard medical students rioted, and the admission was rescinded. Delany went on to be a major in the US Colored Troops during the Civil War but never returned to medicine. Other schools began to respond to abolitionism and sympathy for Black populations by admitting one or two African students during the Civil War. No one was stopping either women or Black people from being health care providers. No one questioned the mother caring for her child or husband; it was the woman caring for a strange (even naked!) man that caused vapors. Likewise, Black people were servants who attended the sick, north and south. But Black men tending white women? Or a Black man coming in the front door as a gentleman doctor ready to see a patient? No, that would not do, according to many. It was intolerable, if for no other reason than letting them formally into the medical profession would lower the status of all white men involved.

While in the present-day United States, women have met and even exceeded the number of men currently in medical training, there continues to be an underrepresentation of Black matriculants in medical schools, relative to their proportion of the US population. Although multiple efforts have been made in the first two decades of the twenty-first century to increase the number of Black medical students in this country, their proportion relative to their share of the general population has actually declined.[13] Valerie Montgomery Rice, MD, now president of Morehouse School of Medicine and crusader for modern reform in health inequities, has taken as her professional mission the medical education of African American students. But, as she emphasizes, remedying modern disparities in the health professions is all about the "pipeline." When she talks about the "pipeline," she is addressing the underperformance of Black students in American elementary and high schools, which leads to fewer attending college and even fewer being ready for medical education.[14]

Why does it matter if the race of the physician or other health care provider matches that of the patient? Two decades ago, a landmark study on racial and ethnic disparities in US health care reported that minorities "tend to receive a lower quality of healthcare than non-minorities, even when access-related factors, such as patients' insurance status and income, are controlled." When focusing on the health care encounter itself, the authors found "evidence that stereotyping, biases, and uncertainty on the part of healthcare providers can all contribute to unequal treatment." How to remedy this problem? "The healthcare workforce and its ability to deliver quality of care for racial and ethnic minorities can be improved substantially by increasing the proportion of underrepresented US racial and ethnic minorities among health professionals."[15]

This book is, in part, an account of how one Black man, whose parents had been born in slavery, managed to "stay in the pipeline" or "climb the ladder" or "jump the many hurdles" that characterized the path from childhood to medical graduation and practice. The 1850 US Census counted roughly 4 million Black people in the nation, slave and free. Again, only fourteen Black surgeons served in the US Civil War, and there were only a handful of identified Black physicians in the United States who did not serve. My study is an exploration of one such "success story." What challenges did he overcome that blocked others who might have followed his course? How did he navigate a narrow and perilous pipeline?

This book's explanation can be broken down into multiple steps: (1) he was born free and survived to adulthood; (2) he was literate, although he grew up in a state (North Carolina) where teaching Black people to read was illegal; (3) he acquired enough money to pursue a medical school degree (a period when his family thus did not have his wages for support); (4) he found a white preceptor to train him; (5) a medical school admitted him; (6) he found employment after completing the MD; (7) he found hospitals that would take "his" patients; (8) he could make enough money practicing medicine to support a family. He also participated in medical school teaching because of the existence of Howard University in Washington, DC. Perhaps we should also add to the list that he did not get arrested for his connection to the John Brown plot, and he did not get captured and "returned" to slavery, as some other free Black males did in the North.[16] This combination of characteristics was both unusual and time-limited. The Civil War opened doors to Black people that would close within a few years, such as employment of Black doctors by the US government and the opportunity to run for elected office in the South. There is no clear and lasting trajectory to success illumined here.

A second component of the biography is the opportunity to watch this intelligent, passionate man react to the overt racism of his day. In the early phases of his adult life he followed nonmedical paths seeking a place to grow and prosper, including time spent on the frontier in Iowa, involvement in antislavery activism in Cleveland, and a foray into Caribbean settlement. The idiosyncrasies of this man's thought reflect one intelligent viewpoint under omnipresent racism. He thought, for example, that Black people suffered less from the diseases of the tropics, such as malaria and yellow fever. While there are now known biological explanations for the differential malaria response, the decreased susceptibility of Africans to yellow fever remains contentious, especially since no modern scientific answer has been found. I reported that this assumption was common opinion in late nineteenth-century New Orleans in my book *Yellow Fever and the South*. Other scholars, such as Kathryn Olivarius, are convinced that this protection is not found among Black populations.[17] It is certainly possible that the "trait" represented childhood-acquired immunity. But my point here is that Dr. Harris believed it to be true. This does not mean that he had any time for the overtly racist medicine of Samuel Cartwright (who assigned the disease of "drapetomania" to slaves who ran away). Certainly, he would have agreed with Black physician James McCune Smith that physiological differences did not account for the poor health of many African Americans; rather, they were ill-fed and ill-treated.[18]

Harris also reported scenes of graphic racism presented by political candidates in 1855 Iowa, as well as the dignity and excitement of Black conventions in Ohio in the 1850s. He was gleeful about horrible scenes remembered from the Haitian Revolution (when Blacks slaughtered whites in creative ways). He recalled instances of slaves being beaten to death, the fear of being forced into slavery like Solomon Northup (recounted in Northup's *Twelve Years a Slave*), the literature on the female octoroon and her sexual licentiousness, and other demeaning and scary facts of life for the (even free) Black man in America. By the end of the 1850s he shared the despondency and fatalism of many free Blacks about life in the country. Harris was deeply wounded by the *Dred Scott* decision (which declared that no Black person could ever be a citizen of the United States). Months later he was on the periphery of the failed John Brown "conspiracy." His despair at life in the United States drove his decision to resettle in Haiti. There he dreamed of an Afro-American empire, where educated Blacks could lead the Caribbean islands to Protestant sobriety, modern farming, and settlement of African peoples in their "proper" clime. His commitment to "serve his people" after the Emancipation Proclamation echoed his brothers' work in teaching and preaching on the Virginia Peninsula. For him, medicine, rather than the Gospel, was the best way to help.

As I approached this project, I sought guidance in other biographies and autobiographies of prominent Black men and women of this period. Some patterns quickly emerged. Most such stories are about the accomplishments of escaped or liberated slaves. Dr. Harris was born free and came from a nuclear family of freed Black people. Unlike Frederick Douglass, for example, he had no thrilling story of escape to tell. Douglass also differed from Dr. Harris in that he made his living by writing and publishing; Douglass produced not one but three autobiographies over the course of his life.[19] While Dr. Harris wrote a self-revelatory long poem and published a travelogue about the Caribbean, he made his living first in the building trades and later as a physician. There is no published diary or autobiography to guide the historian. Another role model for this study was Jacalyn Duffin's *Langstaff: A Nineteenth-Century Medical Life*, which tells the story of an ordinary medical practitioner in Ontario. He kept meticulous notes on each patient, allowing Duffin to discern his reactions to medical innovations while also depicting the range of illness in a small farming community. A third model was Laurel Thatcher Ulrich's *A Midwife's Tale*, which uses the diary of Martha Ballard to describe her life and practice in northern New England from 1785 to 1812. Although both historians are telling the stories of "typical" but not "great" medical practitioners, in both cases they had rich primary sources to guide their studies.

My use of multiple records that provide intersecting details of the life of Dr. Harris moves this study into the realm of microhistory. This methodological strategy of historical research relies on the close reading of primary sources, such as legal documents, letters of all sorts, newspapers, government records, hospital notes, and often quite rare publications. It is easier now, in the age of broad digitization, to find searchable online archival caches; many of these were not even available when I started my quest. Some of the earliest overt microhistories focused on a single trial, particularly those for witchcraft or heresy, to unravel the social networks or belief systems of a given community and time. Paul Boyer and Stephen Nissenbaum's 1974 study sorted out the property and political disputes that underlay the Salem witchcraft trials in colonial Massachusetts, and Carlo Ginzburg made waves in 1976 with his account of a sixteenth-century miller accused of heresy.[20] Thomas Robisheaux continued this tradition by similarly dissecting the community that burned the last witch of Langenburg.[21] This list could be extended to books covering multiple contexts but with the common approach of seeking to understand the lives of persons, events, or phenomena existing in the lower ranks of the social hierarchy. Women, people of color, immigrants, the enslaved, the impoverished, the illiterate—all can be subject to this sort of "capture," if you will.

Microhistory as a method of historical practice is not limited to following one life story, but it has, in practice, significantly overlapped biography. Given the association of "great men" with past biographical practice, biography has at times been rejected by the academy as an "unloved stepchild" of the historical profession.[22] What is old is new again, however, as is often the case. Leaving the "great men" behind, newer biographies have abandoned political hagiography and instead used the structure of biography to explore race, gender, and social formation. As American historian Jessica Hauger argues, "Especially when informed by the ethic of micro historical primary source analysis, Biography shows how deeply historical context shapes a subject's self-concept and relationship to societal structures and sweeping historical processes."[23] This goal underlies every chapter of this volume.

The merger of microhistory and biography has been especially powerful in trying to recreate lives lived outside the white male spotlight: the history of women, the history of subordinated racial groups, and the women who were also people of color. Writing biographies of women has been a key way that historians have sought to resurrect their "hidden" histories, in America and elsewhere.[24] And, as I hope this study will illustrate, a biography grounded in microhistorical sources can illustrate the many multivalent experiences of state-sponsored racism in the everyday lives of mid-nineteenth-century Americans of color, free or enslaved.[25] Often, events are captured in minutiae—a two-line newspaper article, an unusually large hospital requisition, or a marriage license issued in an unlikely place—which reveal a much bigger story.

I present Dr. Harris's life chronologically, from birth to death, as is the custom in biography. Gaps are frequent and guesses are made, although both are clearly indicated as such. Several key questions guide the text. First and foremost, who was he? Or, putting it more accurately, how did a Black man achieve the medical training that put him on that hospital entrance in Richmond? How did he shape and reshape his own identity? What were the barriers to his accomplishments, and what were the enabling influences that allowed him to get there? There were very few African American surgeons in the mid-nineteenth-century United States, what we know of them is limited, and existing biographical work is accordingly brief. Achieving such status required a very difficult path. How did Dr. Harris find his way?

This approach is distinct from the deeply valuable work that looks at African peoples as healers throughout the Western Hemisphere. Gretchen Long's *Doctoring Freedom: The Politics of African American Medical Care in Slavery and Emancipation* is exemplary in this approach. This is an impressive book, but it does not cross my project as much as might be imagined. Her approach is patient-based, not physician-based. She acknowledges that there were some Black doctors in the Civil War and then cites my chapter on this topic in *Intensely Human*.[26] What Long and others do emphasize is the variety of Black healers in the United States before and after the Civil War. Here she joins Sharla Fett's *Working Cures*, Todd Savitt's *Medicine and Slavery*, and a more recent entrant with information drawn from the British records about the transatlantic slave trade: Manuel Barcia's *The Yellow Demon of Fever*. In the tradition of social histories of medicine cited above, these works focus on healers, not specifically physicians. Chris Willoughby and Sean Smith's edited volume, *Medicine and Healing in the Age of Slavery*, also has essays on folk traditions of healing throughout the Atlantic world. The Harris story is somewhat different, as he sought all of the requisite markers of professional attainment. Saying this is not to diminish the other healers—as I tell my history of medicine classes, the primary healers in families throughout history have been the women who have tended their kinfolk, not the doctors called when the usual remedies were not enough.

Returning to the Harris story, it is important to ask questions about distinctive personality formation and life course. What can we identify in his background that explains not only his accomplishments but those of several of his siblings? These questions highlight the values instilled in childhood about what a proper life course involved but also signpost differentiation from that family unit, made all the more necessary given his nine brothers and sisters. Harris reinvented himself multiple times. Sometimes this happened because he made a great effort to change, while at other times such transformation was forced upon him by society or his own biology. This book draws on no particular theory of identity formation. Rather, I think about how he would answer the question, at any given point in time, "Who are you?" In his North Carolina childhood, he was one of the Harris boys, African Americans born free to mixed-race, free parents, who pursued several construction trades. In Ohio and later Iowa, he wanted to be a fully free man and farmer, living apart from his family, with the same rights as whites, but he found instead multiple restraints on that ambition in the 1850s. By 1858 he was immersed in the radical antislavery movement in Cleveland, and a year later he was on the edge of a slave revolution, the failed John Brown insurrection.

J. D. Harris then abandoned the United States in despair (and fear) and turned to creating an agricultural utopia in Haiti or the Dominican Republic. He argued that modern farming techniques would provide great advantages for relocated Black Americans, so that together they would elevate the race and create a Black empire in the Caribbean as a home for African peoples. After publishing articles and the book *A Summer on the Borders of the Caribbean Sea*, he returned to the islands with a group of Black emigrants from the United States and worked to establish a colony for them in the Artibonite valley of Haiti. The Caribbean experiment failed for a variety of reasons, including poor settler skills and rampant disease, and the survivors returned home to the United States.

There, Harris pursued a new profession, one that would allow him to serve his people more effectively than the settlement. He decided to become a doctor. After medical training in Ohio (and Iowa?), he became a contract surgeon for the Union army (1864) and later for the Freedmen's Bureau (1865), with postings in southern Virginia. Those jobs, for an African American surgeon, had come into being only after the Emancipation Proclamation and the formation of Black regiments. Such was his reputation as an educated professional that it was not entirely surprising that the Republicans in Reconstruction Virginia nominated him in 1869 as a candidate for lieutenant governor. Even though this was a maneuver to actually help the other ticket, still he made a respectable showing. At that point he had another new identity as well—he had married a northern white woman who had served as a teacher among the newly freed slaves. After losing the election and at the end of his contract with the Freedmen's Bureau, Dr. Harris and his wife moved to South Carolina, where he garnered a political appointment (from Radical Republicans) as assistant physician at the state mental asylum in Columbia. Run out by the return of the "Redeemer" government there, he retreated with Elizabeth and their first child to Washington, DC, where he joined the new Howard University medical community and served as ward physician for the hospital affiliated with Howard Medical School. The District of Columbia had the largest educated Black community in the country, where the growing Harris family could comfortably fit in. Sad to say, after just a few years he began to show signs of illness. His end, at age fifty-one, was tragic. Under the ravages of insanity and epilepsy, Dr. Harris sank into dementia and death.

Having briefly sketched here the many identities that Dr. Harris assumed over the years, it is appropriate now to consider identity aspects that remained throughout his life. Two key qualities of his person, components always intertwined, were race and class. Given circumstances in antebellum America, race was *the* defining category for freedom and citizenship. Harris had been born free, but all around him were people who had been born enslaved and marked by the same skin color as himself. Some of them were his relatives. A free Black man found guilty in court could be bound over in servitude similar to slavery. And everyone knew stories like that of *12 Years a Slave* in which free men had been kidnapped and forced into slavery. Freedom was fragile for those marked with African blood, and even more so after the 1857 *Dred Scott* decision made it the law of the land that African Americans had none of the rights of white Americans. So, Harris learned that a Black American was a man without a country, a man without legal rights, a man who was not free to exercise his supposed freedom.

There was more to his racial identity than this legalized oppression, however. Dr. Harris drew a line between his people and the "lowest" Blacks still in slavery or sunk in poverty in the United States or the Caribbean. From the history of pre-revolution Haiti, he learned that Haiti then had three legal castes—"free whites," "free mulatto/colored" folk, and "Black slaves." In the United States as well he noticed that the free Blacks were more likely to be "colored" or of "mixed race," because such mixing had led to both their education and their freedom. I should emphasize that this is Harris speaking, not my opinion or the reality. It was his family's story. There were many mixed-race people who remained in slavery. But for J. D. Harris, the lighter skin tone went together with higher education, culture, social standing, and ambitions. His family began as craftspeople; some "rose" to white-collar jobs as preachers, teachers, and, in his case, a doctor. Others remained in the construction crafts such as brickmaking and plastering. But even they probably wore a suit to church on Sunday. In two generations, enslaved persons in his hometown, including his parents, had become middle-class, free gentlefolk. Harris grew up in this world of free mulattoes and prized his specialness. He was probably unaware that the "mulatto tinge" was becoming ever more common among the slaves in the "New South"—Georgia, Kentucky, Tennessee, Mississippi, Alabama, Arkansas, and Texas. Most white fathers did not liberate and educate their offspring with slave mothers; instead, they sold their own children for a profit.[27]

Even for Dr. Harris himself to self-identify as "colored" or "mulatto" had its ironies in later years. From the letters that he wrote from the wards at St. Elizabeths after his hospitalization in 1876, it becomes clear that he was housed in the main building with white patients, not in the "Black wards" elsewhere. J. D. Harris, with his white wife and enough money to pay the private patient rate, was categorized as a white patient. There simply was no category there for "Black middle-class patient" or "Black paying patient." Harris's two children, daughter Worthie and son Thoro, although listed as "mulatto" in census records from their childhood, became "white" as of the 1900 census. Thoro moved to Eureka Springs, Arkansas, after his father's death. There he always passed as white. When his descendants recently visited the town, they were amused to find that in death Thoro was "colored" again. He was the centerpiece of their local museum's African American history month exhibit.[28] J. D. Harris himself never abandoned his African ancestry but clung to the hope of elevating the situation of his destitute and degraded brothers and sisters.

In conversations with my colleagues about Dr. Harris, several questions have come up frequently. "So, what was his significant achievement?" Or phrased another way, "What is he known for?" Well, if known at all, it was because of his book on Caribbean colonization, *A Summer on the Borders of the Caribbean Sea*, initially published in 1860, which was reprinted alongside another contemporary text on the subject as *Black Separatism and the Caribbean 1860*, edited by Howard H. Bell and published in 1970. Multiple libraries have this combined version, and now the volume is also available through online collections. It is the focus of chapters 5 and 6 in this volume. The original book was unfortunately timed, in terms of contemporary influence. Its whole point was that free Blacks had no place in a country with slavery, so they must leave for a place where they could exist as full citizens. The Civil War changed this discourse radically, with the Emancipation Proclamation and the enlistment of Black troops. Now the challenge became for the best-situated northern Blacks to help others in the United States transition from enslaved to free.

I usually answer the query about his significance by saying that he was one of the few African American physicians to serve in the Civil War. This is true but quite incomplete. What is interesting is to see this accomplishment as one of several pathways he followed to find success as a self-supporting adult and to serve his people. The questions are all the more pressing when you realize that he was born in a small southern town where it was illegal to teach Black people to read. What was his path? Who supported him on the way? Who taught him to read, not just English but French? How did he manage to convert from a plasterer to a doctor? What drove him? This is not just a rags-to-riches story but one of repeated self-actualization. One point to emphasize is that society structures blocked him at every turn in prewar America but also evolved along with him, creating, for example, government medical jobs in the army and the Freedmen's Bureau, the South Carolina asylum appointment under the Radical Republicans, and the hospital at Howard, funded by the government.

A second frequent query asks, How can you write a biography without papers, without a diary, without the "J. D. Harris Manuscript Collection" in some library? This has been, admittedly, difficult. Archival sources such as diaries or letters are valued for their direct connection to the creator's mind. Published sources are good but have perhaps been edited or changed to obscure those aspects thought too provocative, erotic, illegal, or politically unpopular. Editor Howard Bell (of the Caribbean book) did not change Harris's text, but he did apologize for Harris equating skin tone with intelligence and capability. And the original publisher of that book cut some angry material that had appeared originally. It would be wonderful to have the original manuscript in the Harris hand, but alas, no.

The third question concerns my theory and method. On the most basic level, I was trained in the school of social history, and particularly the social history of medicine, as noted earlier. But theory crosses method in my granular attention to the ways in which racism hindered Harris at every turn. In recounting this man's life, it is at least as important to see the mountain of racism that blocked his way as it is to celebrate his many accomplishments. He was born in a country and a state where slavery of African people was legal. Many caricatures emphasized that Blacks were more animal-like than white people; they were literally chattel to be bought and sold, just like cows, pigs, and horses. Their lives were seen as oversexed, primitive, barbaric. The men were prone to wild violence, and the women had no restraints on their sexuality. Harris inserted a text proclaiming such degrading stereotypes in his epic poem, putting its words in the mouth of a politician. His scorn drips from the page.

Beyond such wretched images, Harris was exposed to the violence of slavery throughout his childhood, and even in the supposed safety of northern Ohio, where the Fugitive Slave Act allowed men to use force to retain escapees. Historian Daniel Lord Smail has used research on the endocrine basis of dominance hierarchies in apes to argue that such performance of violence on others in the Middle Ages affected those who watched it in ways that reinforced their own subservience to the violent overlords of their era, and a similar biological system likely worked to spread at least the performance of docility among the enslaved Americans.[29] Harris himself had to overcome all of these influences to achieve the self-confidence that allowed him to break through racial barriers. Society told him he was animal-like and degenerate; its violence warned him to stay in his place and not challenge the hierarchy. His courage in pushing against such incarceration is evident throughout his life, as it was in the lives of several brothers who likewise raged against the system. It was, in other words, a Harris family value, one that helped other brothers to succeed as teachers and preachers in spite of such a derogatory master narrative in their birth society. They were comforted and connected by the Bible and the hope of the Methodist faith.

Attention to the specifics of racism is important. Structural racism surrounded the Harris family in Fayetteville, North Carolina. By "structural institutional racism" is meant the embedded laws, cultural norms, and common knowledge of a society that creates a system of discrimination. In the twentieth-century United States, such practices as segregated schools, "redlining" in real estate, voter suppression, and delegated spaces in hospitals and transport all fall under such a concept.[30] For the Harris family in 1840s North Carolina, the overarching shadow of slavery was supplemented by legal restrictions against free Blacks. Historian John Hope Franklin has ably described the increasing harsh laws in the state that limited movement, education, religion, and property ownership. The laws threatened the very liberty of the free Black population and more and more limited the ability to buy enslaved people out of bondage. Such it was that in 1850 the family made the difficult journey to Ohio, where Blacks were still restricted but not in the many harsh ways of their native state.[31]

Even as the Civil War, as well the Thirteenth and Fourteenth Amendments to the US Constitution, transformed the grossest of these legalized acts of discrimination, societal change came slowly. It was not enough, as in Harris's case, to allow Blacks to acquire medical degrees. If no white patient would accept them as doctors, then their practice would be limited to the lowest economic rung in the country. Most health care happened in the home, so it was a matter not just of accepting a Black doctor but of accepting a Black man or woman as visitor to one's house. Black servants were fine, but a Black doctor was accorded superiority of knowledge and class, which was altogether a different thing. Servants came in the kitchen door; doctors walked into the parlor.

Dr. Harris strove to be recognized as a gentleman, especially after he began medical practice. He would have been pleased to know that Ira Russell called him a "gentleman" in his description. Harris wore suits, was educated, and could speak well. Such respectability was a key aspect of his family culture. But when he ran for lieutenant governor of Virginia in 1869, he learned the limits of class to overcome racial divisions. He challenged the segregation of the steamer that would take him from Portsmouth, Virginia, up to Richmond and failed. He was turned away from white hotels and had to lodge at the "Negro" boardinghouse. And while his running mate, a white man who was currently acting governor, treasured the Black votes that Harris would bring, he never invited Harris to his home, the governor's mansion. Harris might have been elected lieutenant governor, and if the governor had in turn been nominated for the US Senate, as some hoped, Harris would then have become governor. But he would still have slept in the "Negro" boardinghouse the night before his inauguration. This point became moot when their ticket lost the election. In the end, Harris lodged in the middle-class white wing of St. Elizabeths Hospital for the insane. Still, he wore his suit coat to walk the grounds and offered asylum doctors his views on therapeutics. In this sense, the hospital offered the comfort of familiar surroundings. He was a doctor, after all, surrounded by patients.

1

The Formative Years

What do we know about J. D. Harris's childhood? What *can* we know? Here the absence of a detailed autobiography is deeply felt. Even his date of birth is a mystery, while his mother's personality is evident only by its impact rather than in "sainted memory." Even without that autobiography, however, we can learn much from the tools of microhistory. Court records are useful, as are newspaper stories and historical accounts of his hometown, Fayetteville, North Carolina. Information comes from the letters of his brothers, written during their time working for the American Missionary Association after the Civil War (see chapter 8). Even the diary kept by a pupil of J. D.'s youngest brother, Cicero, gives some idea of the values taught in the Harris family household. Finally, we see a reflection of J. D.'s experiences in his quasi-autobiographical but overtly fictional poem published in 1856 (see chapter 3). In it he described scenes and people of Fayetteville before the poem's narrator moved on to Iowa. This account leaves many questions but provides a far fuller sketch of childhood influences than is available for other free Black public figures from the 1850s onward. This chapter takes J. D. from his babyhood to the point of his family's departure from North Carolina in 1850.

Joseph Dennis Harris was born, free, in (about) 1833. His home was Fayetteville, where he arrived as the fifth child of Jacob and Charlotte Dismukes

Harris. North Carolina did not record birth certificates in the 1830s, so we are reliant on the retrospective claim in the 1850 census that he was seventeen years old.[1] The Harris family—all ten children, two adult parents, occasional apprentices, and sometimes slaves—lived together in one small house. That Charlotte Harris raised ten children to adulthood amid the unsanitary conditions that prevailed in the Black quarter of a small southern town is impressive and provides evidence of discipline and cleanliness in the household. Throughout his childhood, J. D. was a silent witness to the world about to be described here.

Several themes will be highlighted in this chapter. The social network created by free Blacks first in New Bern, North Carolina, and later in Fayetteville spun a web of support, livelihood, and safety that made survival and prosperity possible. Second, and rivaling the first, was the creation of the family value of "respectability," those features of behavior, dress, personal cleanliness, and occupation that distinguished the household and its offspring. Literacy, education, religion, and sobriety were all cornerstones of this self-construction. Racial identity was of paramount importance in the South; the mixed races of the Harris family had to be delicately negotiated by them and even more carefully considered by the modern historian. Over all of these important aspects of the Harris household looms the powerful, mysterious, and silent figure of Charlotte Dismukes Harris.

THE PARENTS

The origins of mother Charlotte Harris are obscure. Her last name was Dismukes, and she was of mixed race, as witnessed by the *M* (for mulatto) after her name in the 1830 census. She was born around 1808; at age sixteen she married Jacob Harris, when she was already pregnant with her daughter Sarah. Charlotte does not show up in the indentures for Craven County or Cumberland County in the 1810s or 1820s, which means she was not officially bound out as an apprentice in the New Bern or Fayetteville area during those years before her marriage. (Or, such legal documents did not survive.) There are fewer women than men in the indenture papers altogether, although some women were so bound. They might be put to learn the seamstress craft, for example, or general homemaking.

A review of North Carolina wills for the early nineteenth century revealed a (white) George Dismukes who died in Chatham County in 1827. He had multiple slaves and left one named Charlotte to his daughter Sally Haynes. But this was not J. D.'s mother—she had already been a free woman for at least three years when Dismukes died in 1827 (as she was legally married as a free Black in 1824). Still, the concurrence of names is interesting. Might this "slave Charlotte" be Charlotte Harris's mother and her father George Dismukes, who then freed his mixed-race daughter? There is also a white man named Alexander Hamilton Dismukes who edited a newspaper in Fayetteville in the 1820s and was living in nearby Chatham County in later decades (again, according to the census). He had been born in 1797. A further point—one of the Harris children was named William D. Harris, with the D never spelled out. George Dismukes had a son named William. Might William D. Harris be named for his mother's father, William Dismukes? Or for a half-brother, who helped her to freedom? It is possible, but all speculation.[2]

Father Jacob was from New Bern, a coastal town that was a colonial capital, important port, and North Carolina's first urban area. There he was one of many "artisans of color" who worked in skilled trades in an era when free Blacks were much more accepted in towns than they were in rural areas, or would be anywhere in North Carolina in later decades. As historian Catherine Bishir notes, such free urban Blacks found that "in town they were likelier to observe and do business with a wide range of black and white people, to hone their skills and learn strategies from other enslaved and free blacks." They had the opportunities to gather together openly and meet "with people of diverse backgrounds and political views in churches, taverns, and workshops." New Bern, in the decades of the early republic, offered "prime opportunities for blacks to gain their freedom and, especially after emancipation, to participate in political and civic life."[3] Into this world, with its majority Black population, father Jacob Harris grew to adulthood.

Coastal New Bern was a center for craftsmen, who pursued occupations in shipbuilding and repair, house construction, tanning, woodwork, and leatherwork. Craft training was an important societal institution, especially in the lives of people of color. Skilled slaves not only did their master's work but could be rented out to others, earning their own wages and augmenting their master's wealth. According to Monticello historian Annette Gordon-Reed, training "lighter colored" slaves in crafts was a long-standing tradition there. On Thomas Jefferson's plantation, the children of liaisons between white men and light-colored slaves such as Sally Hemings were favored for training in the various crafts that were needed there, like barrel making, harness production, furniture construction, and the multiple skills that went into making a house—stonemasonry, plastering, framing, and so on.[4] Women learned household tasks, such as cooking, childcare, and all aspects of fabric production—weaving, dressmaking, and fine handwork. In the colonial and early republic eras, such skilled craftspeople (men and women) formed the core of free African populations in coastal urban areas of the South.[5]

One local story from the community sagas of New Bern may have made it into the Harris family lore. A free Black cooper and Revolutionary War veteran named Asa Spelman lived in the town and regaled his friends with stories of his exploits during the war, including meeting General George Washington. In 1791 then president Washington visited New Bern, and as the people gathered around him, Spelman ambled up. All were curious to see if his supposed familiarity with the great man was a fable. According to a town memorialist writing a century later, Washington looked at Spelman and cried, "Why Asy! How come you here. I'm glad to see you."[6] Harris may have known this story since childhood, and the importance of Black Revolutionary War ancestors as marking citizenship and dignity figured in his poem written decades later.

New Bern was unusual in its casual approach to enforcing restrictions upon the movements and rights of free Black and enslaved people. Of central importance to this local culture were wealthy white citizens who supported manumission and the rights of free people of color. The spirit of the Revolution with its declaration of the universal rights of man seems to have held on longer here than in other southern locales, finding expression in frequent liberation of enslaved peoples. Many leading whites in New Bern were open to arguments about the evils of slavery and eager to find ways to ease out of it peaceably. Some were politically vocal in the promotion of Black rights.[7] Attorneys among this group represented slaves or free Blacks in court or advised whites who wanted to free their slaves or write wills that would ensure their liberation after death.

In this atmosphere of relative liberality, slaves and former slaves frequently learned to read and write, which was legal in North Carolina into the 1820s. In fact, teaching a child to read was a usual part of the apprentice agreement, so that when children completed their time of training, they should be at least minimally literate as well as skilled. Other slaves and free Blacks taught each other, passing around simple spelling books and readers. Whether Jacob or Charlotte Harris learned to read in this way is unknown, but their literacy is evident in later documents.[8] Overall, Bishir described the community of New Bern in the late eighteenth century as a hopeful early model for the abolition of slavery. And so it might have been, if Eli Whitney had not invented the cotton gin in the 1790s. This machine (and later improved versions of it) made the mass processing of cotton feasible and cost-effective. This in turn paved the way for the huge cotton plantations worked by African American slaves in the nineteenth century, the great generators of wealth that made cotton king and the southern planter elite rich beyond all expectations.[9] Slavery was the linchpin of the extravaganza.

But back to our story. As mentioned, Jacob Harris entered the historical record in 1807 when he was bound, at age seven, as an apprentice plasterer and bricklayer. His master was Donum Montford, plasterer, glassworker, and brickmaker—and a man who had bought his own freedom from slavery just three years earlier. And where did seven-year-old Jacob come from? Harris was one of the most common names in colonial North Carolina, and there is no specific father or mother who can be identified for him.[10] The indenture that bound him to Montford as an apprentice did not call him an orphan or colored (labels that commonly appear in other indenture documents of the time).[11] Was he the son of a white man and his African American partner (slave or free)? Yet another mystery.

New Bern's prosperity dimmed in the second quarter of the nineteenth century, as that of Fayetteville rose. Located on the Cape Fear River, it formed an inland port for the agricultural products that traveled by slow wagon to its market terminus, and from there to the sea. Many of New Bern's resident craftspeople moved to the inland town as it became the locus of new construction and opportunities for craft trades. This motion was accelerated when in 1831 a devastating fire hit the downtown business district of Fayetteville, destroying municipal buildings, local businesses, and more than 600 homes.[12] Disaster for local inhabitants became opportunity for skilled craftsmen with knowledge of masonry, woodworking, and plastering.

THE HOUSEHOLD IN FAYETTEVILLE

Jacob Harris had moved to Fayetteville before the fire, however. He married Charlotte Dismukes on June 17, 1824, in Cumberland County, where Fayetteville is located.[13] He had also apparently fallen on some hard times as well, for his name appears in a "sheriff's sale for taxes" in a newspaper advertisement of January 8, 1829. This was "1 lot imp[roved] Hillsborough street," listed as worth $121.[14] Harris may have been able to clear his tax debts, as he sold a lot on Hillsborough Street, north of modern-day Chance Street, to Joseph Hostler in 1833 for $200. By the 1840s the family lived on the corner of Hillsborough and Moore Streets, a block or two south of the Hostler lot.[15] In the 1830 census the Harris family had six people in its fold: Jacob Harris, Charlotte Harris, and children Sarah (b. 1824), William (b. 1827), and Mary (b. 1828). In addition, a teenage male lived in the house, possibly an apprentice, although there is no paperwork for him, if so, in surviving indenture records.[16]

The great fire of 1831 must have given Jacob Harris more work than he could handle, as plastering and bricklaying would be key to the construction of new homes and commercial buildings. In that year Harris took on two apprentices to learn his trade, Owen Clinton Artis and William Burnett, both boys aged fourteen.[17] The next year he took on yet another, Cicero Richardson, who had been sent by friends in New Bern to apprentice with Jacob. A note that accompanied Cicero (and served as his "papers") attested to his freedom. When African Americans traveled, they had to be ready to prove that they were not runaways, especially in the climate of fear generated by Nat Turner's rebellion the previous August.[18]

Richardson's case illustrated the webs of connection that tied the free Blacks of Fayetteville to those of New Bern. Richardson's note was directed to white lawyers and politicians in Fayetteville whose family had owned Richardson's grandmother and freed her when she was fifty. His grandmother's name was Caty (Catharine) Webber, who was also friends with Donum Montford (Jacob Harris's apprentice master) and John C. Stanly, another prominent free Black man in New Bern.[19] Jacob and Charlotte named their fourth daughter Catharine Webber, attesting to the connection. As we do not know Jacob's origins in New Bern, it is tempting to speculate whether his relationship to Caty Webber was that of mother and son. In any event, Cicero Richardson became an important figure in the Jacob Harris household. He married Sarah in 1841, and three years later Jacob and Charlotte named their tenth and last child Cicero Richardson Harris.

The apprentice bond for Cicero Richardson reveals another set of business and friendship connections for the Harris family. Apprentices were bonded by the state to the master, usually until their twenty-first birthday. This served several purposes. It functioned as occupational training, guaranteeing the young person would acquire skills that he or she could use to become a self-supporting adult. It was not uncommon to bind orphans to apprentice masters, thus relieving the state of the need to provide for their support. Small children might be bonded over into this situation. The master had to promise to "produce" the apprentice if called upon by the court, or pay a penalty of $500. The point here was to make sure that the master maintained discipline and kept the apprentice from running away, generally reducing the risk of teenage vagrancy. The master was also responsible for housing, food, and teaching the "art and mystery" of the master's craft. The indenture for Jacob Harris himself, age seven, promised also to teach him to read and write. By the 1830s the forms for the indentures of free colored youths excluded that clause, as North Carolina had discovered that literate apprentices could read incendiary political materials.[20] Still, when a master took on an apprentice, he had to sign a bond promising to complete his responsibilities toward the apprentice and attest that he would forfeit $500 if he failed to do so.

Several such bonds survive in the state apprentice records for Jacob Harris in the role of apprentice master. In each case the bond had cosigners, although all stated that Harris would be the master. For Burnett in 1831 the cosigner was John E. Patterson; for Artis, the cosigners were Patterson and Hiram Robinson. Although my original hypothesis was that these additional names would be those of white men who acted to buttress Jacob Harris's respectability, this turns out to be true only of Hiram Robinson, a local white physician. In the case of Cicero Richardson, the two cosigners were George W. Ragland and Matthew Leary. Leary and Patterson appear again in later apprentice bonds. According to census records, Patterson was a free man of color, born in 1804; Matthew Leary was also a free man of color, born in 1802. Ragland was likewise African American, born into slavery but purchased and freed by Matthew Leary. Leary's grandfather Anton Revels fought in the Revolutionary War, and he may well have been another source of military stories for young J. D. Harris. Leary and Ragland went into business together as saddlers and harness makers. According to an account written by his descendant, Leary helped many slaves buy their freedom.[21]

Jacob Harris named his second son after Ragland and was some sort of kinsman to the Ragland family. This information came from a court document related to a fight over George Ragland's will. The exact date of Ragland's death is unknown, but the will was written, signed, and witnessed in 1835 and produced in a court dispute of 1838. The dispute apparently turned on questions of Ragland's acuity when the will was made, and the subsequent court battle pitched Ragland's wife against his two sisters. One of those sisters, Charlotte Huntington, contacted Jacob Harris and contracted to sell him her share in any potential positive outcome of the suit. This was filed with other land deeds in the county courthouse. In typical legalese, it begins with the phrase "Whereas the relations of said Charlotte are slaves generally and whereas Jacob Harris aforesaid one of her relations is a freeman of colour and hath ever been kind to her..." Slaves could not inherit property, so she chose Jacob as the recipient. How Jacob was related to the Ragland siblings—who were freed slaves—is unknown but intriguing. She granted to him, in return for one dollar, all rights she might have in the lawsuit. Her other reason for settling this was that she was "now becoming advanced in years and to some extent incapable of attending to her interest in the estate of the late George Ragland her brother." So although we do not know how old the Raglands were in the 1830s, they were likely older than Harris himself, who was only thirty-six in 1835.[22]

Matthew Leary remained a close business associate into the 1840s and served as executor of Jacob Harris's will after his death in 1847. There seems to have been one period of disaffection between them over a business deal, however, found in a curious set of deeds from 1846. Jacob Harris was listed as selling a piece of land to Benjamin Robinson, the clerk of court, for $300. This was a lot Harris bought in 1840 for $400. The sale was part of the settlement of a debt that Harris owed to Matthew Leary. But the same day a second deed indicated the first one was null and void, as Harris had now settled his debt to Leary. Apparently, the initial sale was done to guarantee that Harris would pay the debt, and then once that was settled the sale was nullified and the land returned to Harris.[23]

The Harris family continued to grow, with George born in 1831, J. D. born around 1833, Hannah Brimage in 1834, Catharine in 1836, and Robert W. in 1840. Who were these children named for? There was a free man of color named Joseph Dennis in the 1840 census in Fayetteville. Historian John Hope Franklin mentioned him, quoting a white citizen as saying in 1840 that Dennis was "a mechanic of considerable skill and has frequently been in my employ."[24] Brimage as a middle name for daughter Hannah probably relates to the fact that Jacob Harris took on a Thomas Brimage, age seventeen, as an apprentice in 1837. While she was born three years before he came as an apprentice, the apprentice relationship itself may have been a marker of the pre-existing connection between the two families. In the 1840 and 1850 census records for New Bern and nearby towns, there are several free families of color named Brimage, all of which adds up to the possibility that Jacob was friends with people named Brimage during his youth in New Bern, named his daughter for a woman in the family, and also took one of their sons as an apprentice.[25] Perhaps these namesakes served as godparents for the children, informal guardians in the event that the children should become orphans or otherwise be in need of aid. Overall, it reveals a continuing web of social relationships that connected New Bern to Fayetteville and the "colored" artisans to each other's families.

This web of obligation and mutual support shows that the free Black community was rich in the sort of wealth known as "social capital."[26] These people lived together in the Black quarter, supported each other in court, and likely tided each other over with short-term loans as needed. These craftspeople also had white contacts—the people they had done work for who could attest (or not, as the case may be) to the fact that the family was well disciplined, that the workers were sober, that the project was finished and the result as expected. This sort of "reputation banking," if you will, meant that as long as the family members stayed in Fayetteville, they were known and recognized as locals with a solid, positive identity. Many parental values also come into play here. Was it important that the children could read? Did the parents send the children to high school or even college rather than push them to become early wage earners? Did the family model hard work, discipline, mutual respect, and religious observance? There is no direct evidence as to what was taught in the Harris household, but the outcomes point to the presence of such values.

Social capital can also refer to emotional support, and this family worked hard to keep that emotional bond even when the family had to move out of North Carolina. Since they were all literate, letters flowed back and forth. J. D. seems to have chosen locales, when he was old enough, that put him in proximity to his family. One exception was his breakout move to Iowa, which was perhaps in part an attempt to establish a separate identity from that of his encompassing family. In chapter 3 we shall learn that the western enterprise did not go well, and J. D. returned to his mother's house, by then located in Cleveland. His trips to the Caribbean were also made without family members, but upon failure he again returned to his mother's home. He had a safe haven there in which to lick his wounds and decide on next steps. Once his medical training was complete, he went to the Virginia Peninsula in the mid-1860s, where his brothers had just begun teaching and preaching to the freedpeople. After losing an election in 1869, J. D. moved on to South Carolina (with his new wife) to the company of his brother William's family. When he was desperate to escape from St. Elizabeths mental hospital in DC, it was his brother Robert who received the furtive missive begging for help and who at least tried to come to his rescue. All of which is to say that his family was an important source of intermittent financial, social, and emotional support that shored up his various endeavors throughout his life.

By 1840 it appears that Jacob Harris presided over a household of at least eighteen people: he and his wife, eight children, four apprentices, and four slaves. J. D. Harris was seven years old. The census for 1840 did not report individual names, apart from the head of household. We can identify the apprentices from indenture papers, but the slaves are known only by their ages—two males under ten, one female under ten, and one female between the ages of ten and twenty-three.[27] Jacob Harris was identified as apprentice master for eight apprentices in the 1830s; there were four teenage males in the household in the 1840 census. If William D. Harris (b. 1830) was counted in the under-ten list and Robert Harris (b. 1840) had yet to make an appearance and thus be counted, that leaves the four teenage slots to be occupied by apprentices. Two of Harris's known apprentices were clearly too old—apprenticeship ended at twenty-one, so Owen Artis and William Burnett were likely out of the house (although Artis had not gone far—he witnessed Jacob Harris's will in 1847). Calvin Jackson or Thomas Brimage (both age twenty) might still have been in the household. James Fore, David Williams, and George Williams, all teenagers, were very likely in residence. That leaves the identity of the "24–35 year-old" male. It is tempting to assign this spot to Cicero Richardson, former apprentice and soon-to-be son-in-law (he married Sarah Harris in 1841), although his apprentice bond listed him as "13 or 14" in 1831, which puts him just on the threshold of twenty-four in the census year. In any event, it was a crowded dwelling.

What to make of the four slaves? As John Hope Franklin pointed out, free Blacks might own slaves for the same reasons that whites did—to advance their owners' economic well-being by the value of their labor, whether on farms or in workshops. Such owners can be identified, argued Franklin, by their extensive property holdings and their "inactivity in the manumission movement."[28] For example, the famous Black cabinetmaker Thomas Day used slaves for thirty years to assist in furniture production; other free Blacks acquired agricultural land and put their slaves to work farming. But more common was the purchase of slaves for benevolent reasons. In families where one or more members were free but others remained in slavery, it was common for the freedpeople to purchase relatives with the goal of ultimate liberation. Courts did not always allow such manumission, so the family members became virtually free while still legally being slaves.

We know that the Harris family, while free, likely had family members who remained in bondage. Remember that in the court plea of Charlotte Huntington, herself free, she mentioned that most of her kin were slaves and that Jacob Harris was her kinsman. None of the four slaves listed in the Harris household in 1840 was listed in Jacob Harris's will seven years later; slaves were property and normally would have been specifically deeded, as George Dismukes did in his will thirteen years earlier. It is doubtful that Jacob would have just lumped them together with "all my possessions" in the will. Also, three of the four were younger than ten, making them of little value as workers at that point in time. I suspect these children had either been informally placed in the household for training by their masters or were kin purchased with an aim of ultimate manumission. Matthew Leary's descendant claims that his ancestor purchased many slaves and freed them.

Perhaps these children had been purchased by Leary or similar benevolent masters and placed in the house to learn skills. J. D. Harris never mentions them in his later writings.

While it is possible that the slaves had been put in the Harris household to learn skills by their actual owners, Jacob Harris did own at least one slave himself. In an 1845 newspaper notice, a man named John McCaskill warned others not to buy a "note," which was part of a business deal involving Needham Russell's hire of a slave for twenty-five dollars who was "the property of Jacob Harris." McCaskill had "stood security" for the hire. The note was of no value, announced McCaskill, because "the conditions set forth in the note have not been complied with on the part of Harris."[29] The outcome of this dispute is not recorded, but the slave had been stood as capital to secure the loan, just as a horse or cow might be. A 1949 account of the Harris family, which draws in part on family member knowledge, said of Charlotte Harris, "Her late husband had set a fine example of buying cruelly persecuted slaves and giving them the opportunity to work out their freedom on easy terms."[30] Maybe so.

FAMILY CULTURE

This household, with its disparate and multiple members living in a crowded space, is distant from the common experience of affluent Americans in the twenty-first century. It is useful to call upon the work of historian John Demos to help us understand it. Demos studied family life in the Plymouth colony in the seventeenth century, using court records to understand the aspects of family culture in some of the earliest villages in the Americas. There is obviously much that differs between Plymouth in 1650 and Fayetteville in 1840, but some aspects are similar, and perhaps his analysis, based on the family life course theory of psychiatrist Erik Erikson, may shed some light on the Harris family experience.[31]

Like the Harris brood, the Pilgrims lived in small houses that contained large families, often including servants or apprentices. Demos remarks on several aspects that may be relevant here. One is that in large families, there is no sharp demarcation between children and adults, as the family may range from infants to older teens, all under one roof. In Plymouth there was a demarcation, though, between young children, up to about age six, and older ones, marked at times by the fact that children over six might be sent out to live with another family and learn a craft or otherwise go to work. Jacob Harris began his apprenticeship in New Bern at the age of seven. One imagines that his sons and daughters, who mostly stayed in his own household to learn their skills, likewise began to work in earnest in that time range of six to eight years. Given all the work to be done in the home, it seems likely that even younger children would be given simple tasks of cleaning, washing, and helping with food preparation. And the older children were responsible for watching or teaching them at times.

Demos points out that in Plymouth the family had multiple functions that are more typically carried on outside of the household in modern America. First, the family home was a business, a workplace. Whether the work in question was farming or artisanal, still the family unit was the business unit. Boys learned their father's trade, and girls learned women's tasks, such as weaving, candle making, cooking, and so on. Sarah Harris, the oldest Harris child, was listed as a printer in the 1860 census. This label, in conjunction with the fact that a man named Dismukes edited the local paper in Fayetteville, might suggest that Charlotte Dismukes Harris knew the printing trade and shared her knowledge with her daughter. Sarah might even have been hired out to work on the Fayetteville paper run by her possible kinsman. The first three boys were all plasterers and brick masons, the skills that Jacob Harris contracted to teach his apprentices. Seventeen-year-old J. D. was a blacksmith in the 1850 census, although still living with his mother. His father may have arranged for him to learn that trade outside of a formal apprentice agreement, although it is never again referred to in census or family records. Together, these children brought added value to the household economy, just as in a farming family the teenagers would have worked the land, tended animals, and otherwise contributed to the overall prosperity of the family. The Harris family, with its ten children, created wealth as a family unit, for the family unit.

A second function that Demos highlights is that the family was both a school and a vocational institute. By this he meant that in the absence of formal schools, which were rare and transient in the early Plymouth colony (as well as in Fayetteville), children were taught at home. Their vocational training was provided by Jacob for the boys and by Charlotte for the girls. The teaching of reading, writing, and arithmetic likely fell to Charlotte Harris, and perhaps to the two oldest girls as time went on. Someone taught all those children to read and write, not just minimally but fluently, with accurate spelling; the best information we get on the subject is brother William telling an American Missionary Association official that he had "educational advantages moderate or as good as could be obtained in N.C. where I was raised."[32] He went on to describe himself teaching regular and Sunday schools but without detail as to location. At this point William Harris was living in Delaware, Ohio, and these schools where he taught were probably there. Certainly, it is true that there were few educational opportunities of any sort in North Carolina in the 1830s, for Black or white. For the Harris family, it seems likely that at least their initial literacy was acquired at home.

As we shall see in chapter 6, J. D. Harris knew French well enough to act as a translator while working in Haiti in the early 1860s. The English literacy of his family is itself intriguing; the fact that someone also taught him French is an even mightier mystery. What follows is speculative but offers possible sources for his French fluency. Dismukes is an uncommon American name. It may have evolved from Des Meaux, a name carried by some French Huguenots to the United States, according to Ancestry.com.[33] Another origin of French speakers in Fayetteville might have been refugees from the Haitian Revolution or other immigrants from the francophone Caribbean. Another French-speaking influence was a woman known in Fayetteville as "French Mary." Tracking her via Ancestry.com, we find that Mariette Scholastique Huilliad (recorded as "mulatto") married Louis Mimorel in 1816 in Guadeloupe; their daughter Juliet (born eight years earlier, in 1808) married Jacob Leary after her family moved to Fayetteville and became mother to Matthew Leary (mentioned earlier as a business partner and friend of Jacob Harris) and grandmother to J. D.'s friend Lewis Sheridan Leary. According to one Leary family reminiscence, "French Mary" was a cook who could prepare grand meals in the French style. When the Marquis de Lafayette came to visit Fayetteville in 1825 during his tour of the South, "French Mary" prepared the banquet and spoke with the general in French.[34] One final possible French connection was via a French-speaking refugee colony in Wilmington, North Carolina, which had fifty-four whites and thirty mulattoes in 1794. Having fled the Haitian Revolution, many of them were destitute but gradually began to find work teaching the French language, cooking, dancing, and fashion of their privileged island colony. A French-language refugee press also emerged in multiple coastal settlements in the 1790s.[35]

Continuing with Demos's explication of the family's function in the Pilgrim era, the next duty of the family was to convey religion. The family homestead was a mini-church. This is not to claim that there were no church structures for regular attendance but that the family hearth was a principal place for the conveyance of religious instruction and Bible reading. Religious belief was so pervasive among the Harris siblings that it seems all but certain that Charlotte Harris conveyed this religious perspective to her children. From William's letters (again), we learn that he had a poor view of the teachers sent to New Bern after the Civil War, when comparing their fervor with the religious commitment of his own missionary colleagues. "I visited the home of many teachers several times," he wrote in consternation, and "saw not a Bible, heard not a prayer, indeed they have no family altar erected."[36] Presumably, this stood in contrast to his home of origin, which had created a standard of religious propriety in his mind.

A fourth family duty was to discipline; there could be no other acceptable source of such social control in the setting in which they found themselves. First, as Demos emphasized, any family group in which a large number of people lived in a small space had to learn to contain intra-family aggression. In the South there would have been more opportunities to escape the confines of the home as the environment allowed more days when being outside was tolerable (compared with frosty Massachusetts). But this free Black family knew the price of any sort of bad behavior outside of the home, especially if it called family members to the attention of police. The ruling whites could be harsh in their punishments and even decide that a free Black child should be "placed" outside of his or her own family into conditions just short of slavery. Control of emotions and appropriately subservient behavior toward whites were paramount for survival, and surely this was beaten into the Harris children.

These family dynamics of business and social structure would change radically in the next generation. As the Harris siblings moved into white-collar occupations, their income may actually have decreased with the rise in status. We are told by family legend that Charlotte Harris moved her family to Ohio in order for the younger children to go to high school. Clearly there was a family tendency toward leaving artisanal labor for the white-collar professions—teaching, preaching, doctoring, law. It is possible that this shift would have been opposed by Jacob, who had done well in the house-building trades. But with him dead in 1847, Charlotte had an open field to transform her sons' opportunities toward the sort of "elevation" that was apparently a family value (and one shared by Black progressives in Ohio, as we shall see). And this change in turn led to shifts in the value of children, toward the more modern model, where children go outside the home for school and contribute minimally toward building the family's wealth in their youth. William's daughter Lottie, for example, attended Wilberforce College until he could no longer afford to send her there (and sought a teaching position for her with the American Missionary Association). Only Sarah Harris Richardson would give birth to offspring in numbers to rival her mother's—nine—and it may be relevant that she was married to Cicero Richardson, who, more than any of Jacob Harris's biological sons, followed the pattern of housing construction that put sons to work in the family business and made him moderately wealthy in Cleveland.

The function of the family changed dramatically in just three generations. The parents of Jacob and Charlotte Harris may well have included slave mothers and white fathers. There was no nuclear family in the first generation but rather the unstable mix of slave mother plus children, who were all subject to persistent slavery, sale, or liberation at the whim of the master. In the family with Jacob and Charlotte at the center, a traditional large family unit centered on artisanal production emerged and created wealth. In the next generation, J. D.'s, the family moved from skilled labor to white-collar work (in part) with clear progress toward the notions of "elevation" or "up from slavery" that mid-nineteenth-century rhetoric praised.

J. D.'s youngest brother Cicero Harris continued this tradition as a preacher and teacher to the next generation. The young Charles Chesnutt, reading books in Cicero Harris's household in 1874, found *Hand-Books for Home Improvement*, which he quoted at length in his diary. It emphasized the importance of being clean, to the extent of requiring a daily bath, with a special focus on the feet and hands. The nails should be carefully cut and cleaned, especially before sitting down to table or going into company. Such characteristics were not ones that a manual laborer could maintain, but Charles Chesnutt, pupil of the Harris brothers, could see that they were clearly part of the expectations of this newly white-collar generation.[37] Also, these middle class aspirants had to learn to speak like white people. J. D.'s younger brother Robert Harris reported from his freedmen's school in Virginia in the winter of 1865 that "learning to read with them is like learning a new language, so different is their language from that in the books. I find it beneficial to have an exercise in articulation at every recitation."[38] The recently freed slaves had to learn "proper" English pronunciation before they could know how to sound out written words. The path to "elevation" was indeed a steep one for such children.

These various aspects—education, proper speech, cleanliness, and so on—can be clustered under the phrase "respectability." Respectable families disciplined their children and taught the value of hard work. Respectable families read the Bible, abstained from alcohol, and were polite in their work and social interactions. Respectable people, as Chesnutt was taught by Cicero, washed their hands before coming to table. Robert Harris would later express amazement at the wild religious frenzy of dancing and singing that he saw among newly freed slaves in Virginia. It was, he feared, closer to paganism than to quiet Methodist teaching. Aspiring Black families had to perform respectability in order to make a claim for middle-class admission.

Historian Erica L. Ball describes what happened next when free Blacks found so many doors closed to them, despite achieving such markers of respectability: they turned to Black congresses and voted for declarations of abolitionism and state constitutional reform. But "once prominent free blacks understood the intransigence of white racism," they turned to other measures. Abandoning "the politics of respectability," they took up "more radical, aggressive forms of abolitionist activism, independent institutions, black nationalist ideology, and ultimately emigration efforts."[39]

Once J. D. Harris and his brothers left North Carolina, they joined the political antislavery and antidiscrimination institutions in the North. Such outspokenness would have been dangerous in North Carolina, but in Ohio some of them became downright "uppity" over time, engaging with the John Brown conspiracy and then escaping to the island of Santo Domingo to explore emigration possibilities for Black Americans. Cicero Richardson, sister Sarah's husband, was a known Underground Railroad conductor. Sarah was a printer in 1860 for an unknown newspaper. Perhaps it too was on the radical side. Two of her sons fought in the Civil War with the US Colored Troops. Rising through politics and revolution was a Harris family practice. J. D. would take that much further during and after the war. These family characteristics gave appeal to life in the North, but equally important was the "push" from southerners who wanted those free Blacks gone.

In his account of free Blacks in North Carolina in the antebellum era, historian John Hope Franklin titled his last chapter "An Unwanted People."[40] Franklin depicted a trajectory of the increasing oppression of free Black individuals, from the colonial period to the 1850s. In the early republic free Blacks could vote; some had earned their freedom by fighting in the American Revolution, although none were allowed to serve in the War of 1812. But as their numbers grew and fears of slave revolts escalated in the 1820s and 1830s, the relative tolerance of the free Black population gave way to paranoia and growing limitation of rights. The legal standing of free Black people become increasingly constricted. In 1826 the legislature decreed that justices of the peace could bind free Black children as apprentices if their parents were not taking sufficient responsibility for them. Initially apprentice masters were required to teach their charges to read and write, but the law was changed in 1838 so that it no longer applied to Blacks. If Black persons became debtors, unable to pay their due, then the court could hire them out to work off their fines and debts. The involuntary servitude had a limit, but still, white debtors were not similarly treated. In 1831 the legislature limited the movement of free Blacks from their home counties and declared that if they left the state for more than ninety days they could not return. If they traveled to another town, even within their own state, the bounty hunters might capture them, claim their papers were forged, and sell them into slavery. All these steps were in at least partial response to the slave uprisings of the 1820s and 1830s, with the common goal of limiting the ability of free Blacks to foment rebellion.[41]

Educational opportunities were likewise increasingly circumscribed. After 1832 it became illegal in North Carolina to teach a slave to read. Laws were introduced in the state legislature in 1834 and 1835 to forbid free Blacks from teaching others to read, but the laws could not be enforced. Given that incendiary tracts such as David Walker's *Appeal* were seen as key to inciting rebellion, this control of literacy was an important tool in the fight against freedom. It is unclear how and where many free Black people did acquire their education. Historian Franklin noted that "the education of free Negroes in North Carolina after the eighteen thirties is one of the most puzzling problems in the history of North Carolina. . . . There is no doubt that there was considerable amount of clandestine teaching of free Negroes."[42] The clergy were one source of such teaching, although after 1831 free Black men were forbidden to preach in public, which limited the ability of such men to earn a living. Again, the fear of insurrection drove these restrictions.[43]

The pressure on free Blacks increased in the 1850s. As the *Goldsboro Patriot* declared, "We hear but one opinion expressed, not only by the press of our State, but by everyone with whom we converse, in respect to free negroes. All are unanimous in the opinion that the approaching legislature ought to pass an act to remove them beyond the limits of the State." While some whites supported the scheme that helped free Blacks to immigrate to Liberia, this newspaper had a simpler solution: "Let the North have them. . . . On the head of Northern fanatics rests the responsibility."[44] Franklin's description of the Liberian emigrants from North Carolina in the 1850s applies to the Harris family and the many others who fled to Ohio as well. "It is no mere accident that the majority [of those who emigrated] was from the towns. Doubtless it was in those urban centers that the free Negro was least welcome and that he, in turn, saw the boldest manifestations of hostility to him." Thus the most skilled people were the most likely to go. "The urban free Negro . . . had made his presence felt in the skilled trades and had provided his family with some decent social experiences. When he began to feel the pressure of law and the community bear down upon him . . . he fled his beloved State . . . and went to a strange and inhospitable land."[45]

The Migration to Ohio

Sometime in 1850 seventeen-year-old J. D. Harris and his family traveled from North Carolina to Chillicothe, Ohio, in covered wagons. Mother Charlotte would have purchased the wagons and necessary supplies using the money yielded from Jacob's estate, and those funds likely also gave her the money to start again in Ohio. All ten Harris children left North Carolina, although they may not have traveled together or at the same time. The oldest girls were married with children of their own: Sarah with husband Cicero Richardson and their four children, and Mary with husband James Williams and their two children. The late September sale of the Harris family home on Hillsborough Street was advertised alongside that of James Williams, which was around the corner on Frink's Alley. It is likely that the families had left by then, given the need to avoid snow while crossing the mountains in late fall. Still, the September sale provides a definite date for their end time in Fayetteville.[1]

Historians of immigration talk about factors that push people out of their native land and factors that draw them to a new world. Charlotte Harris, as matriarch of the Harris family, left no written records explaining why they left. But some information survives in family legend. A descendant reported in the late 1940s that Charlotte was determined that her younger children should have a formal high school education and saw only closed doors in

North Carolina.[2] If indeed this was a principal reason for the move, it attests again to a family culture that highly valued education and the transition to "learned professions."

Other testimony comes from the diary of Charles Chesnutt, whose sister Lillian married J. D.'s nephew Garrett. Chesnutt was a well-known African American novelist of the late nineteenth century. He was born in Cleveland, where his free Black family had also migrated during the 1850s, but after the war the family went home to Fayetteville. There Chesnutt studied under two of J. D.'s younger brothers, Robert and Cicero. He was with Robert Harris during the final months of Robert's illness and mourned the death of his teacher in 1880. That spring Chesnutt was talking to Dr. Haigh, a white bookseller in Fayetteville, about Robert Harris.

"The conversation then turned on his family; and finally on the colored families who left Fayetteville before the war—in the fifties," reported Chesnutt. Haigh sighed and admitted, "Those," said he, "were our best colored people. It was a loss to the town when they left." Chesnutt responded, defending not only the Harris family but his own, "Yes, but they couldn't live here. Things were getting too warm for them. You had taken away their suffrage; the laws were becoming more and more severe toward free colored people; and they felt that their only safety lay in emigration to a freer clime."[3]

Chesnutt expanded on the fear that drove his parents and their friends to leave the state. "They didn't know how soon they themselves would be made slaves. They had been deprived of every safe-guard of liberty. If one were smitten in the face by a cowardly ruffian, he could not retaliate. He could be swindled of his property, defrauded of his earnings, and could not testify in court of law to the justice of his cause." It is likely that Chesnutt heard such declarations in his childhood. While he was born in 1858, the justifications for flight must have been frequently recalled. "With such a gloomy prospect is it strange that he should leave?" Chesnutt continued. And then he turned the conversation to the present day. "'As for my part I can't see how intelligent colored people can live in the South even now.'—And I went on to state my reasons why;—the existing prejudice—the impossibility of a rise in the social scale, etc." Chesnutt contrasted the situation in the North, which offered not only opportunities to rise but also cultural advantages in the arts, sciences, and literature. While his listener warned that disruption of the social hierarchy was dangerous, Chesnutt countered that society would regulate itself. Here and elsewhere in the diaries he expressed ideas that were either imbibed from his Harris family mentors or shared between his own family and the Harris siblings. Unlike the hostile southern climate, northern culture offered freedom and opportunities for education that would allow the social advancement of the colored race.[4]

THE ROAD TO OHIO

We have no direct knowledge of the Harris family expedition to Ohio, except the aftermath that proved it happened. What would such a journey have been like? We can borrow from John Mercer Langston's autobiography to get some idea. Langston was born in Virginia in 1829, the son of a white planter named Ralph Quarles and a mixed-race woman named Lucy Langston who had been born a slave but was freed by her master and partner, Quarles. In his autobiography Langston described her as an Indian woman, from the tribe of Pocahontas, with a "slight proportion of negro blood."[5] Quarles freed her and would have formalized the connection in marriage, but that was not legally possible (or so reported their son). Quarles had three sons by her and no other offspring. In his will he left his estate to the boys, doing "all that he could" for them. Langston became a family friend of the Harrises in the mid-1850s and knew J. D. and his wife in DC after the Civil War. His brother Charles Langston will likewise appear later in this story, promoting antislavery work in Cleveland in the late 1850s.

John Mercer Langston's biography is remarkable.[6] He was the first African American lawyer admitted to the bar in the state of Ohio and later the first admitted to the US Supreme Court. During the Civil War Langston recruited Black troops for the famed 54th Massachusetts Regiment (and likely encouraged the enlistment of J. D.'s nephew and namesake, Joseph Richardson, for that unit). After the war Langston served the Freedmen's Bureau as an inspector and then moved to Washington, DC, where he was founding dean of the law school at Howard University. After service as the American minister to Haiti, he returned to Petersburg, Virginia, where he acted as president of Virginia Normal and Collegiate Institute (later Virginia State University, one of Virginia's historically Black universities). In 1888 he was elected to the US House of Representatives, the only Black congressperson from Virginia during the postwar era, and the last for another 100 years. The poet Langston Hughes, his great-nephew, was named for him.[7]

For the moment let us focus on the difficult journey that John Mercer and Charles Langston made from Virginia in 1834, following a road that the Harris family likely joined somewhere near Wytheville, Virginia, on the way to Ohio in 1850. Both groups of emigrants would have to cross the Appalachian Mountains and then the Ohio River to reach the free state of Ohio. The Langstons left Virginia in October 1834, bearing legal documents that established that all in the party were free. Otherwise, they might have been accused of being runaway slaves, imprisoned, and sold into slavery. Much like the Harris family, the Langstons bought two covered wagons and teams of horses to transport them across the mountains. One carried the Langstons and the other a group of freed slaves from the plantation who were traveling with them to Ohio. It was a difficult trip, and the Harris family journey sixteen years later was likely similar. As John Mercer Langston remembered, "Besides being mountainous and rugged, it lay across a country largely without comfortable and accommodating stopping-places for travelers situated as these were." That "situation" was that they were Black or colored, and most inns or taverns along the way would not admit such people. So, they pitched tents and camped out at night.[8]

One anonymous reader of this manuscript suggested that the Quakers in North Carolina might have been one resource for the traveling Harris family and other free Blacks leaving the states where slavery was legal. By 1800 strains of antislavery thought had emerged among Quaker writers, alongside their persistent pacifism. As we have seen, the community of New Bern, North Carolina, had, like Tidewater Virginia, included a trend of freeing enslaved people in wills, especially when those freed were kin to the master's family. But this tolerance dissipated in the nineteenth century as fears of slave revolts caused a tightening of controls on both free Blacks and freedom of speech against slavery. As historian Ryan P. Jordan has noted, "Southern white opposition to Quaker anti-slavery sentiment and the concern for free Blacks accompanying it ultimately forced thousands of Friends out of Virginia, the Carolinas, and Georgia and into Ohio, Indiana, Michigan, and Illinois in the years from 1810 to 1835."[9] One response of the Quaker community was to organize caravans of free Blacks to accompany them to the West, especially to Ohio. Free Black people who could read and preach and teach were especially in danger in North Carolina, although they were not particularly welcomed in the free states, either.[10] Cincinnati received many African Americans fleeing slavery in Kentucky; these new workers competed with working-class whites for jobs, and rioting broke out against them in 1829. Similarly, Indiana and Illinois had already passed laws discouraging Black migration into their lands by the 1830s. One ship carrying ninety-three free Blacks bound for colonization in Africa was met by an angry mob in Philadelphia in 1832.[11] It was one thing to support the liberation of Black people from slavery, but quite another to find a hospitable community for them, even temporarily. As one Virginia Quaker noted, "Where were the resources for deporting half a million people? And where would we send them?"[12]

The Quakers are often linked to the Underground Railroad, a term used by the *New York Times* in 1853 to "describe the organized arrangements made in various sections of the country, to aid fugitives from slavery."[13] But as historian Jordan has argued, what began as a response to the evils of slavery in the late eighteenth- and early nineteenth-century American South grew more nuanced and complex as the century went on. There were Quakers who held slaves themselves and had a vested financial interest. However, many more despised slavery but saw no way to liberate and incorporate them into American society. They took a watch-and-wait attitude, or even actively opposed abolition, for the moment. Thus, they did not uniformly support the illegal manumission of slaves or their covert transfer out of the slave states.[14]

In the past two decades historians have come to emphasize the role of free African Americans themselves in helping escaped slaves travel to states or countries where they would be safe. Historian Keith P. Griffler has reoriented the historical gaze from the white humanitarians helping the slaves to escape to the African American communities and institutions in the free states that created the "railroad" from the Kentucky border through Ohio and on to Canada. There was not one route but many, each with nodes formed by safe houses, barns, and church basements. As Griffler says in his preface, his work "demonstrates that African Americans were central to the development and operation of the Underground Railroad."[15] Cheryl LaRoche concurs; she combines the tools of archaeology and history to map the many paths African Americans took from slavery to freedom. She particularly emphasizes the role of historic Black churches. "Ministers, such as [Bishop] William Paul Quinn, and their wives, in addition to congregations of interrelated families, acted as major forces for social change."[16] The freedom struggle became integral to the work of independent Black churches, such as the African Methodist Episcopal Church, the Baptist Church, and AME Zion Church. "The independent Black church, as the institutional, family, and religious center of life in small communities, centralized the struggle for freedom," LaRoche declares.[17] Wherever there was a cluster of Black farms and shops, there was also a church binding the community together and ready to assist the traveler.

The Langstons crossed the Ohio River by ferry at Gallipolis and at last stood on the ground of a free state. They left the freed slaves of the party at a "negro settlement" nearby and went on to Chillicothe, where "they found themselves in their battered and worn carry-all, with horses reduced in flesh—all, persons, animals and conveyance bearing a wretched and forlorn appearance—entering the famous, beautiful city of Chillicothe, once the capital of the State of Ohio." So too would the Harris family arrive years later and, like the Langstons, find friends from home. Chillicothe was a common destination for those leaving Virginia and North Carolina for a new life in Ohio.[18] But even in this free state Langston was insulted in his travels, as in stopping at an inn where he was told "we do not entertain n——s!" Langston labeled this verbal assault "an experience more deadly than poison."[19] The Harris family likely suffered similar humiliations.

The large Harris family followed this same route during their emigration nearly sixteen years later. Sister Sarah Harris Richardson had her fourth child, Alexander, somewhere along this rocky trail to Ohio. My imagination wants to populate that campsite with the sounds of her labor mingling with crying children (her three-year-old twin boys were in the group, perhaps being comforted by their older brother Jacob), creating a general climate of melee and misery. They may have crossed the river at Gallipolis as well, or at other narrow points in the river nearby, into southeastern Ohio. This was one area often used by escaping slaves following the Underground Railroad. It was the quickest route into Ohio from North Carolina and western Virginia.

While we have no direct record of the Harris family interacting with the African Protestant churches in Ohio during their trek, we do know that the small church communities were there along their path. Sons William and Cicero became AME and AME Zion ministers, respectively. When Robert and Cicero needed references in order to work with the Freedmen's Bureau as teachers after the war, their ministers from Ohio wrote the letters. The African Protestant churches would have provided the Harris family with immediate sympathetic aid, as well as helped them become settled. The Harris family were not escaped slaves, of course, but free Black Americans. Even so, the family still needed sustenance, friendship, information, and community structure, such as they had left behind in North Carolina. The church connections of the Underground Railroad would have made them welcome.

The Harris family first settled in Chillicothe and then moved to Delaware, Ohio, in 1854 before arriving in Cleveland by 1857.[20] William bought a farm in Delaware, Ohio, that was still supporting his family in the 1860s. "And it was in Cleveland that the younger Harrises received the education which had motivated the migration of their family from North Carolina to Ohio," concluded family historian Constance Daniel in the 1940s.[21] J. D. Harris arrived in Ohio when he was seventeen or eighteen; he left Ohio for Iowa when he was twenty-one or so. What happened to him in the interim? It is impossible to say with certainty, but we can reconstruct something of his political transformation by comparing the content of the poem he published in 1856 with known free Black activism in Ohio during that time period. Such activism increasingly centered on "Colored Conventions" that verbalized the many changes needed in the legal rights of Ohio's Black population. The Langston brothers, Charles and John Mercer, were key figures in these institutions from their instauration. J. D.'s brother William attended one such convention in 1856, when J. D. would have been in Iowa. Given the centrality of the Langstons in these events, John Mercer Langston's writings continue to offer a window into the political world that radicalized Harris upon his arrival in Ohio.

THE COLORED CONVENTIONS AND RISING POLITICAL SENSIBILITIES

In 1848 Black leaders in Ohio met for the first time in formal convention to call for reform in the state. Charles Langston (who also had a college degree from Oberlin) was one of the organizers, and Frederick Douglass and Martin Delany were visiting dignitaries who urged the colored Ohioans to action. Their central theme was the need to "elevate" the Black population. To the group this meant recommending to "our brethren throughout the country, the necessity of obtaining a knowledge of mechanical trade, farming, mercantile business, the learned professions, as well as the accumulation of wealth," all of which they saw as the "essential means of elevating us as a class."[22] While one delegate protested that menial work was not shameful and was necessary for some, the overall push was for education and "rising" into middle-class occupations. Accordingly, one of the conference resolutions proclaimed the "occupation of domestics and servants among our people is degrading to us as a class, and we deem it our bounden duty to discountenance such pursuits, except where necessity compels the person to resort thereto as a means of livelihood."[23] They were drawing a delicate line here—not just urging education and the learned professions but allowing farming, skilled crafts, and any kind of business to count. One wonders where the Harris family, with its plasterers and blacksmiths, would fall on this scale of respectability. Did exposure to such ideas in Ohio push J. D. Harris toward medicine as more honorable a profession than the skilled craft work of his youth? Perhaps.

When the convention next met in 1849, both Charles and John Mercer Langston were present, representing Ross County (which includes Chillicothe). Also in attendance were William Howard Day and Lawrence Minor of Lorain County, home of Oberlin. (Harris would call out Day in his *Love and Law, South and West* poem, and calls his hero therein "Minor Larry.") Lawrence Minor was mentioned as a signer of the report of this convention;

I could find out nothing else about him. The convention discussed the long list of inequities that afflicted Black men in Ohio. They were taxed to pay for public schools but could not send their children to them. The same was true for various public asylums, which would not admit Black people. The law that said a Black person entering the state had to pay a bond was still on the books and at times enforced. They could not vote, serve on juries, or join the militia. (One exception to this latter restriction was for mixed-race men who could show that they were more white than Black; J. M. Langston and his full brothers were "white enough" to vote in Ohio once they reached twenty-one years of age.)[24]

The convention also addressed an issue that would come to dominate J. D. Harris's life a decade later. Should they stay or should they go? And if go, then where? Mr. George R. Williams was in favor of all free Black men leaving the United States. "He said that he did not want to look up to the white man for everything. We must have nationality. I am for going anywhere, so we can be an independent people." Others said that they should stay, fight for their own rights, and work to free the slaves. John Mercer Langston proclaimed that as much as he loved his country, he was willing "to leave it, and go wherever I can be free. We have already drank too long the cup of bitterness and wo[e], and do [you] gentlemen want to drink it any longer?"[25] In this debate the delegates had joined a larger conversation about Black emigration since the end of the 1820s, when the American Colonization Society was founded to assist the movement of Black Americans back to Africa, particularly to Liberia. By 1850 many free Blacks saw this group as a tool of slave owners, who wanted to expel free Blacks to keep them from forming an abolitionist network. But others said that free Blacks should find a new home outside of the United States—somewhere in Indian Territory, in Canada, in Latin America, or in the Caribbean. Such a settlement would be led by Blacks and offer freedom from the injustices of American society.[26] J. D. Harris would become a leader in the pro-Haiti movement by 1859. By then John Mercer Langston had become his friend, and whether or not Langston still held to these radical views, it seems likely that he at least looked upon Harris's ambitions with sympathy.

The convention met again in 1850, and John Mercer Langston was even more prominent in the proceedings (at the mature age of twenty-one, he was a college graduate and rising orator). He exhorted his fellow attendees to form the Ohio Colored American League to promote the elevation of the colored man, the abolition of slavery, and the legal acquisition of full citizenship rights. During the following year Ohio would hold a constitutional convention, he pointed out, and the Colored Convention should push hard for full colored enfranchisement and legal rights under the law.[27]

At the 1851 meeting the Fugitive Slave Act of 1850—part of the compromise that admitted California as a free state, limited slavery in the territories, and settled the borders of Texas—was uppermost on the delegates' minds. It forced officials in free states to assist in the acquisition of runaway slaves on the word of a claimant that the persons were not free. The suspected slave had no rights to legal representation or jury trial, and anyone caught helping a runaway was liable to fines. In practice this meant that any Black person in a free state could be claimed as a runaway and taken south of the border into slavery. One famous case of such kidnapping was that of Solomon Northup, a free Black man from upstate New York who was kidnapped in Washington, DC, in 1841, was sold into slavery in Louisiana, and finally escaped in 1853. He recorded his ordeal in a memoir in that year (and 160 years later a movie based on his story won an Academy Award). Northup's story only became widely known two years after the convention that is under consideration here, but it exemplifies fears that ran through the free Black community even before the 1850 Fugitive Slave Act made it even easier for them to be kidnapped and sent into the hell of slavery.[28] John Mercer Langston said of it, "No enactment ever given birth to by the American Congress has created so much dissatisfaction and excitement, as the Fugitive Slave Law of 1850.... It is a hideous deformity in the *garb* of law." There could be no doubt, Langston proclaimed, that "by it all the great bulwarks of Liberty are stricken down."[29] Harris and his family were in Ohio by this time and likely were familiar with the outrage and fear expressed in this assemblage.

In 1852 the convention named John Mercer Langston its president. His summary of important issues would echo in the works Harris would write later in the decade. "The subjects which we are to consider are of great importance," Langston told the gathering. "The education of our children—the Agricultural interests of our people—the temperance movement among us—the course which we are to pursue during our stay in this country and plan of emigration which we shall adopt if we see fit to go out of this country, are matters for our most calm and deliberate consideration." The conference discussed emigration at length but opposed such a move to Africa. The temperance movement, as one marker of respectability and self-control, was a cause J. D. Harris took up as well, at least in his forties. Again, the group urged elevation and self-respect. One resolution read "that they (the colored people) should aspire to be the equal of the 'Saxon,' equal in intelligence, wealth, enterprise, commerce, mechanism, arts and science." Harris would give the

"Saxon" an explicit and unflattering role in his poem about race relations that would follow in a few years. The convention also expressed solidarity with the "oppressed Hungarians and German Socialists," seeing one cause against tyranny, be it expressed as American slavery, Russian serfdom, or the crushed Hungarian peasant.[30] These men were finding a global voice in the cause of freedom.

In 1853 the group convened again, this time with speeches by William Day, John Mercer Langston, and H. F. Douglass. These three men are mentioned together in Harris's poem; it seems likely that he either attended this convention in Columbus (fifty miles from his home in Chillicothe) or else heard about it in detail from friends or published reports. Themes from prior years persisted, with a strong statement that birth in the United States gives citizenship, and thus according to the US Constitution they were citizens and should have full rights thereof. William Day read an account of colored Americans in the wars of 1776 and 1812. Military service likewise demonstrated citizen status.[31]

These ideas formed the basis of an argument John Mercer Langston crafted as a memorial to the General Assembly of Ohio the following year, upon direction of the convention. Many of his ideas would appear in the Harris poem. Langston's petition asked that the General Assembly of Ohio take "appropriate steps for striking from the organic law of this State, all those clauses which make discriminations on the ground of color." He drew on a variety of evidentiary sources to demonstrate that Black people were citizens of the state and deserved full rights as such. "We are men, native born, and born free. We have inherent rights," he asserted, including the elective franchise. He pointed out that when the US Constitution was written, free Black men could vote in New York, Pennsylvania, Massachusetts, Connecticut, Rhode Island, New Jersey, Delaware, and North Carolina. Black men fought in the Revolution and the War of 1812. General Andrew Jackson himself praised the Black soldiers who fought with him and said they should have the same reward as whites. Langston also pointed out that they were taxpayers. Taxation and representation should go together. Black people were striving for education and elevation and deserved equal treatment under the law.[32]

At an 1854 meeting of the National Emigration Convention of Colored People that met in Cleveland, a man spoke who had been a soldier with General Jackson; he showed off his numerous scars, echoing Langston's (and later Harris's) proclamation of wartime service as a mark of citizenship. Still, this convention resolved that the Fugitive Slave Act, which had led to the "frequent seizure in the North of colored men, women and children, who are sent into slavery," had destroyed their love of the United States. It had "alienated our feelings toward this country; dispelled the lingering patriotism from our bosoms," and made us "regard as our common enemy every white, who proves not himself to the contrary." The convention considered arguments for the immigration of free Blacks to Canada, Mexico, Haiti, or other islands.[33] During this year J. D. Harris decided to leave Ohio and move to Iowa. Did he think things would be better there? The push to find a better place, so evident in his poem, was strongly expressed in these conventions.

While J. D. was in Iowa, the state conventions continued to meet. In 1856 his brother William D. Harris was listed as a delegate for Delaware County, Ohio, and elected secretary. In the proceedings of this convention at this point, all we hear about William is that he had been charged with presenting an address written by the Ladies Anti-slavery Society of Delaware, signed by Sara G. Sta[n]ley. They cited the story of the Spartan mother who charged her son to come home with his shield, or on it! No surrender! The delegates should be equally courageous and steadfast, they declared.[34] Since John Mercer Langston was also at this meeting, he presumably made the acquaintance of William, and perhaps heard about his brother, still off in Iowa. The 1857 meeting echoed similar themes to prior gatherings. The group again petitioned the legislature with text written by Langston declaring, "We are native born citizens."

It is time, finally, to hear the voice of J. D. Harris. This chapter has illustrated details of the home that nourished him, body and soul, and revealed something of the political climate into which he entered in Ohio (with Iowa to come). Using the concept of social capital, the chapter reveals the complex network of social support available to the Harris family in Fayetteville and the newfound social network of Black Protestant churches that would have eased their passage into Ohio and suggests that political organizations such as the Colored Conventions would offer the young J. D. another source of ideas and succor. But first, he went off by himself and received a noxious lesson about country and his place within it.

3

Poetry and Politics

More than a decade ago my friend Jill Newmark of the National Library of Medicine sent me a document attached to an email and asked, "Is this your guy?" It seemed that in 1856 one J. D. Harris, MD, published *Love and Law, South and West: A Poem*, under the imprint of Charles Scott in Chicago.[1] "That's not him," I told Jill. It could not be the same J. D. Harris. Harris was a common name, and "J. D." could also represent many name combinations. Fayetteville and Cleveland were his known locales in the 1850s, and his MD would not come until 1864. But as I read the text, it became obvious that the work was indeed by the subject of this biography. It is dedicated to "my brother, Wm. D. Harris," and it mentions George R. Harris—another brother. Events in the poem happen in and near Harris's hometown of Fayetteville.[2] The poem praises the beauty of an "octaroon," a light-skinned mixed-race girl—not a likely choice for a white author (unless she dies tragically at the end).[3] Above all, the themes of freedom and citizenship that echo through the pages are repeated in Harris's later work on Haiti. This is our fellow, all right.

    I use this epic poem to explore the mind of the young man who wrote it and his experiences in the last decade of antebellum America. It is admittedly an unreliable craft for crossing the choppy seas of the 1850s or determining biographical facts. It is fiction, yes—but it is fiction inspired by emotions and events that populated J. D.'s daily world. He was following that common dictum for new authors: "Write about what you know." Using a variety of sources from and about the 1850s, we can at least attempt to sketch the young man's perspectives that will later emerge more clearly in his mature writings. The fact that he cites his brother as a source about the slave uprising late in the poem indicates that he felt the need to offer testimony about the accuracy of the events portrayed therein. To him, the poem was "true" even as it was also fiction. So, with such caveats, let us explore this poem as an entry point into his young adult mind.

The poem has a classic fairy-tale structure. A pair of young lovers are separated. The male suffers a variety of trials, which he overcomes. The fair lady is endangered by a villain who seeks to steal her from the hero. The hero returns just in time to slay the wicked one and save his love. All this imaginary narrative is intertwined with a political tract that condemns the many inequities suffered by free Blacks in 1850s America, not only in the slave South but also in the states of the Midwest. One wonders why Harris did not just write a political tract. Perhaps he was impressed by the power of *Uncle Tom's Cabin*, Harriet Beecher Stowe's famous novel that humanized slaves and made their plight visible to the sympathetic reader. He was likely familiar with a variety of proslavery writings that depicted the free Black person as destitute, miserable, and pining for slavery. By placing his characters amid the lines of a fairy tale, complete with a prince and princess, he has the reader imagining his light-skinned, free Black protagonists as similar to the beloved characters of familiar stories. The poem is not a lost literary masterpiece, and it had limited circulation, but its aims were grand.

As described in the previous chapter, in 1850 the Harris family traveled in covered wagons over the Appalachian Mountains into the promised land of "free" Ohio. J. D. Harris was seventeen and probably quite muscular, given that the 1850 census listed him as a blacksmith. They would have camped most of the way, as public lodging would not take in Black families, even in Ohio. It is likely that other free Black Fayetteville families came as well, escaping the increasingly hostile environment of their home state. Traveling in such numbers offered some protection against slave catchers. The family stayed in Chillicothe for a few years, then moved to Delaware, Ohio, in 1854 and finally to Cleveland in 1857.[4] In 1854 (or thereabouts), J. D. left his family to strike out on his own. He moved more than 100 miles farther west, where he was listed in the 1856 census of Delhi, Iowa, as a plasterer. Why did he leave? There is no direct information. But through this remarkable book of poetry, we gain our first access to his motivations, passions, and deep frustrations.

The theme of the poem is "love and law," and one candidate for the anonymous preface writer is John Mercer Langston, the first African American lawyer in Ohio whose diary was mined in the last chapter. Harris knew Langston by 1858 and remained friends with him into the 1870s, when they both lived in Washington, DC. Harris may have gotten to know Langston through a series of conventions held by free Blacks in Ohio as early as 1851, conventions that argued for equal rights before the law. The first convention (1851) and the third (1853) occurred in Columbus, just fifty miles from the Harris family in Chillicothe, or thirty from Delaware. The second, in 1852, was in Cincinnati, a hundred miles distant. Any of these meetings might have fired up the young Harris concerning the rights of free Blacks as citizens of the United States, rights that by law ought to have included voting, testifying in court, free public school education, and freedom from harassment by those bent on capturing fugitive slaves. Remember that public speech on such topics was barred in North Carolina. How exciting it must have been to see African Americans speaking their minds, in public, about such radical ideas! Toward the end of his poem Harris mentions a triad of antislavery Black leaders by last names—(Charles and/or John) Langston, (William H.) Day, and (H. F.) Douglass. All three of them were prominent in the 1853 convention, which focused on questions of citizenship and rights for colored Americans. If Harris did not attend one of these meetings, he seems to have read about them. The Ohio Anti-Slavery Society was one product of the meeting.[5]

Some notion of the sort of radical ideas disseminated at these meetings can be gathered from the list of resolutions passed by the 1853 conference. For instance, "Resolved, that the Bill introduced into the Ohio senate, lately, 'To prevent the further settlement of Blacks and Mulattoes in Ohio,' is diabolically worthy of its author." Not limiting their proclamations to such invective, they went on to take a radical legal stand. Resolved, "That while we will cheerfully keep and support every good law enacted to govern American citizens, we will never obey this Bill, should it assume the form of law, as we feel it to be at war with our self-respect, as well as with the great principles of justice." They likened it to the hated Fugitive Slave Act, which was obviously (to them) unconstitutional and should be "resisted to the last."[6] There is no direct evidence that Harris was there to vote on these resolutions; certainly, he was not listed as one of the representatives from Chillicothe (Ross County). But he may have read the report or otherwise been influenced by it. The emphasis here and in other Black antislavery rhetoric on the rule of law and the danger of bad laws shines through his poem about law in the West. Perhaps he left Ohio because he thought Iowa offered a more liberal landscape.

IOWA IN THE 1850S

Iowa became a territory in 1838 and a state in 1846. It may have appeared to offer all the shining hope of the frontier that Harris expresses in his poem. I have found nothing to explain why he went to Delhi, Iowa, in particular. The town was organized in March 1847 in Delaware County, forty miles due west of Dubuque. It began with great hopes of prosperity, but the railroad passed it by, and today it has fewer than 500 inhabitants, 99 percent of whom are white.[7] In 1856, though, it had 1,144 residents; 6 were from North Carolina and 32 from Ohio.[8] Perhaps one of those people was the connection that drew Harris. What is striking is that there was only one other person listed as "mulatto": Moses Robinson, a cook from Virginia. Harris boarded with the white Stone family, who came from New York. Farmer Andrew Stone, the father, lived with his wife and four children. Also present in the household were E. C. Taylor, a physician from Vermont, and his wife. There was also a twenty-year-old man named John A. Marvin (spelling of last name not certain), also from Ohio. His occupation was listed as surveyor, and he had been there only one year (as had the Taylors). Harris might have traveled to Iowa to join a free Black community, such as existed elsewhere in the state, but instead he chose this lily-white township. Was he perhaps running away from the law, or from family conflict, or from a love affair gone bad? There is no way to know. It does seem likely, from the poem, that he saw in Iowa a "bright radical star" of hope for freedom and justice.[9]

The first cluster of free Blacks in Iowa settled in Dubuque, where about seventy-two Blacks had landed by 1840, many of them working in the lead mining industry. Open violence against them, coupled with the decline of the lead mining trade, led them to migrate elsewhere, including to Muscatine, a settlement eighty miles to the south, which was the center of lumber milling, with a steamboat stop. Sixty-two Blacks lived there in 1850, mostly in independent households. Prominent among these was Alexander Clark, a literate barber. Born in the mid-1820s of emancipated slaves in Pennsylvania, he attended grammar school in Cincinnati before moving to Iowa. Light-skinned and outspoken, he was the leader of free Blacks in the state, and it is tempting to believe that Harris knew him. Clark might even be the author of the poem's preface. Clark first emerged in the historical record when he helped defend a former slave entangled by the Fugitive Slave Law.[10]

In terms of political attitudes toward slavery, abolitionism, and free Blacks, Iowa was divided. In both its territorial and state constitutions, slavery was forbidden, but many settlers moved there with their slaves in the early years of the settlement. Very few free Blacks lived in the state, but there was great fear that if Iowa legislated equality for Blacks, then it would become a magnet for African Americans. Some 115,000 enslaved people lived just over the southern border in Missouri. The whites in the southern counties of the new state largely originated from southern slave states and brought their attitudes, if not their slaves, with them. Settlers from New England, New York, and Pennsylvania were more likely to be *against* slavery, although not necessarily *for* an open-door policy toward Blacks. Such feelings were evident in the first Iowa "Black Code," passed in 1839. It declared that public schools were for whites only, voting was reserved for white males, the militia was not to enroll Black men, and no Black or Native person could testify against a white person.[11]

During the 1840s and 1850s, the status of Black people in Iowa, including fair-skinned mixed-race people, was repeatedly debated in the territorial and then state legislature. Some argued that Black peoples should be excluded altogether and those present should be forced to leave. But antislavery sentiment was building too, especially among settlers from New England. The national Compromise of 1850 was popular in Iowa because it promised peace, even if the strengthening of the Fugitive Slave Act meant some racial strife. The state assembly passed a law in 1851 that forbade the further settlement of Black and mixed-race people in the state and said that current Black residents could not buy property there. Due to a confusing clause about the publication of the new bill, it was and is not clear whether it became law. But it spurred the "colored citizens of Muscatine county," led by Alexander Clark, to petition for its repeal. The petition was tabled when it reached the floor of the House, but it marked the beginning of African American organized political action in the state.[12]

By 1856 the political balance in Iowa was tipping in favor of "Free-Soil" politicians, the nascent group that would become the Republican Party in a few years. They had the political numbers to repeal the Black Code, and that repeal passed. Alexander Clark saw his chance and again tried to get the 1851 exclusion law repealed, but it was again shunted to committee.[13] This is the time that Harris was in Iowa, and his bitterness may have emerged in part from this defeat. Whether he was still in Iowa in 1857 to see the success of the convention that revised the Iowa Constitution is unclear. Issues about currency and credit had impelled the need for revision, but questions about race and slavery were a major topic of debate. Harris may have intended his poem, published in 1856, to speak directly to this dialogue. A petition from fifty-five citizens of Delaware County (home of Delhi) argued for the full voting franchise for all races and the right to witness in court, which the representative from that county refused to present. Ultimately the new constitution was written with the word "white" struck from the article on suffrage. But that aspect of the constitution's modification was put to a separate vote. The new constitution was barely approved (51 percent), but the decision to make suffrage color-blind failed, with 85 percent of Iowans voting against it.[14]

With this background, let us move on to the poem itself.

THE TITLE PAGE

The title page of *Love and Law* lists the author as J. D. Harris, MD. Harris had been a seventeen-year-old blacksmith in the 1850 census and a plasterer in the 1856 Iowa one. Both of these designations are consistent with his origin in a family of skilled craftspeople. So, where did he get the MD designation? It is possible that he found a location for medical training in early 1850s Iowa, but if so, why was not that identity noted by the Iowa census taker? One answer is that in Iowa he was boarding with a family, and the head of household provided the answers about his tenants. J. D. could have thought himself a doctor, or at least a doctor-in-training, while his landlord saw him as a skilled laborer. J. D. is listed as being born in Ohio, further evidence that someone other than J. D. answered the census taker's questions.

A second possibility presents itself upon looking at that Iowa census report. Also living in the household was Vermont physician E. C. Taylor.[15] Perhaps in the company of Dr. Taylor, J. D. hatched the idea of training in medicine and indeed started learning from him. It is likely that Taylor had a medical book or two with him, ones that J. D. might have read. Taylor could have taken him along as an assistant in visiting some cases when construction work was slow. Such relationships could be casual, especially on the frontier. But all of this is just guesswork. When writing his brief medical autobiography a decade later, J. D. made no mention of medical training prior to 1863. When he published the poetry volume, though, he saw himself on track for a medical career and thus tacked the MD on his name with bravado. Others around him were reaching to the white-collar professions—his brothers to teaching and preaching, while his friends John Mercer Langston chose law and Charles Langston learned dentistry. J. D. may have aspired to medical training in the mid-1850s but had no way to reach it from Delhi aside from the title page of his book.

In the 1860s J. D. would claim that he had a medical degree from a school in Keokuk, Iowa, although given his timeline then he had very little opportunity to actually attend such a school. Might he have studied medicine formally in Iowa in the 1850s, giving some claim of legitimacy to his MD degree? What was the state of medical institutions in Iowa in that decade? There were seven physicians in Delaware County who formed a medical society in 1856, including E. C. Taylor. All initial members were "regular," meaning none followed the homeopathic teachings of Samuel Hahnemann or ascribed to the botanic/Eclectic school of practice.[16] There were no laws regulating the practice of medicine in Iowa at that time, so forming such organizations was one step toward classification of practitioners as mainstream and legitimate. With similar ambitions, twenty-five physicians had formed a statewide medical society six years earlier, inspired by the formation of the national American Medical Association in 1847.[17]

One aspect of professional uplift was the founding of a medical school. The one in Keokuk began in Illinois, crossed the river to Davenport, Iowa, and then moved to Keokuk in 1850, where it officially joined with the recently created State University of Iowa as its official medical department.[18] In 1876 a report on the school included the claim that it had 915 alumni. The requirements for the MD in that year were that the student be twenty-one years of age and of good moral character and attend two full courses of medical lectures, the last of which were actually at the college. The lectures were sixteen weeks long. Or, as an alternative to this requirement, the candidate could show evidence of four years of reputable practice (certified by a competent physician). In any event, he must have three years total of medical study, including the lecture terms. Finally, having taken a written exam and paid his fees, the school would issue a diploma.[19]

Keokuk is 165 miles from Delhi, but it is possible that J. D. saved enough money to travel there for a course of lectures in, say, 1857. The school had seventy students attending in 1854–55 and seventy-five the following year; did the light-skinned J. D. "pass" as just another student? This was no diploma mill—one report claimed that the winter session included more than 600 lectures. If Harris went, he would have needed both the lecture fee money and cash for housing and food, which seems improbable. But he may have become familiar enough with Keokuk's requirements to choose it as his medical school in 1864.[20] The most that can be said, from the claimed degree after his name on the title page, is that the idea of medical training took root during the Iowa stay.

THE PREFACE

Love and Law, South and West begins with a brief unsigned preface. Its contents give us some indication of the author's point of view but none of direct identity. The preface author noted approvingly that herein "the charms of poetry are enlisted in the sufferings of the oppressed, and in vindication of the rights of mankind." He then quotes from W. A. Alcott, "It is necessary for young men to aim high, were it only to accomplish little."[21] William A. Alcott (a cousin of the more prominent Bronson Alcott) wrote books that recommended young men seek self-improvement, a perspective that accords with sentiments urging education and elevation that were common at the Colored Conventions in Ohio. This might point to John Mercer Langston or another leader in that group as the author of the preface.

Later lines in the preface offer more clues. The writer praised Harris for using "the charms of accent, the music of versification, and the license of poetic fiction, to impress more forcibly some of the evils that flow from the institution of Slavery, and the monstrous injustice of those laws in our State that proscribe a man of color, and make the different shades in men's skins the test of qualification for the enjoyment of the rights of a freeman, and particularly of the elective franchise."[22] In Ohio (but not in Illinois or Iowa), a man who could establish that he had more than 50 percent of white blood could vote. Since the poem explicitly mentions Iowa, which was undergoing all the political upheaval of the mid-1850s, Alexander Clark could also have been the author. He could certainly speak knowingly about the situation "in our State" of Iowa.

Was the poem intended as an intervention in ongoing political debates? Almost certainly. It was published in Chicago, then a hotbed of abolitionism. I have not been able to find out anything about the printer, Charles Scott. There were abolitionist newspapers in Chicago—the *Western Citizen* (1842–53) and the *Free West* (1853–55)—but Charles Scott was not associated with them. Illinois had passed a new constitution in 1848 that forbade free Blacks from coming into the state. As in Iowa, free Blacks were not allowed to vote, serve in the militia, or serve on juries. So, the message of the poem could have easily been adapted to the Illinois case. Senator Stephen Douglas argued that free Blacks should be kept out because otherwise Kentucky and Missouri would free decrepit, aged slaves and send them over the border for

Illinois to care for. This was yet another argument against the ingress of free Blacks who sought a homeland.[23]

INTRODUCTION TO THE POEM

Five characters feature in this eighty-four-page poem. The hero is a poet named "Minor Larry," who appears to have many characteristics of Harris himself. What does the name mean? There was a Black political activist in Cleveland named Lawrence W. Minor, who might have attended the early 1850s "Colored Conventions" in Ohio and caught Harris's attention.[24] Or maybe Harris was simply tired of being told he was a minor, as he was just twenty-one when he traveled to Iowa alone. Larry writes poems, he travels to the West, he rails against injustice, and loves a fair lady. Larry is described as "beardless," with dreamy black eyes and skin of "sunny hue," which is a poetic way of saying that he is "high yellow" or mixed-race. He is a "nature-loving rover."[25] The heroine is named "Carolina Belle" or, shortened, "Carrie Belle."[26] She is lovely, black-haired, black-eyed, and, the poet rhapsodizes,

> Tinted, just enough to show
> That complexion which we know
> Oft in quadroon beauty glows
> Brighter than a blooming rose!
> Small of form and medium height.[27]

The poet gives her an aquiline nose, beauty spots on her cheeks, ruby lips, pearly teeth, and raven "[t]resses [that] fall around her neck, / Such as queen of fairies deck." She has dimples, a slender waist, a lovely singing voice, and a neat foot prone to skipping "o'er the green."[28] An ideal of perfect girlhood.

Harris draws here on the tradition of the "beautiful quadroon" (or "tragic quadroon"). His hero, Minor Larry, finds that Carrie's beauty is amplified by its rosy tints. Other works of the 1840s and 1850s United States highlighted the tragic outcome of such women. In some stories they end up betrothed to their own brothers (for their father's identity was kept secret); another plotline had the woman discovering her "taint" only when a baby was born darker than it should be.[29] But for Harris, his mixed-race heroine is beautiful, happy, and in the end joyfully reunited to her true love, Minor Larry, whose skin likewise bore a "yellow taint." Harris's mother and sisters were thus placed in the company of a happy heroine, not condemned to tragedy by the color of their skin.

In the supporting cast are two men and a witch. Carrie Belle has a brother named Winslow, labeled "the reformer" in the dramatis personae. Also important is Curtis Cory, the "Poltroon," an evil local man who holds Carrie Belle as his ward. Finally, in the last pages, we meet Old Peggy, a witch who lives near a tumbled-down mansion.

While this book is about love, the title indicates that it is also about law. The author uses this poem not only to present a traditional hero who struggles against odds to win a fair maiden but also to rail against the many injustices that challenge free African Americans in his time. This is not just an antislavery work but one that challenges the Black Codes of northern states, including Iowa. The free Black man was not safe in his own country.

The poem is overly florid and at times tedious. I am not presenting it here as great literature but rather as the outpouring of a young man barely out of his teens who longed for heroism, for greatness, for love. He sought a country where he was welcome, a place where he could be fully equal to the other men in his community. Instead, all around him he saw the horrors of bondage and the cruelty toward emancipated Blacks who were, in fact, only partly free. J. D. Harris was full of anguish and did his best to make the reader feel it too.

The story begins in North Carolina, near his childhood home. Nostalgia glows from his lines.

> Hail thee! Hail, thou fairer land,
> Carolina's coral strand,
> From the Blue Ridge tow'ring high,
> Like a pillar of the sky!
> To her eastern ocean shore,
> And the grand Atlantic's roar,
> Blessings rest forevermore.

With the emigrant's maudlin memory, he longed for this "Eden of the sunny States!" set in "[f]air creation's finest clime."[30] It was cold in Ohio and even colder in Iowa. He missed the southern warmth of his boyhood home, even as he wrote in exile from it. The more specific setting was the Cape Fear River, which flowed through Fayetteville, carrying flat towboats, lumber rafts, and fleets of oystermen.[31] Harris looked on that river in his youth; perhaps his description of the

> hardy working man,
> Leaning back, as best he can,

Distancing a Yankee's dream,
Poles the flat boat up the stream

was autobiographical.[32] He had worked near that river but now dreamed of heading downstream, out to the ocean, and away to the free North.

Then Harris focused upon a hillside overlooking the river with mockingbirds, cypress, weeping willows, and a cooing dove. They are near "the celebrated springs," where people seek "health and pleasure."[33] Visiting springs was a common pastime in an era when water was seen as particularly restorative of health. Historian Matthew Perry noted about Fayetteville, "The scenes of [Charles] Chesnutt's conjure stories were laid between the Lumberton Road and the Wilmington Road around the old mineral spring which was once considered to give out waters of great mineral value."[34] It is interesting that Chesnutt, whose sister married J. D.'s nephew, set his conjure woman on the same grounds as the witch in Harris's story. Maybe that area was a known "spooky hollow." Or perhaps Chesnutt had read *Love and Law*.

It is the month of May, and a May Day celebration is in progress. The maidens are dressed in white with flowers and bright kerchiefs, celebrating the "Queen of [the] May." Our hero is passing by when the queen herself reaches down to pick a flower by the Cape Fear River and tumbles in! Of course, he dives in and saves her. And naturally they fall in love in that instant. "Peerless beauty! How she seems Goddess of his daily dreams!"[35]

In the next chapter the fair maiden is identified as Carolina Belle. Her brother, Winslow Belle, is with her. Harris describes him as

[f]aultless, saving in his pride;
Pride was not a fault, but came
Native as his father's name!
In his bosom glowed a fire
Patriots alone inspire,
Was connected with a band,
For the glory of their land![36]

Since we know that Carrie is an octoroon, presumably her brother is as well. Like John Mercer Langston, Winslow has a powerful white father of whom he can be proud. And like Langston and other Black politicos in Ohio, Winslow Belle burns with patriotic fervor. Harris probably had two white grandfathers; it is possible that he too was proud of his white ancestry. Certainly, he struggled to know what country was his to love. It was a theme deep in his thoughts and actions as he searched for a homeland.

Abruptly the brother and sister, who are reading together, are interrupted by the wicked Curtis Cory, who is the guardian of Carrie Belle (although not of Winslow, which may be an indication that he had reached his majority). Cory is apparently white, the default skin color of his time. While there is no indication that Harris had ever been a ward—his mother still lived and the family was together—his friend Langston had been. And there had been charges about the management of John Mercer Langston's affairs while he was still a minor (and suspicions that the guardian might steal his inheritance). So the evil guardian may have been a stock figure in Harris's world. Still, this guardian wants more than Carrie's money—he wants her womanhood. Unwelcome, he plops down with the Belle siblings and urges them to continue with their reading.[37]

The text in question is a poem by Minor Larry called "Going West"—a poem within the poem, in other words. It is a love song to western travel, the explanation why he must leave the beautiful Carrie Belle and go away—just as J. D.'s family had left lovely North Carolina for the snows of Ohio. After a series of verses establishing that the sun, moon, and stars travel west, not to mention the bird and the bee, Minor Larry reveals his love for "[t]he free and the plenteous West." "[H]ome of the free," it is, "[t]he great and the glorious West." And Minor Larry proclaims his destiny to be in the "lands of the West."[38] Carrie is clearly pleased by his lines, causing evil Cory to sneer, "Fie, fie for the *Poetaster*."[39] But Carrie is ardent in the cause of Right over Might, saying that

[e]ven now we may foresee
Onward march of Destiny—
Truth and justice through the land.[40]

Cory sulks as Carrie and Winston enjoy a night partying with their friends. The next day Carrie professes love for Larry in the privacy of her room, while Larry's thoughts run along the same lines. So true love is established, just in time for a classic separation of the lovers. Minor Larry vows to return to claim his bride.[41]

The next day, Larry says farewell to his childhood home. "Adieu to ye, scenes of my childhood; my home / Will ne'er be forgotten where'er I may roam." He sings the praises of the trees, the birds, and "thy sweet sulphur spring." Smells of flowers, the sound of the creek, all reveal "[t]here's a heaven above and a heaven below."[42] J. D. Harris left North Carolina reluctantly, it is plain to see. And did he leave a girl behind as well, hoping later to return and claim his bride? Or was Carrie Belle just a figment of his teenage longing for love and beauty, the perfect queen of the May? We will never know.

Minor Larry's poem sets up the "West" as "great and glorious." Yet by the time this poem was published in 1856, Harris had good reason to know that Ohio (part of the "West" in his day) was not a paradise, and he had in fact pushed farther west to Iowa. The "Going West" poem nestled within his broader *Love and Law* story was presented to show Minor Larry as naive and fooled by false promises (as his family had been?). Harris was picking up on a song published in 1852 and sung to the tune of "Oh! Susanna." It appeared in William Lloyd Garrison's *Liberator* and thus likely circulated among the free Blacks in southern Ohio. It echoed the themes familiar from the Ohio Colored Conventions by countering the hope that Ohio might be "the home of the free." Titled "Away to Canada," this work by Joshua McSimpson was the song of an escaped slave who first landed in Ohio but now was heading farther north.

> Ohio's not the place for me;
> For I was much surprised . . .
> Her name has gone out through the world,
> Free Labor, Soil, and Men;
> But slaves had better far be hurled
> Into the Lion's Den.
> Farewell, Ohio!
> I am not safe in thee;
> I'll travel on to Canada,
> Where colored men are free.[43]

In Canada, the song proclaimed, a man was a man by law, unlike the fearful country where the Fugitive Slave Act ruled. Simpson's hero was an escaped slave; Minor Larry a free Black. He heads for the unspecified West, traveling by steamer on the Cape Fear River, down to the ocean at Wilmington.

As he says goodbye to North Carolina, Minor Larry also faces squarely the evil of slavery in his homeland. Larry looks warily on the scary ocean waves but concludes that he would rather drown than risk becoming a slave. What he sees next reinforces this horror. On the riverbank he sees an overseer whipping a "[m]aiden with uplifted hand." The slave

> [q]uivers as she sees the flash,
> Stinging from the burning lash!
> Falls, imploring, on her knees,
> By submission fails to please.

The woman turns to her slave husband for help; he attacks the overseer, and both slaves are soon killed.

How to overthrow the State,
O! to God they cry! They pray!
For a guide to freedom![44]

This is a radical question indeed! The revolutionary is emerging within the world of fantasy.

Next, from the deck of the steamer he sees a military unit march in a square with banners, bugles, and speeches. It is the Fourth of July, and the orators speak of "[t]his day [that] gave birth to freedom!" But nearby a slave auction is also happening. Harris interleaves the two events. He indicates the auctioneer's words in italics and the patriotic speech in roman print. "*How much! how much! five hundred do I hear?*" is followed by "But we as citizens are proudly blest"—as if one is coming in the right ear and one in the left. Next comes "*He's going! going! cheaper than the rest,*" paired with "The immortal Jackson! kindled our fame." The stanza continues, alternating the auction in all its gruesomeness ("*Just feel what limbs, and finger in his mouth!*") with the orator's conclusion that southerners should band together against the North and "[l]et the Union go." "Huzzah! huzzah!" cries the political crowd, shrieking, "The laws! the laws! and God protect the right."[45] It is a heartrending depiction of the deep conflict between the Declaration of Independence and the persistence of chattel slavery. Just in case the reader was slow to catch this point, Harris titled this chapter of the poem "The Mockery." Fayetteville was home to a large slave market and also had a parade ground suitable for patriotic display. This contrapuntal performance rings with tragic dissonance.

Having contrasted in "call and answer" fashion the slave auction with the Fourth of July political speech, Harris next moves the action to a neglected burial ground near New Orleans. He has Minor Larry traveling by boat from Fayetteville to the mouth of the Mississippi and then up it to Iowa. Since Harris himself started to Iowa from Ohio, the locations here are more imaginary than most. In a burial ground near New Orleans Minor Larry meets an elderly veteran of the famous 1815 Battle of New Orleans who tells a tale of courage and betrayal. The bravery of Black troops made the British soldiers tremble and retreat, leaving the Mississippi "dyed in gory red." General Andrew Jackson had promised the Black troops, recruited from among slaves and the free, "equal rights, and dowry the same" as that for white men who fought with him. The Black troops celebrated the great victory, only "[t]o learn their hero's promises were lies!" The narrator urges the reader to listen no more to the aged veteran, "[b]ut draw a curtain o'er the Orleans plain, / And shut the feeling ear against the clanking chain."[46]

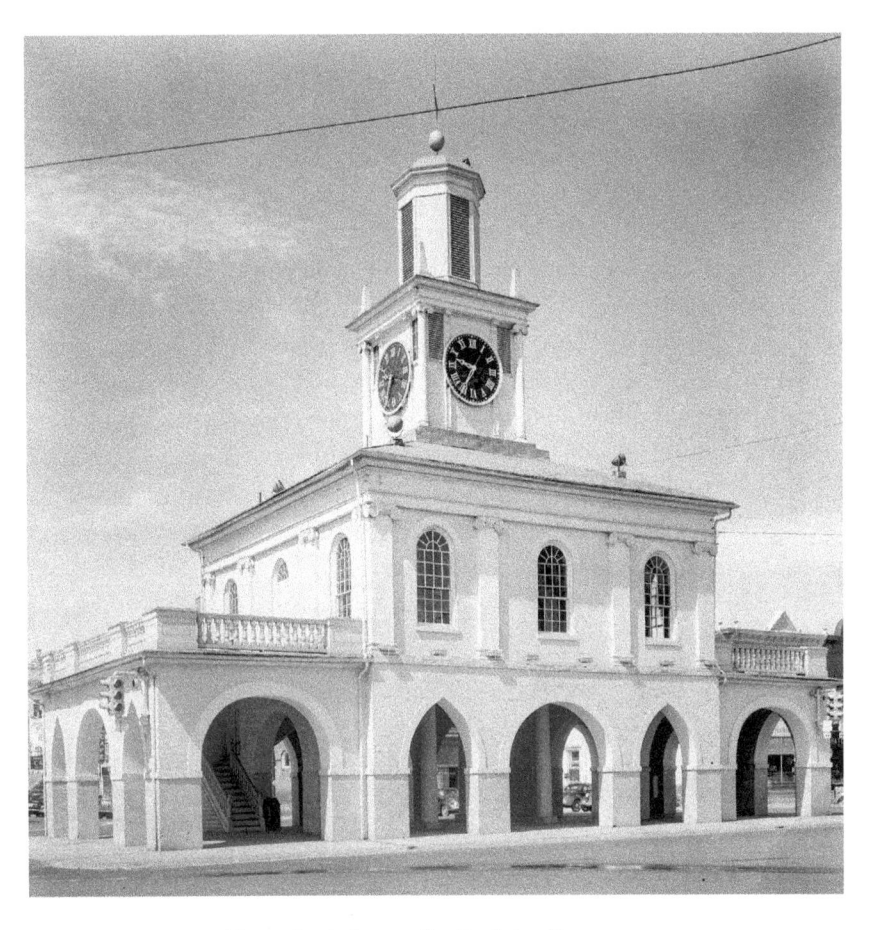

Public market in Fayetteville, North Carolina, ca. 1930.
Courtesy of Library of Congress.

Historian John Ernest has described the challenge for African American writers in the nineteenth century to create their own historical narratives to counter the glossy, happy, white triumphalist account of America from the Revolution to 1860. They knew the South's immense prosperity was built on both the expulsion of Native Americans and the lash of slavery.[47] Harris contrasted those stories here—emphasizing that Black troops fought in the Revolution and yet are sold like cattle. In a later text he counters the myth of the great Columbus discovering the New World with nostalgia for the aboriginal Caribs and condemnation of the slave system introduced by Europeans. Harris extolled the Haitian slave revolution of 1792, refuting the prevailing narrative of his time that it (and later liberation of the slaves in

Jamaica) had ruined the islands so altered. While one commentator chided Harris for errors in his Haitian account, historian Ernest countered that "the history Harris does present, reckless though it is, draws attention to its own recklessness, and questions the nature of historical understanding itself."[48] Blacks must, in other words, write their own histories.

In the next chapter, titled "The Alarm," Minor Larry suffers the indignity that all free Blacks feared the most.[49] He is taken up by the night watchman of an unknown "slavish city," perhaps still imagined as New Orleans or farther upriver in Natchez or Memphis. An exchange follows, with the guardsman ordering, "Hold there! give the pass and name," and Larry responding, "Pass! I bear no badge for shame!" The guardsman is assuming that Larry is a slave and asks for the kind of identification badge that allows for free movement of a slave around the city and the specific pass that dictates the purpose of the trip. Larry declares his free status. The guardsman says that since Larry has no pass, he and his men will take him into custody. Larry promises to respond with his strong arm, but the man says that he acts by virtue of

> the law alone...
> T'is the law that we obey,
> When to prison thee convey.

Larry responds that the law is "a mockery." The man threatens to call on twenty more to help him, using a noisemaker called an "Alarmer."[50] Harris is emphasizing here that it is "the law" that imposes this injustice; "the law" is the executive arm of a state that oppresses his people, even though their fathers fought to bring the country into being.

Larry lies in a prison cell, considering his fate. He sees and hears the action at the whipping post in the prison yard. If he cannot prove his free status, then he is doomed to "be sold a slave forever." Many days and nights pass, with Larry bound in a cell, sure that slavery will be his lot. And he the son "of such a sire, / As had breast a foreign fire." Here Larry claims a father who had fought the British, although J. D.'s real father would have been too young for the War of 1812. Larry is also unhappy because his true love has not written him. He prays to God for release but admits that he cannot forgive his captors. He had given up hope when the guardsman bursts in, crying "Fire! fire! flee! the slaves arise!" Somehow Larry gets out of his cell and onto a river steamer.

> Up the Mississippi now,
> Does the steam propeller plow,

For my hero's barque is free,
And the West he soon shall see.[51]

THE WEST

"Hail, the West!" He is finally there, the place that "[w]ears a face that tells she's free!," where the fields of grain shine like "a plain of sweeping fire!" or, as "now / Wrapt in waveless seas of snow!" He sings a love song to the shining prairie.[52] He meets friendly people and goes to work, earning his living. "For the West, aside from law, / Is a land without a flaw!" To this paradise, though, came the "[t]he infernal, slavish yell / Bursting from the vaults of hell!" He discovered the "Western Code" stained this paradise, a statute law that prevented the Black man from enjoying his full liberties.

> Thus the minstrel [that is, Harris] found a fate
> In the great, young hawk eye State!
> Yes, Iowa!

Harris has a footnote at this point referring to the Code of Iowa, which guaranteed freedom of speech and voting rights for whites. And "[e]ven Ohio! Freedom's queen, / Stands half hid behind the screen," denying equal rights for all. Harris calls on the "noble men, and free" to hear him; for "[f]rom thee claim, from thee expect, / Not thy sympathy, but respect." No pity, but rather "[w]hat we demand is what is right."[53] Once again he is emphasizing that the injustice and prejudice is codified into law. Structural racism, indeed.

The next chapter, "Servility," depicts Minor Larry reaching a crisis of anguish and despair over the fate of political freedom for Black men in Iowa. The scene is a political rally. A "mean-souled wretch" who is "a fool, an ill bred dunce," struts before the crowd. The man proclaims that if Blacks were free, they would "retrograde / To their old barbaric trade," namely, cannibalism. Harris has the politician limn a grim scene, in which a passing Saxon discovers that the liberated Blacks have a living man "scathed by fire" and then laid on the board "serving meats on festal day"; the man bleeds as his limbs are pulled apart. An asterisked footnote on the page claims that "there is a book published by a northern man, entitled 'Slavery,' to which the Author here alludes." Or if the Saxon could escape from those savages, he would find another "[b]y the speed uncivilized" standing ready to attack with a bow and arrow. This, says the speaker at the rally, is how the world would be if governed by Black people.[54]

POETRY AND POLITICS

The book Harris calls out here is a particularly nasty proslavery screed by Josiah Priest, who was indeed a northerner, born in Unadilla, New York, in 1788. Priest first published the book in 1843 under a long title that began with the word *Slavery* and then revised and expanded it as *Bible Defence of Slavery* in 1852. In both versions Priest brought forth detailed analysis of biblical texts, backed up by classical references, to argue that Blacks had been either savage or slave throughout recorded history and not even partially civilized until they came in contact with "the white race." This was, Priest believed, because they bore the curse of Ham, the son of Noah who was punished for looking on his drunken father's nakedness. Priest likewise supposed that the American Indians were incapable of civilization and argued that the Cahokia Mounds near St. Louis must have been built by visiting populations from Europe or Asia, or even the descendants of Noah, as perhaps the ark came to rest on American soil.[55]

Priest described the persistence of cannibalistic practices in nineteenth-century Africa with the same lascivious eagerness that he brought to the orgiastic fertility practices supposedly carried on by Jezebel and her like in ancient Sodom. (Jezebel and her court were Africans, in Priest's version of history.) Blacks of all biblical nations, Priest believed, exhibited "lewdness, of the most hideous description," including man on man, man on beast, and man on woman, whether sister, mother, or neighbor's wife.[56] Having established that the Black man's penis compared in size to that of the ass, he opined, "The baleful fire of unchaste amour rages through the negro's blood more fiercely than in the blood of any other people."[57] Such proclivities were not limited to Africa but bred in their biology. "In all ages, the character of the race appears to be the same—their nature predominates."[58] Priest was sure that "were it not for the restraints of the Christian religion, and the salutary laws enacted under its influence in America . . . they, as a people, if left to themselves, would be guilty of the same things as anciently, for their natures are ever the same."[59]

Here, then, is the argument that Larry hears—even Blacks with the patina of order and civilization would, inevitably, revert to their core savage nature. Sexual license would be accompanied by even worse actions. "The horrid and heart-appalling practice of *cannibalism* has, in all ages, attached more to the African race than to any other people of the earth," Priest proclaimed.[60] He described executions among "Negro" peoples in Sumatra, in which the criminal was tied to the stake and happy executioners cut away parts while he was still alive.[61] After describing other places and times when such activity was witnessed by appalled Westerners, Priest concluded that over three millennia of history had demonstrated that Blacks persistently practiced "the dreadful crime of eating human flesh, as an article of food; not from necessity, nor on account of the requirements of their religion, but wholly from the common desire of that kind of food, the same as dogs or any other carnivorous animal." Such behavior was evidence of "absolute mental and practical degradation, as is found over the whole earth, among the negro race, whether in a civilized or a savage state."[62] Priest was not alone in making such arguments, which persisted in American culture well into the twentieth century.[63]

Having presented a "southron" spouting the vilest arguments possible against racial equality, Harris reverted to his main theme.

> O ye States professed free!
> How much longer shall we be
> Bound down by your shameless laws,
> Forced upon us for no cause?[64]

The poet then points out that Black people are

> Being robbed, as we foresaw,
> By a fiend with tiger claw,
> Backed up by Iowa Law!

Has he actually been robbed and been denied proper representation in court because a Black man could not testify against a white? Not enough information here to say. Harris does have Larry rise to respond. "Larry rose to speak in place, / On the merits of the case." On the politician's speech? Or on a court case that he is promoting? Unclear. But what happens next is not subtle.

> [A] half-bred Irishman,
> Hating men of scarce less tan,
> Said, "I say, you lawless cheat,
> I know how your stamp to treat;
> And near me if you repeat
> Ideas, I will learn thee what
> Is thy place, thou hast forgot."

Larry turned to the man "as the hot blood in him burned," but the justice of the peace called a halt to the fracas.[65] Note that the Irish are as tan as Larry is. Yet such immigrants fight as white.

When Larry reached home, he was with "[b]itter anguish overcome," the "[f]eelings of his heart betrayed." And did this just happen one time? "O no, / Ever and anon 'tis so." Only a man "of hardest steel" could remain unfeeling in the face of such insults. Larry ponders suicide as an alternative to living in this dastard world." But then he prays and turns against such a plan, even though he has no friends to help him. Instead, Larry swears a vow:

> He that insults me, he that does impose,
> Without a cause, on me his hellish laws,
> Shall feel my steel! and dogs shall lap the blood.

Larry continues,

> I am determined. Let the villain snare
> Once more my peaceful pathway, if he dare;
> Then, O sweet vengeance! then will I begin
> To feed this flame that burns me so within.[66]

This is the center point of the poem, the apogee of fiery rage against the *law* that binds him even as Harris was living in what he thought would be a land of liberty. He had instead found that Iowa, like Ohio, had plenty of men who defended or at least tolerated slavery, who helped the slave hunters acting under the Fugitive Slave Act, who voted for Black Codes that restricted voting and other legal rights. Iowa, sweet Iowa, had betrayed him. It was no country for free Black men. Even as he vows vengeance against the boorish Irishman, he walks away, literally and metaphorically. As he lies awake, mulling over the previous day's humiliation, his spirits begin to lift. The sun dawns in the East and with it a return to optimism.[67]

Our hero is bolstered by remembrance of several sources of hope in his life. The first is to call on God on high,

> whose praise is sung
> As devoutly by the tongue
> Of the linguist of each race,
> And perhaps with equal grace.

In the "intellectual sphere" he draws strength from the free Black political figures he knew in Ohio:

> Sing of Douglas[s], Langston, Day,
> And of all the bright array
> Who, with genius, wit or lore,
> Light the way for many more!

These prominent leaders of the Colored Conventions still believed that petitions and speeches could change the law. Harris viewed these men as the stars in his firmament, stars to follow to victory. There is hope, in other words, in politics bringing a change in the laws.[68]

Most exciting to our hero's low spirits, though, is a letter from "his fairy, / From his loved, his idol Carrie."[69] His rhapsodic response is to describe his trials in metaphor, to confess his despair, but then to dismiss his grim thoughts and turn to a determination that they should fight together against the evils of their world.

> It will be noble, Love,
> For us to labor here to elevate
> The humane standard of the laws of State,
> So darkly desperate;
> And O, the joy may never be repressed,
> When Freedom sings the glory of the West![70]

Having ended his letter to Carrie with these words, Harris abruptly changes the scene to an unnamed city of the slave states, where Carrie's brother, Winslow ("the reformer"), has moved. The chapter, "The Slaves Arise!," begins with the author asking his readers whether they had ever awoken from a nightmare, having heard wolves howling round or seen demons dancing, graves bursting, the lower regions of hell released upon the land. If so, says the author,

> Faintly then you could surmise,
> Of the terror and surprise
> That is startled by the cries
> Of the slaves! "The Slaves Arise!"

The cry has gone up in the city where Winslow lives, although it turns out to be merely a rumor. The whites gathered up some of the slaves, who were beaten into confessing their comrades' names. Then, "the rulers of the place, / Dyed themselves in the disgrace" and had sixteen men bound and killed by "their rotten-hearted lords." The murderers, as Harris dubs them, cut the captives' throats and stuck their heads on poles. At this point there is a footnote that reads, "The Author has this as related to him by George R. Harris, Esq., as the closing scene of a late rumored slave insurrection."[71]

What insurrection did George allude to? George Harris was two years older than his brother and a Methodist preacher. So, at the time of this poem's publication, he was twenty-five years old. He had been in Fayetteville with the Harris family in 1850 and likely traveled with the family to Ohio in that year. Herbert Aptheker, historian of slave revolts in the American South, identified only one uprising in North Carolina in the 1840s and 1850s.[72] According to an October 1851 report in the antislavery newspaper the *Liberator*, "The people of Pitt Co., N.C. have been much excited the last week or two with a rumor of servile disturbances." Several Black men who were suspected of "concerting schemes for an outbreak" had been arrested. Some had been punished and released, while others were still in jail.[73] Pitt County is home to Greenville, and it is quite possible that George had heard about these events in nearby Fayetteville. But while the "suspicion" aspect of the event matches the poem's depiction, there is nothing in the Pitt County account to match the harsh retribution depicted by the poet's lines.

The scene described, of panic and rapid retribution on the innocent, did happen in North Carolina, but it was in 1831, not the mid-1850s. Harris is conflating past and present. In August 1831 Nat Turner led a slave uprising in Southampton County, Virginia, which spread panic farther south.[74] As one historian of these events, C. E. Morris, noted, "Two weeks after the rebellion in Virginia, racial chaos swept across southeastern North Carolina."[75] Rumors sprang up everywhere of 100, 200, 2,000 slaves on the march, and communities rapidly organized militias, rounded up their women and children, and viewed Blacks, slave and free, with fevered suspicion. One free Black man entered Halifax County, and on mere suspicion of his allegiance to Turner he was shot and killed and his head was put on a pole.[76] Whites were terrified, and the Blacks even more so. Again and again suspected Blacks in multiple communities in southeastern North Carolina were beaten for confessions, and some did not survive the torture. An unknown number of Duplin County Blacks were executed, with at least one man burned at the stake. As historian Morris noted (and Harris would certainly concur), "The punishment showed that whites had little compunction or mercy in squelching even a rumored insurrection."[77]

Harris continued his account of the slave uprising with the sad story of Winslow's death at the hands of a mob. He was the victim of the cry, "The Slaves Arise!" The men who killed him suffered from their deed, for "now [they] are crippled, drooped, or dead." The poet wants more, that the murderers be brought before the law and branded with the letters *M. S.* for manslaughter, as was the custom in North Carolina. "Burn him till he 'scapes the fate, / Saying thrice, 'God save the State!'" One suspects that Harris actually saw this done, but in any event he is describing how the law *should* act for such a murder, not how it actually acted when a white man killed a Black person in a time of slave uprising panic.[78]

The poet pauses and says, "Need we now philosophize, / For a moment moralize?" He has shown what havoc a false alarm can bring. But

> [f]ear they well the day must come,
> Frightful to their safeless home;
> Death and darkness, hand in hand,
> Sweep in terror through the land.

The slave revolt was coming, or the spark of abolitionism would lead to the overthrow of the system. One thing that will guarantee this outcome, the poet warns, is to keep kidnapping free Blacks under the Fugitive Slave Act.

> One thing know we, the best way
> That the South herself can slay,
> Is t'continue to enslave
> Free, intelligent and brave,
> Persons of another State.[79]

In the next chapter Harris returns to the fate of Carrie Belle, now bereaved of her brother and parted from Larry, from whom she has heard not a word. Her guardian, the evil Cory, has stolen Larry's letters and ridiculed him as a faithless lover. Cory also, to increase Carrie's dependence on him, has defrauded her of her income, leaving her penniless and now alone without a protector. His goal is transparent—to force her into his arms. Carrie refuses him over and over and finally seeks employment at the cotton factory, where she can earn enough to survive. She goes to the factory and looks in the window.[80]

Harris then describes the miserable condition of the white factory workers. He surely was familiar with the proslavery argument that northern wage laborers in factories were worse off than the southern slaves, who were guaranteed housing and food. But Harris argues here that the slave system impoverishes southern poor whites. "Know ye the effects of slavery / Fall on all alike." He describes these white cotton mill workers as "poor wretches, pale and sallow, / Mixture like of wax and tallow!" answering the bell of the factory's morning call. Even here, the beauty could not find work. Trudging home, in despair, she is kidnapped by "the villain Curtis," who throws her on his carriage floor as it clatters away.[81]

The reader may be surprised to know that there were antebellum cotton factories, but Harris is likely drawing on personal observation of mills in the Fayetteville area. Southern cotton mill culture emerged most vigorously in the late nineteenth century, but there were factories as early as the 1820s in eastern North Carolina. The area was rich in cotton production, and eastern rivers allowed transportation to the coast and beyond. Processing raw cotton into yarn or even fabric elevated its market value while making it more compact for shipment. Yet there were barriers to this industrial process. Mills had to be situated on streams fast enough to turn a mill wheel, and such spots tended to be rural, requiring the factory owner to build housing for the workers. Some mills, such as the McDonaldson factory in Fayetteville in the 1830s, initially used slave labor.[82] But this led to problems. When slave prices were high, it became cheaper to hire poor whites than to rent Black slaves. And, some argued, slaves did not work well with machines and were not as reliable as teenage white girls. Although at least one experiment tried working white and Black girls together, it quickly became the practice to racially segregate the mills, with Blacks excluded from the workforce, whether slave or free. Hiring free Blacks would have "demeaned" the work in white eyes, and then there was the problem of housing them in mill villages or otherwise encouraging terms of equality, however poor the situation.[83] Mill workers were either white or Black slave—there was no place for a middle category such as Carrie Belle, a free octoroon who was "brighter than a blooming rose."[84]

Harris's depiction of the paleness of the workers was likely also due to his personal observation. Unlike the usual sun-exposed white farmers, these young women worked twelve-hour days, five days a week, and nine hours on Saturday—and all for a wage that ranged from twelve to thirty-seven cents a day.[85] No wonder they were pale and sallow! There may have been some irony in his description of these wage slaves as so white, given the preoccupation of the time with skin tone and all its meanings in terms of citizenship. That Carrie Belle was not pale enough for such grim work was a commentary on both the misery of white factory work and the lack of any place for the free Black person in North Carolina. Harris, like John Hope Franklin, illustrates here the wretched hopelessness of the "unwanted people" in the state of his birth.

At the beginning of the poem's next chapter, lo! our hero appears, jumping out of a carriage pulled by two white horses. He opens Belle's cottage, but it is empty. "She was gone! and no one knew where. / Shocked! he stood as if he grew there." Then he remembers Cory's treachery. At that point, the poet introduces the witch, "Old Peggy." And a proper witch she is, who could travel through keyholes or turn into a black cat that would leap astride someone's back and ride the unfortunate through the air at night. She has pointy teeth and eyes "like two blazing moons upon the midnight raising." This witch lives in a shanty that is near an old, deserted mansion, which was so haunted with "sounds of blood and thunder" that only Old Peggy would venture inside.[86]

Larry suspects that Carrie is imprisoned in the house and heads toward it. On the road he meets a tall, athletic woman riding a horse, who blows a horn

> that sounded to him
> Like the howl, infernal yell of
> Hounds of hell that he heard tell of.

Larry labels her the devil's daughter and gives chase when she races away toward the house. The woman turns and draws a dagger. Larry shoots her with a pistol hidden in his pocket. She falls and dies. Larry rips off her white headdress and finds the wicked villain, Curtis Cory![87]

Larry races into the house, throwing open doors, going room to room looking for Carrie Belle. Not finding her, he goes to the shanty of Old Peggy. He rails at her, calls her a witch, and demands answers. Spare me, she asks, saying that she was no witch but the remnant of the servants of the great house whose master was murdered by bankruptcy. She had kept guard since. Today, a man had brought a groggy maiden to her and paid Old Peggy to look after her. So, "Where then is she?" Larry roars. Peggy replies that she went to check on the girl and found her gone. The maiden had escaped out the window by means of a ladder made of strips of cloth. Larry threatens to kill the old woman, thinking she is lying, but Carrie Belle just then jumps from her hiding place, crying, "Stay!" And they lived happily ever after, with "old Peggy, now called Aunty," to look after them.[88]

The poem closes with a plea to politicians in Iowa and probably in Ohio as well.

> Ye, who o'er these pages read,
> Who would further trace the thread
> Of the lovers, of their fate,
> Either of the laws of State,
> We will tell you now, they are
> In a Western State, afar
> From their native code, that says,
> Having left there "ninety days,"
> They may not again reside
> By the novel Cape Fear's tide.
> West! we leave them, for we must,
> By the laws of justice, trust
> That you, Reader, will, ere long,
> Number one among the throng

> Who, erewhile of southrons prate,
> Turn to your own laws of State,
> And the base eradicate!
> Let us not renew the strain,
> But when thou hast met again
> In Assembly, may we see
> That thy laws are truly free.[89]

Harris hoped that the poem would inspire the legislators of the free states to rescind the Black Codes that limited individual freedoms in the midwestern states. But the most important law was the federal one, the Fugitive Slave Act, which endangered every Black person in the free states. He had found little improvement in Iowa, and by 1858 Harris was again in Ohio and active in an antislavery group in Cleveland. There he met John Brown, who offered a new direction for this fiery hero's ambitions.

To reprise the comments made in the poem's introduction about racism, it is clear from his words that Harris experienced the many ways that his race was physically and mentally demeaned in his public landscape. Rape, brutality, murder—all were condoned by the state. He could have internalized it, believing it proper that the whites ruled supreme and so forth. But his response was not submission. He was enraged, and not just at individuals but at the *law* itself, which excluded African American rights and promoted African American slavery. Even in the so-called free states, the Black man met nasty condemnation of his race as primitive, animalistic, and hypersexual. Harris was a young hothead, some might say, but one determined to find a path to the reform and betterment of his people.

4

Revolution in Cleveland, 1858-1859

It is hard to read the events of the 1850s without knowing the Civil War is imminent. This foreshadowing can create a "prelude to the great conflict" tableau out of every action—even though, of course, the actors in the 1850s dramas knew only that their times were fearful and turbulent. The Fugitive Slave Act of 1850; the congressional struggle to balance the slave states against the free, as in the Kansas-Nebraska Act; John Brown's strikes against slavery; the *Dred Scott* decision; the split of the Democratic Party into northern and southern wings; the rise of the Free-Soil Party; and the emergence of the new Republican Party defined by opposition to slavery's extension—all presaged the coming disruption. Abraham Lincoln famously proclaimed in 1858, "A house divided against itself, cannot stand. I believe this government cannot endure, permanently, half slave and half free."[1] Why not? Because that criterion of division, slave and free, refused to stay binary and within hard borders. Each region was defined by its inhabitants, and people can move.

J. D. Harris and his fellow free Blacks in the North were enraged by the increasing encroachment of the slave power on their political efforts to increase the civil rights of free African Americans. The gatherings of "colored citizens" across the northern states continued to petition the government for voting rights, public education for their children, and in general for the recognition that their hard work and taxes should earn protection by their governments, federal and local. J. D. Harris was radicalized by two major acts of uprising, acts that demonstrated that the Black men and their supporters were willing to take up arms against the slavocracy: the Wellington rescue of a runaway slave and the John Brown raid in Virginia. He was also motivated by the seeming futility of political action to expedite reforms. He and many free Blacks concluded that it was time to leave the hostile and dangerous United States.

Historian Andrew Delbanco, in his monograph *The War before the War*, has highlighted the importance of escaped slaves in tearing down the imagined wall between the two very different societies that composed the United States in the 1850s. Northerners who might have believed slavery was a benign institution or at least something that was none of their business were horrified when they saw slave catchers dragging an escaped slave from hiding as that person screamed for mercy and rescue. "Fugitives from slavery ripped open the screen behind which America tried to conceal the reality of life for Black Americans," argues Delbanco.[2] And it was the Fugitive Slave Act of 1850, meant to help balance the powers between the regions and make the admission of free states from new territories palatable, that lit the fuse of the coming conflagration. While the right to recapture escaped slaves was embedded in the Constitution, the 1850 law gave it teeth. The captured Black person could not speak in court, even about contested identity. No exonerating circumstances were allowed, no matter how brutal the owner's prior treatment. Local authorities had to act on the side of the slave owner, and sheltering an escaped slave became a criminal act.[3]

At the Colored Conventions in Ohio through the 1850s, the participants aired multiple grievances, including insecurity of property, the denial of voting rights, the inadequate provision of schools for their children, and their prohibition from juries. The very fact that they could petition for reform and publish their proceedings indicated freedoms granted only outside of slave states. One reason free Blacks fled states like North Carolina was to get away from the "pattyrollers," the slave patrols who might kidnap free Blacks and sell them into slavery. The Fugitive Slave Act fractured the putative safety of the North. Slave catchers could manufacture documents claiming a free Black person in a free state was actually a runaway slave, and if legal papers could not be produced on the spot proving otherwise, then that hapless individual could be sold into slavery. This famously happened to Solomon Northup, whose story was well covered in northern papers when revealed in 1853;

now it could happen to anyone with dark-hued skin anywhere in the United States.[4] The federal marshals' service was required to help the slave catchers, and local law enforcement was helpless to block the taking. Northern citizens had become unwilling servants of the southern slavocracy and witnesses to the horrid violence of slave "management."

The Supreme Court *Dred Scott* decision in 1857 aroused the free Black community in the North even further.[5] The case involved an enslaved man who had been taken into the free state of Illinois by his master and then later returned to a slave state. Dred Scott's attorney argued that since slavery was illegal in Illinois, Scott had become a free man once he entered its borders. Chief Justice Roger B. Taney delivered a lengthy verdict justifying his opinion that Scott was still, rightfully, a slave. And he denied the power of the federal government to prohibit slavery in new states and territories. One line in his decision became particularly infamous, as it denied that African Americans could *ever* become citizens, since the framers of the Constitution thought them not quite human. They were, said Taney, "beings of an inferior order, and altogether unfit to associate with the white race." As historian Don Fehrenbacher concluded, "The effect of Taney's statement was to place Negroes of the 1780s—even free Negroes—on the same level, legally, as domestic animals."[6] If that was the opinion when the Constitution was framed, then it persisted in every line of the Constitution that dealt with the question of citizenship, Taney argued. The slave was "an ordinary article of merchandise and traffic." In a gross overreach of legal precedent and the contemporary laws as enforced, Taney concluded that African American persons were "so far inferior, that they had no rights which the white man was bound to respect."[7] Slave or free, they were not human beings to be protected by the American system of government.

A key question in the *Dred Scott* decision was whether Scott could, by entering the free soil of Illinois, acquire citizenship and hence protection under the Constitution from unlawful search and seizure. Did state citizenship imply automatic federal citizenship and hence coverage under the Constitution? Taney denied that this was possible, as at the time of the Constitution's acceptance the definition of individual states' "citizens" had been subsumed under the national standard. J. H. Van Evrie, contemporary publisher of the printed edition of the decision and a notable racist in his own right, drew conclusions in his introduction to the text that boiled down the key points, just in case the reader lacked the time to wade through its dozens of pages.[8] "The facts in the case are all very simple, distinct, common-place, and the conclusions from them plain and unavoidable," he began. This opinion would go down as an "epoch in our civil history... a land mark in American civilization." Only white men were encompassed by the language of the Declaration of Independence. Granted, there had been doubts expressed lately in some locales about whether free Blacks could become citizens. "This confusion is now at an end!" he roared. The decision has "defined the relations, and fixed the status of the subordinate forever—for that decision is in accord with the natural relations of the races, and therefore can never perish. It is based on historical and existing facts, which are indisputable."[9]

The denial of citizenship in the United States led to an obvious quandary. What was the legal status of Black persons? What if, unlike the cows and horses whose status they supposedly shared, they should want to go abroad and receive a passport from the country of their birth? President James Buchanan, in office from 1857 to 1861, applauded the *Dred Scott* decision when it appeared two days after his inauguration. He ordered his secretary of state, Lewis Cass, to issue no passports to those of African descent. "A passport being a certificate of citizenship," Cass wrote to one supplicant, "has never since the foundation of the government been granted to persons of color." Therefore, Cass concluded, no change in policy need follow the *Dred Scott* decision. The supplicant in this case was Dr. John Rock of Massachusetts, and Senator Henry Wilson of that state vouched for his probity (despite his color), but to no avail. The newspaper reporting these events noted that a man cannot "safely or conveniently travel upon the Continent without a passport or a protection from some recognized government." After the newspaper pointed out multiple persons of color who had received passports in the past, putting the lie to Cass's statement, it argued that Cass was covering up the administration's real motive, which was to "degrade and oppress colored men in every possible mode." The newspaper concluded, "To our mind, the most disgraceful feature of the Dred Scott decision is that which takes away from *American Citizens*, travelling in foreign countries, that shield of mutual protection" provided by a passport.[10] A more famous American suffered a similar fate in 1860. The American minister in London denied Frederick Douglass a passport to visit Paris "on the ground that [the consulate] do not recognize persons of color as citizens." So, the French consul obliged instead, creating "a fresh cause for European jeers at American Democracy."[11]

THE WELLINGTON RESCUE

Although it is easy to imagine J. D. Harris reading about the *Dred Scott* decision and its sequelae with mounting anger, there is no direct evidence of his reaction until he himself became an international traveler a few years later. But the free Black community in Cleveland and neighboring Oberlin (which offered Harris respite from the most virulent racism of more southern locales) was itself shattered in the fall of 1858. Oberlin College had admitted Black students for years, as well as white ones, and the Oberlin-Cleveland area was a popular destination for escaped slaves who found there a safe haven. In fact, Oberlin residents liked to boast that no fugitive slaves had ever been captured and returned from their hospitable town. When slave catchers came after John Price, a Black man staying in Oberlin who had recently escaped from northern Kentucky, the town rose in the man's defense. The captors had taken him to the town of Wellington, where they aimed to catch a train. A mob of abolitionists from Oberlin surrounded them and the hotel where they waited. John Price was freed and fled to Canada.

The rescuers crowed about the success of their civil disobedience: "The Fugitive Slave Law 'can't be did' in this part of the [Western] Reserve at least," said one.[12] The federal grand jury of northern Ohio, ruled by the Democratic proslavery governments of the country and the state, brought indictments against thirty-seven men, charging them with aiding and abetting the Price escape in defiance of the Fugitive Slave Act. Local abolitionists on the list included Charles Langston, Ralph Plumb, John Copeland, and Lewis Sheridan Leary. The prosecutors wanted to try lawyer John Mercer Langston, the most outspoken African American in the region, as well, but since he was absent on business, they had trouble making any charges stick.[13]

Charles Langston was the second rescuer tried once the case came before a jury. After conviction, the judge asked whether the defendant wished to speak as to why punishment should not be meted out to him. On May 12, 1859, Langston rose and gave a stirring defense of his case and the antislavery cause. "Being identified with that man, by color, by race, by manhood, by sympathies, such as God has implanted in us all, I felt it my duty to do what I could toward liberating him," he declared. Langston made clear that the shadow of the *Dred Scott* decision hung over the proceeding. Despite the risks, though, "I supposed it to be my duty as a citizen of Ohio—excuse me for saying that, sir—as an *outlaw of the United States* [much sensation]." If a man was not a citizen, what was he? He was at least a concerned bystander who wanted to know whether a proper warrant had been presented. And Langston questioned in his own case whether the jury trying him was a jury of his peers. Such things were standards of English law passed down to the people in their colonies. Oh, but he forgot: "Black men have no rights which white men are bound to respect." These words are printed in bold in some typescripts of the speech; perhaps they were shouted. In any event, the crowd erupted in loud and prolonged applause. The judge gave him a "lenient" sentence—a $100 fine and one month in prison. And Charles Langston had become a civil rights hero.[14]

THE "COLORED MEN OF OHIO" ORGANIZE

Two months after the Wellington rescue (but before the trials), the "Colored Men of Ohio" met in Cincinnati, with both Langston brothers in prominent leadership roles. J. D. Harris had not been present at the previous year's meeting, but in 1858 J. D. appeared among those mentioned as doing the convention's work. Charles Langston succeeded his brother, John Mercer, in the president's chair. He appointed a group of men, including J. D., to be members of a nominating committee to name permanent officers for the convention. This group confirmed Charles as leader and appointed J. D. Harris as one of the secretaries. In an initial statement the group again articulated the broad range of inequities that afflicted Black people in America. Despite the principles in the Declaration of Independence, "millions of our brethren are publicly sold, like beasts in the shambles," they complained. "They are robbed of their earnings, denied the control of their children, forbidden to protect the chastity of their wives and daughters, debarred an education and the free exercise of their religion." Following the *Dred Scott* decision and the events of the Wellington rescue, it was even more obvious that "they may be hunted like beasts from city to city, and dragged back to the hell from which they had fled," and "the Government which should protect them, [was instead] prostituting its powers to aid the villains who hunt them." J. D. may have been the secretary who recorded those words; we know from his prior writings and future actions that he took them to heart.[15]

Nowhere was the safety of Black people guaranteed. Granted, as the conventioneers noted, "we cannot visit large portions of our country in pursuit of health, business or pleasure, without danger of being sold into perpetual slavery, the shores of neighboring States being more inhospitable, than the bleakest or most savage shore that excites the mariner's dread." Still, there had been some semblance of safety in northern Ohio. Convention speakers reminded their hearers that "in our own State of Ohio, while we are permitted a partial freedom, we are subjected to iniquitous and burdensome legislation. We are refused the right to vote; we are refused a fair trial by jury; we are refused ... [the] honors of office; we are denied equal education." Should one of them fall into lunacy or pauperism, only the jails existed for refuge.

The conventioneers called, yet again, for constitutional reform in their home state.[16]

Charles Langston had spoken directly to the ways in which the *Dred Scott* decision affected the liberty of free Blacks. They were not citizens; they had no rights; they had, in effect, no country. The convention debated the meaning of this outcome. Said one resolution, "If the Dred Scott dictum be a true exposition of the law of the land, then ... colored men are absolved from all allegiance to a government which withdraws all protection." Should we stay and fight, or emigrate? the delegates debated. Representative E. P. Walker raised the country of Haiti as an "example of proper independence" for colored people and urged emigration. J. D. Harris was among the discussants, although his specific views were not recorded. Later that day he responded to a man who argued that successful emigration required large numbers of people, as well as "energy, fortitude, [and] self-sacrifice." Harris "proposed to show that we had numbers on the continent, sufficient, if concentrated, to force freedom and respect from our oppressors." In other words, in November 1858 Harris was proposing armed uprising in the United States. He may well have agreed, at that point, with the man who spoke after him who "thought emigration, as a panacea for the ills that afflict us, was an unmitigated humbug." Harris had seen the failure of politics in Iowa, the failure of politics in Ohio, and armed force displayed against his friends in the Wellington rescue. He was ready to go to war.[17]

Harris resonated with the growing militancy of the group. One resolution reflected the group's strong feelings about the events of the Wellington rescue: "We tender to the noble men of Lorain county who rescued John Price from the bloody hands of a heartless slaveholder, and ruffian Deputy US Marshal and his mercenary posse, our most hearty sympathy and grateful thanks. We pledge them our sacred honor that whenever the opportunity comes, we will imitate their worthy example." The conventioneers wanted to be clear—"we love law and order, ... we venerate the Declaration of Independence, and the Constitution of the United States," but "we trample the Fugitive Slave Law and the dicta of the Dred Scott decision beneath our feet, as huge outrages." Harris was not the only man there ready to "force freedom and respect from our oppressors." In the same audience was one John Brown Jr. of Franklin County; his father had earned quite a name for himself in Kansas and had new plans afoot, as would become evident in coming months.[18]

The convention went on to create the Ohio Anti-Slavery Society, complete with constitution. J. D. joined the process as a member of the executive committee. And he handed over one dollar in dues after signing the document. His brother-in-law Cicero W. Richardson of Cleveland was also mentioned as part of an outreach committee for Cuyahoga County tasked with seeking members and donations from their home turf. Similarly, Mrs. C. Harris and Miss S. Stanley of Delaware County (where brother William had a farm) were assigned to a committee to organize in that district. Miss Stanley was the sister of William's wife; Mrs. C. Harris was J. D.'s mother, Charlotte. So, the Harris family connections were increasingly active here. J. D. Harris himself became the "corresponding secretary" of the Cuyahoga County Anti-Slavery Society.

JOHN BROWN'S RAID AND THE CLEVELAND CONNECTION

The fires lit by the Wellington rescue raged in the summer and fall of 1859. The focus continued to be on liberating individual slaves, and their hero was John Brown Sr., who had led an expedition into Missouri and freed six slaves from a farm just across the border. Brown had plans for a bigger raid, one that would raise the slaves in Virginia and conquer territory for a new nation. He even wrote a constitution and had it signed by conference attendees in Chatham, Ontario, a town populated by self-emancipated slaves. But he could not rouse those people to go with him to Virginia. Through his son John Brown Jr. and Jr.'s friend J. D. Harris, Brown tried to reach converts through the Cleveland Anti-Slavery Society mailing list. Then, on October 16, 1859, John Brown Sr. led eighteen men in a raid that captured the arsenal at Harpers Ferry, but they were easily overcome by the arrival of US Army troops.[19]

In the papers found within John Brown's "carpet bag" after his capture were letters from Cleveland that refer to J. D. and his friends. Most direct was a letter to John Brown's first lieutenant, J. Henrie Kagi, written August 22, 1859. Its author, "J. D. H.," announced, "I wrote you immediately on receipt of your last letter, then went up to Oberlin to see Leary; I saw Smith, Davis and Mitchell; they all promised, and that was all." Harris was exasperated with the lot of them. "Leary wants to provide for his family; Mitchell to lay his crop by, and all make such excuses until I am disgusted with myself and the whole negro set—God DAM 'EM." Leary was Lewis Sheridan Leary, boyhood friend of Harris and son of the man named as executor of his father's will. Mitchell is probably I. Mitchell, listed in the Colored Convention documents of 1858. Smith was James Smith; the first name of Davis is unknown to me. Harris lamented the absence of Kagi, who he believed was more persuasive. "If you was here your influence would do some thing, But the moment you are gone all my speaking don't amount to anything." He promised to persist. "I will speak to Smith to-day. I know that Mitchell hadn't the money, and I tried to sell my farm and everything else to raise money, but have not raised a cent yet."[20] This is the only reference to Harris owning property at that time, in these papers or elsewhere.

J. D. went on to mention his friend Charles Langston, famous orator of the Wellington rescue trial. "Charlie Langston says 'it is too bad,' but what he will do, if anything, I don't know. I wish you would write to him, for I believe he can do more good than I." This is the second time in the letter that J. D. expresses his impotence, and the third if his reference to making excuses indeed applies to disgust with himself. Harris asked Kagi to write to Charles Langston immediately, and "I will give up this thing to him. I think, however, nothing will inspire their confidence unless you come. I will, however, do all I can." Then in a postscript he noted, "Charlie goes to see Leary to-day." J. D. was in a tizzy. He was cursing his friends and even himself. In the end, the delaying Leary would go and die with John Brown, and J. D. would stay home.[21] Harris did not mention the other free Black man from North Carolina, John Copeland Jr., who would participate in the Harpers Ferry raid. The letter makes it clear that Harris had been assigned the task of contacting this list of people to get their support. Perhaps Copeland had already agreed.[22]

The letters and other documents with John Brown were widely circulated in the press after his capture. While some have identified the letter writer as J. H. H., in congruity with the signer of the constitution in Chatham, the *Cleveland Plain Dealer* "outed" J. D. H. as Joseph D. Harris of 162 Ohio Street in Cleveland, on November 1, 1859.[23] This was the Harris family home (his brother Robert wrote letters from that address in 1864). Other letters likewise clearly allude to him. John Brown Jr. wrote to Kagi from West Andover, Ohio, on September 2, 1859; he was on the road, about seventy miles east of Cleveland. Of their contacts in Ohio, he said, "Friend L——y at Ob—— will be on hand soon. Mr. C. H. L——n will do all he can here, but his health is bad. J. D. H I did not see, but L——n thought he would be right on." The first person referred to is Lewis Sheridan Leary, the second Charles Langston, and the third J. D. Harris. John Brown Jr. said that James Smith "is marrying a wife and therefore cannot come." John Mercer Langston "sympathises strongly, and will work hard."[24] Another letter, this from L. S. Leary to Kagi on September 8, 1859, reported that "I have not seen J. D. H. since I received [your letter via Charles Langston], but have heard from him. Nothing delays me more than want of means. I have been unhealthy for some time, but have grown quite well." After referring to John Copeland Jr., who did end up joining Brown's raid, Leary said that he had seen a Mr. P[lumb?], who could perhaps help him.[25]

Harris had a key role with this group. John Brown Jr. wrote again to Kagi from West Andover. He told Kagi that his letter of September 2 was received, and he would "hasten to lay its contents before those who are interested." Lacking modern means of reaching his social network, he turned to helpful men who would assist in spreading the information. Leary reported, "Through those associations which I formed in C—— [Cleveland] I am through the corresponding sec'ys of each, able to reach each *individual* member, at the *shortest notice* by *letter*." J. D. Harris, corresponding secretary of the Cuyahoga County Anti-Slavery Society, was one such amplifier of the John Brown endeavor.[26] Harris and his friends used code phrases in their correspondence, at the suggestion of John Brown Sr. Brown Jr. used such coded language when he referred to working on the company business, finding workers and shipping supplies. In an undated memorandum found in his papers, Brown Sr. directed, *"Be careful what you write to all persons. Do not send or bring any more persons here until we advise you of our readiness to board them."*[27]

While the Wellington rescue had done its part to radicalize these men, it also had a sequela—less available money within the abolitionist community. Ralph Plumb wrote that "our people have been drained of the last copper to pay expenses for the Oberlin trial, and are now sued by Lowe for $20,000 damages for false imprisonment." Plumb had lost money due to his imprisonment and said he was going to Missouri in a few days to see about property there. "If I could possibly do so I would send you the required amount, but in my opinion it will not be possible to raise it."[28]

Brown did ultimately recruit two followers in Cleveland. John Copeland and Lewis Sheridan Leary, both born in North Carolina to free parents, left Oberlin on October 10, 1859, bound for John Brown's farmhouse about five miles from Harpers Ferry. Both men were familiar with Brown's success in "stealing" slaves from southern plantations in Missouri ten months before and believed that was the plan here as well. They knew nothing about raising the slaves, arming them from the Harpers Ferry storehouse, and invading Virginia. In fact, to the end, former slave Dangerfield Newby thought he had a chance to rescue his wife and daughter who were still enslaved on a Virginia plantation.[29] Once the Harpers Ferry scheme had failed, US marshal for Northern Ohio Matthew Johnson headed to the Virginia jail where Copeland and Leary were held, seeking connections between these men and the Wellington rescue "conspiracy." He found that Copeland had seen Charles Langston before he left; he had sought financial help from the Plumb brothers, and Mary Sturtevant likewise supported his journey.[30] They were tied to the broad circle of abolitionism in Cleveland and Oberlin, but Johnson already had most of those names. Although John Brown's plans for the raid were made independent of events in Cleveland, there is no doubt that this network of angry Black men and women added fuel to his fire. It did not work out, of course. Even his son John Brown Jr. did not join him at Harpers Ferry, much less Charles Langston, J. D. Harris, or the dozens of people who rallied around John Price. Armed conflict was perhaps a bit too much for these budding radicals.

J. D. HARRIS AND EMIGRATION

Harris found a different outlet for his idealism and racial fervor in 1858. He became a convert to the idea of free Blacks leaving the United States and finding a new homeland where they would be in charge. Here his ideas came into congruence with those who wanted to "get rid of" the Black populations that might be freed by a successful abolitionist plan. And the idea had support among some white politicians. For Harris, something had to be done. Appealing to politicians to change policy was getting nowhere. So, in other words, it was time to leave. The South enslaved his race; the North did not welcome free Blacks and even assisted slave hunters. There was nowhere in the United States or its territories for Black people to make a home, even if slavery was abolished. And Canada? Canada was too cold!

In the late 1850s, Francis Preston Blair Jr., Republican congressman from Missouri, began proposing a radical resolution of the "slave problem." Although Missouri had been admitted as a slave state in 1821, slaves made up a smaller portion of the population than elsewhere in the South. Independence, Missouri, was the well-known gateway for pioneers heading west, and many European immigrants, including the Irish and the Germans, settled in the northern areas of the state. Blair had considered promoting abolition of slavery in Missouri, as the state in many ways was more aligned with the politics of Illinois and Iowa than with the Deep South. This prompted him to think deeply about what to do with the imagined freed slaves. In his first major speech to the House of Representatives in January 1858, Blair spoke in detail about recent political events in Central America, including William Walker's invasion of Nicaragua.[31] While approving of Walker's ultimate capture by the British, Blair did feel that Americans could do much better at managing the countries of Central America than their current administrators. Black Americans—freed from slavery but imbued with American values and know-how—would make ideal leaders.[32]

This would solve the present problem of the growing free Black population in both the North and the South, Blair argued. "For, whether as a slave or a free man, the presence of multitudes of the Black race is found to be fatal to the interests of our [white] race; their antagonism is as strong as that of oil and water." But, he continued, he proposed "Central America—tempting in gold and every production of the tropical soil . . . with a climate innoxious only to the Black man," as a natural homeland for American Africans. Why, he proclaimed, its existence as an outlet would promote the gradual end of slavery through voluntary manumission. By saying the land was "innoxious," Blair was emphasizing that white people could not live or prosper in such torrid and plague-ridden lands, but Blacks could be comfortably at home there. J. D. read this speech and probably found the arguments of some interest. But it was Blair's next speech on the subject a year later, *The Destiny of the Races of this Continent*, which really grabbed his and the public's attention. The first speech had long quotations from British orators and was otherwise turgid; the second one was faster, sharper, and more accessible.[33]

"I dare not speak for all the States, but for that in which I live I can assert that there is a strong feeling among the masses to absolve Missouri from the shame of countenancing the slave trade, foreign or domestic," Blair proclaimed to an audience in Boston. "But there are difficulties in accomplishing this last point, that the people of the free States do not seem to estimate," he warned. Nearly half of the free states forbade the emigration of freed slaves from the South. Those people, however much against slavery, "should understand why it is that almost every man repels any scheme of emancipation which would let loose a hundred thousand negroes in Missouri, either to prey upon the community as paupers, or to become competitors with free white labor for wages." Any state that abolished slavery will want to remove them once freed; that was one of those self-evident truths in Blair's mind.[34]

Blair made several racist arguments to bolster his assertion that white people did not want to have Black people in their communities. First, any interbreeding among them would "carry degradation," with the families "running out" over time. The "half-Breeds" are not strong and the line does not survive, he claimed. Likewise, hybridizing the government "must prove a failure in the end." The "semi-civilized tribes on our Western frontier" would sell out and join their kindred in Mexico. Reminding his audience that the US government had removed Indigenous peoples from the East, as they could not live among the white population, Blair similarly argued that all Black freedpeople should be removed. "By the gradual transfer of four millions of our freedmen to the vacant regions of Central and South America," they would make themselves "a rich commerce, growing spontaneously," while harvesting the forests of mahogany, the dye stuffs, the medicinal plants, and all the various fruits, as well as reopening the mines for gold and silver. These people would naturally fall "under such a dependency of the United States" and look to it for protection, he believed. "It would, in fact, become our India."[35]

This was a plan of great moral power, according to Blair, one that would give the country honor in the eyes of the world. Black people would escape the social subordination inevitable in the United States and settle happily in the "terra caliente of the continent," where "the Negro alone can reclaim the vast level plains and pampas."[36] In this argument he oddly eliminated the Indigenous inhabitants in the region from consideration. White people found the tropics notoriously unhealthy, but Black populations were, in this aspect, superior to the Caucasian race. The tropics were their natural habitat. In the letters that followed Blair's published essay, one Alfred V. Thompson of Cincinnati reported that he and his family had gone to Liberia in 1842 along with a group of 225 Black Americans but came home when disease had reduced their number to 85 or 100. But instead of arguing against further emigration plans, he believed that colonies in Central America would be healthier, and he volunteered to go.[37]

Ignoring such fears of disease, Blair was confident of success. "Can any doubt the American-born and American-instructed African, carrying with him the intelligence, the industry, the progressive impulse, acquired by all engaged in the agriculture of this county, would fail to carry success with them?" Imagine him with voice raised and fist hitting the podium with that line, speaking to an excited crowd. Our Blacks will be superior to their Blacks and Indians and will certainly prosper, thought he. So, he was razzing up the American spirit of exceptionalism while not stopping to think that the 4 million aforementioned freed slaves might not carry the traits supposedly shared by the farmers of the free states. But never mind, American spirit would permeate the tropics, he believed, and make them suitable dependencies of their Mother America.[38]

The second letter included with the printed version of the *Destiny* speech was from J. D. Harris, responding to the earlier congressional speech of 1858 and its call for the acquisition of land outside the United States for the "settlement of the freed colored people." He assured Blair "that the thinking portion of the colored people appreciate your efforts in that direction, for while it is evident the white and Black races cannot exist in this country on terms of equality, it is equally certain that the latter will not long be content with anything less." The fact that the freed Black would demand equal rights was not quite Blair's argument; he focused more on the evils of miscegenation and violence. But Harris was talking about an incipient revolt; his people were "fast Beginning to rebel" against the federal and state laws that limited their freedom. Yea, "even while I write, in consequence of a late fugitive slave case, this spirit is spreading to a marvelous extent." We want to be the ruling power of our own nation, said he. Canada would not do. He beseeched Blair to bring the matter before Congress again and then volunteered his services should the proposition proceed so far "as to need an agent among our people," either to instruct them or to carry out initial plans or expeditions. "Begging to be remembered as one who feels the present embarrassing condition of his race," Harris declared himself to be "willing to sacrifice his time, his comfort, and his life, in order to create for [his people] a higher and more ennobling position."[39]

In early June 1859, J. D. Harris began to put words into action as he planned to spearhead the immigration of free Black Americans to a better home in Central America. He published a notice in the *Cleveland Morning Leader* that the Central American Land Company was thereby established in order to "use every effort to give practical effect to the propositions submitted to Congress" that a new Black homeland be found outside of, but close to, the United States. Harris was the "General Agent" for Cleveland, and the two other listed agents were H. F. Douglass of Chicago and R. A. Harper of Georgia. The president, secretary, and treasurer were, respectively, Joseph Wilson, Justin Holland, and J. H. Morris. The identities and hometowns of these gentlemen were not further specified. Holland was a free Black man from Virginia who became known as a classical guitarist, but at this time he was active in "the Colored Citizens of Cleveland" and in promoting immigration to South America. The common names make it difficult to identify the other two.[40]

In his notice about the Central American Land Company, Harris explicitly aligned it with the "colonial policy advocated in Congress by Messrs. Blair, Doolittle, and King." Like them, he said, "we believe it to be the destiny of the colored race to occupy the tropics of America, and that the establishment of a colony in that direction would lead to the choicest and most inestimable results." Harris apparently ignored the negative aspects of Blair's oratory—that the end of slavery would fill the country with millions of impoverished, inferior Blacks who would be a massive drain on society—and emphasized only the positive aspects of such a plan for the Black people themselves. Perhaps this is the concept that Harris signified when he wrote that emigration would be "calculated to convert that which threatens so much evil into good." Still, Harris was ready to go, and he had a plan.[41]

The offer made by Harris to Blair, presenting himself as an agent, was now expanded under the planned company. "We propose to send out as early as the first Day of December 1859, a delegation of colored men as Commissioners to select a permanent location, purchase the land, and upon their return sell the same in suitable quantities to such persons as wish to establish themselves in a free and independent country." Consider the monetary needs and flow here. These commissioners needed travel costs, not just to one location but several, in order to choose the best site. They had to find land for sale, with enough adjacent acreage for emigrants to build homes and farms. After putting money out for land purchase, the agents had to come home and find willing and financially able persons to make the great journey. It was a tall order. To further the company's legitimacy, Harris listed multiple quotations by prominent men who supported the idea of Black emigration (although not the Harris plan in particular). Apparently, Harris had failed to get any money from Blair and the Congress, as the next step was to "issue certificates of shares [in the land company] of fifty dollars each, feeling comfortable that it will challenge the favor of every true American and prove also a profitable pecuniary investment."[42] Whatever else one may say about him, this twenty-six-year-old man of little means had chutzpah!

The officers of the Central American Land Company posted a disparaging notice regarding the company and its Cleveland agent ten months later. "In the month of June, 1859, a publication was made through the 'Morning Leader' of this city, announcing the formation of an association under the title of 'The Central American Land Company,' to which the names of the undersigned were appended, severally as President, Secretary, and Treasurer, and the name of Mr. J. D. Harris as General Agent—Although this publication was made prematurely, it was not deemed of significant consequence to require public explanation, and was so suffered to pass." It is not clear what "prematurely" means here; had the three men not actually agreed to participate? In any event, the company had made no land purchases yet, due to "circumstances." But now they heard that Harris had been in St. Louis and elsewhere, "making collections of money, for which he represented to be for promoting the object of the said 'Land Company.'" This he was not authorized to do. They did have one of their number (Holland) query Harris directly on the subject: Was he collecting money? "He answered, distinctly, that *he had not.*" Just to make the situation crystalline, the trio concluded, "We deem it proper to add, that the 'Central American Land Company' herein referred to, has never had any active existence, and that we now formally absolve ourselves from any and all connection with it."[43]

Although this venture never got off the ground, Harris continued to be involved in emigration schemes. He was not the only Black leader to promote such measures; Martin Delany, James Theodore Holly, and, briefly, Frederick Douglass himself all saw emigration as the answer to the Black man's "unwanted" status in the United States. Historian Floyd Miller's volume on Black nationality, emigration, and colonization surveys the decades-long efforts to move the Black people of the United States to homelands outside of the country where they would supposedly thrive in circumstances similar to their African countries of origin. Such schemes aroused both support and opposition, although leaving the United States was looking particularly attractive in 1859, given the many insults free Blacks had suffered over the previous decade.[44]

Harris soon shifted his gaze to Haiti as a desired Black homeland. A central figure in Haitian immigration around 1860 was James Redpath, an enterprising Scottish-born American abolitionist who hired Harris to promote his ambitions. Redpath bargained with the Haitian government to set up an emigration scheme that he would organize from the American side, with agents appointed to gather emigrants and guide them to new settlements in Haiti. The Haitian government, then headed by President Fabre Geffrard, felt the need for more agricultural workers and offered inducements for them to come. The Haitian government paid ship passage, provided land, exempted emigrants from military duty, ensured freedom of religion, and offered citizenship after one year.[45]

In the spring of 1860 Harris took ship for Haiti, or, more accurately, the country now known as the Dominican Republic, "the Spanish side" of the island. It was, at the time of his trip, claimed by Haiti as part of its land mass. Who paid for this trip? This is not clear. President Geffrard may have funded his passage on the expectation that Harris would become a positive publicist of the emigration prospect. The *Weekly Anglo-African* newspaper published the early correspondence from his trip and probably paid something for it. He was not fully a "Redpath man" when he set sail in the spring, but by November 1860, a *Cleveland Morning Leader* piece alleged that he was "now Agent of the Haytian Bureau of Emigration for the State of Ohio." This was Redpath's shop. The use of "now" suggests that he was a Redpath man now, but he was not before.[46]

The *Leader* article begins with the statement that Harris had recently given a local lecture. "Readers will recollect that Mr. J. D. Harris, a respectable and intelligent colored citizen of Cleveland, has for some months past been practically engaged in awakening an interest among educated and enterprising men of his race on the subject of forming a colony and emigrating to the West India Islands, or some portion of Central America." The paper described Harris as a "slightly colored" gentleman who was the "duly authorized agent of some twenty-five families of said State [Ohio], recently arrived here, intending to select a location and make arrangements for planting a colony, etc." Perhaps they helped pay for the trip. Then the paper reported that Harris found a patron on the island named Mr. Pastorisa, who owned a "lovely tract of land" that would be suitable for the twenty-five families to settle upon. "Mr. P. is a person of much wealth and influence on the north side of the island," said the newspaper story. Finally, "The place is healthy, the soil productive beyond parallel and well adapted to the culture of tobacco, coffee and sugar."[47] So here is yet another possible patron for the trip—Mr. Pastorisa—and it gives a much clearer picture of why and where he went.

In the next two chapters we shall follow Harris as he searches for his Caribbean dream of free Black nationhood, and even empire. But let us pause in December 1859 and think of him reading about the following event in Haiti. Historian Laurent Dubois tells the story:

> In December 1859, an elaborate official funeral was held in the cathedral of Port-au-Prince. The Haitian president, Fabre Geffrard, oversaw the proceedings, while the head Catholic priest of Port-au-Prince officiated a high mass. In the nave of the church was the coffin, draped in black, lit up by candles and decorated with an inscription naming the deceased as a "martyr" for the cause of the Blacks. After a rousing eulogy, it was carried to a cross at the edge of town by a large procession that brought together many of the town's most prominent citizens. But the coffin was never placed in the ground, for it was empty.[48]

The funeral was for John Brown, who had been hanged by the State of Virginia a few days earlier. Brown had never been to Haiti, but the country's leaders saw him as *the* abolitionist freedom-fighter against the nasty slave power to their north. We do not know what Harris thought of Brown after the catastrophic end of his mission. Saint or fool? Unknown. But I do think it highly likely that when he heard about the Haitian government funeral, it must have reinforced for him that this was the place to build a new life and career, safe from the hatred, not to mention the nooses, of his native land.

5

The Anglo-African Empire

As the cold winds of November howled off Lake Erie in 1859, Harris pondered his fate. His anger about American slavery was unabated, but attempts at political and revolutionary change appeared to show that bastion was unassailable. Harris's passion needed a new direction, and he was not alone in this dilemma. Earlier in the month, Boston abolitionist Wendell Phillips delivered an oration in Brooklyn that expressed a growing radicalism within the northern abolitionists. *The Lesson of the Hour* appeared after John Brown's raid but before his martyrdom at the will of Governor Henry A. Wise of Virginia.[1] For Phillips, "the lesson of the hour is insurrection." Indeed, said Phillips, "the last twenty years have been insurrection of thought. We seem to be entering into a new phase of the great moral American struggle." Phillips developed this theme that abolitionism—thought outrageous only a few decades before—was now increasingly seen as moral and just.[2] Newspapers in Charleston, South Carolina, mirrored this sentiment, calling for southern states to secede, as "the South must control her own destinies or perish."[3]

Phillips linked the John Brown insurrection—for thus did the abolitionist newspapers label the Virginia invasion—to the uprising in Haiti. He urged his audience to "recollect history. There never was a race held in chains that absolutely vindicated its own liberty but one. There never was a serf nor a slave whose own sword cut off his own chain but one—blue-eyed, light-haired Anglo-Saxon, it was not our race." Commerce, Christianity, and law, said Phillips, gradually liberated the European serfs. "Despised, calumniated, slandered San Domingo is the only instance in history where a race, with indestructible love of justice, serving a hundred years of oppression, rose up under their own leader, and with their own hands abolished slavery on their own soil."[4]

Imagine J. D. Harris reading those words and getting more and more fired up. It is unknown how he came across the speech. Perhaps he was there, in Brooklyn, to hear it. Or he found it reprinted in a sympathetic newspaper, or picked up the pamphlet that circulated broadly among the abolitionist community. It is possible that his friend James Redpath, who hired him to work on Haitian emigration, showed it to him; Redpath included the speech in his collected essays and documents about the John Brown raid called *Echoes of Harper's Ferry* (published after April 14, 1860).[5] As another sign of the connection between John Brown and Haiti, Redpath dedicated the book to the county's current president, Fabre Geffrard.

By March 1860 Harris used lines from the Phillips speech as the epigraph for an essay of his own, a marker of how deeply he was touched by its fiery message. His subject was the "Anglo-African Empire," and Phillips's words had clear relevance.[6] Now, if attentive readers take a quick look at the notes, they will see that the author of this essay is "H. H. S." It is hard to see these initials as applicable to our subject Harris. But two points establish the identity.

The first comes from the magazine's editor, Thomas Hamilton, who said in a comment at the end of the essay, "The above paper was written by an enthusiastic defender and magnifier of the 'mulatto race.'" After agreeing that such an attitude might be controversial, Hamilton defends his practice of printing a wide range of opinions as appropriate, both as having "intrinsic value at present" and because it "will become [a] matter of historic interest to those who may come after us."[7] After discussing the content of the essay, Hamilton goes on: "The writer of the essay, Mr. H., is a native of North Carolina, and was playmate of the heroic LEARY, who fell nobly at Harper's Ferry. . . . Mr. H., yet under thirty, has already been a pioneer in our great West, and would still be there, were it not for the fact that the construction put by a pro-slavery government on the pre-emption laws renders the title of a colored man to the public lands imperfect." All of these details correspond to J. D. Harris. And then Hamilton tells us that Mr. H. is now in that part of "Hayti" held by those of Spanish descent. "He goes there to look out a home for himself and like-minded associates, whom the stringency of our laws and the inexorable influence of caste are driving from the West."[8] The second indication, if one is needed, that Harris wrote this magazine article is the fact that he appended it to his essays about his visit to the Caribbean in the book published under his name late in 1860. There the attribution H. H. S. is gone, and the essay is reduced by several pages.

Harris was attuned to his times, times of hope and despair. He had experienced so much loss—his childhood home, the failure in Iowa, his friend Charles Langston's imprisonment for the Wellington rescue, his friend Lewis Sheridan Leary's death, and the collapse of John Brown's imagined slave insurrection. Yet Harris dared to hope, with Phillips, that despite the darkness of the hour, Brown's ideas of abolition and freedom might yet live. "Do these things mean nothing?" he quoted Phillips as asking. "What the tender and poetic youth dreams to-day and conjures up with an articulate speech, is to-morrow the vociferated result of public opinion, and the day after is the charter of nations." Harris was one of those tender and poetic young men who had dreamed of freedom in the West and now dreamed even bigger. He would join his people in building a great Anglo-African empire in the Caribbean.[9]

Harris began his article by arguing that the "controlling influence of the great commercial staple of our Southern States" drove an interest in the production of cotton in the Caribbean and Central American regions. Slaveholders in the South were already moving their chattel from the worn-out lands of Virginia to new cotton lands in Mississippi, Arkansas, and Texas but were hungry for yet more land of the subtropical sort suitable for growing one of the most valuable crops in the world.[10] Southerners, fueled by "the filibustering propensities of Southern fire-eaters as the unerring and immutable laws of destiny," felt it inevitable that the slavocracy should take charge of Cuba, Santo Domingo, and Central America, where slavery could once again thrive and cotton production expand.[11] In mentioning the filibusterers, Harris showed his familiarity with William Walker and others who led guerrilla expeditions to conquer parts of Mexico and Central America. Their goal had been to create new American slave states to counter the expansion of free states on the northern plains and the Pacific Coast. Historian Robert May calls this drive "the southern dream of a Caribbean empire" and emphasizes that the crown jewel of this new cluster of slave states was to be Cuba, with its persistent slavery and high agricultural production. In fact, one of the first aims of the Confederacy was to plan a conquest of this island, although that idea was shelved once war with the North began in earnest.[12] Harris was thus borrowing an argument from the southern leadership, to prepare the way for his radically different vision.

Harris then turned to the question of what the fate of the free Black population of the United States should be, because, he argued, "nothing is more certain than that the people are to be free." Hinton R. Helper's idea was "most absurd and ridiculous"; Helper had proposed mass transportation to Africa. "It did not occur to him that they were men, and might not want to go," said Harris. "At least it did not occur to him that they were *men*." He applauded the idea of sending a small number of Black people from the United States to Africa to promote civilization and spread the Gospel, but the prospect would do little for the millions who remained in North America. Harris argued that the "growing disposition among colored men of thought [is] to abandon that policy which teaches them to cling to the skirts of the white people for support." They were instead talking openly about emigration as a means "to better their condition," and Harris found such conversations admirable. It is time, Harris proclaimed, to discover at last "what is to be the final purpose of American slavery—[what is to be] the destiny of the colored race after slavery shall be abolished."[13]

Harris then launched into a discussion of what he labeled "the colored race," his preferred label for peoples with mixed white and Black heritage. "The history of Hayti and Jamaica, and of the American tropics generally, indicate[s] the propagation of the colored race," he began. "This is simply calling things by their right names, for which the compiler of these facts expects to be ... infinitely abused, feared, hated, and all that attends the discovery of truth generally." Even though whites can live in the Caribbean, he noted, they cannot "keep up their numbers," except in a case like Cuba with "a recent flood of emigration on a large scale from Europe." Yet the colored race "is perfectly adapted to this region, and luxuriates in it; and it is only through their agency that some small portion of the torrid zone has been brought within the circle of civilized industry."[14] Harris then proposed to prove this fact by evoking the history of the islands.

First off, Columbus found people much like "our Indians," and through abuse and persecution they died off. What followed? "Africa became the hunting-ground of the slave pirate for hardier and more enduring slaves." He described the African peoples' torturous passage, ripped from their homes, branded and whipped, and finally landed in a place where they faced a lifetime of bondage. This "state of wickedness" persisted in the British colonies until Parliament, in an act of "justice and magnanimity," freed all British slaves in 1838. This law "restored the liberties of eight hundred thousand of our fellow-men." In italics Harris then proclaimed that this act "*left them in possession of superior claims and circumstances to those from which they had been originally removed.*" In spite of the American slanders that claimed Jamaica had been ruined in the process, the former slaves had in fact used their exposure to Western civilization, such as it was, to create a new and admirable land. "Lands having been provided and schools introduced, happiness began to smile, prosperity re-appeared, and the whole country was redeemed from what had been a field of terror to what promises to become the very garden of the Western world."[15]

Harris moved on to one of his principal maxims for the future of the Black man. Again, in italics he announced, "*For any people to maintain their rights, they must constitute an essential part of the ruling element of the country in which they live.*" Relatively few whites made their home in the tropics, but those wielding power there had "sustained themselves by their superior wealth and intelligence." But there was no need for the persistence of this white hierarchy, he said. "As the colored people rise in intelligence, their white rulers are pushed aside to make way for officers of their own race. This is perfectly natural." To make himself clear, Harris drew an analogy to ethnic immigrants to the United States and their voting patterns: "Norwegians elect Norwegians, Germans elect Germans, and colored men elect colored men, whenever they have an opportunity." This was, he pointed out, already happening in Jamaica, where the Parliament was equally divided and various executive positions were held by Black men. "It is fair to assume," he concluded, that "within a few years of the date of this paper, there will be not a single white man throughout the West Indies occupying a position within the gift of the people." This was particularly true in Haiti he crowed, "and no white man, not even old Uncle Judge Taney himself, has there any rights that Black men are bound to respect."[16] Echoing and inverting the *Dred Scott* decision, Harris hammered home that where Black men controlled the government, the government protected their rights—unlike, sadly, the situation persisting in the United States.

Harris then turned to correspondence from "a retired merchant of Philadelphia, a man of large thought and liberal views, having an experience of fifteen or twenty years['] residence in Hayti, in response to certain letters asking for information and advice." This merchant published his answers in a pamphlet titled *Remarks on Hayti as a Place of Settlement for Afric-[A]mericans; and on the Mulatto as a Race for the Tropics*. While Harris might seem to imply that the author answered him personally, this seems unlikely. This publication was attributed to one Benjamin S. Hunt or Benjamin Peter Hunt in library catalogs; Hunt's collected papers at the Boston Public Library call him Benjamin P. Hunt.[17] His 1877 obituary noted that he was born in

Massachusetts but lived much of his life in Philadelphia. He was known, it said, as "one of the earliest, most ardent and constant advocates in this city of the rights of the negro, rights now universally admitted, but the vindication of which, at the time Mr. Hunt began his work, exposed their defenders to all the terrors of social ostracism."[18] Hunt particularly took on the equal access of Black people to public streetcars and, after the enlistment of Black troops in the Civil War, the provision of care for their orphans.[19] (Hunt left his large collection of books on the Caribbean to the Boston Public Library, including an annotated, handwritten catalog of the collection. Of the Harris book *A Summer on the Borders of the Caribbean Sea*, Hunt commented, "Mr. Harris was a mulatto, originally from North Carolina. He endeavored to describe what he saw in the Dominican Republic, Hayti and the Bahamas, but his powers were not equal to his opportunities.")[20]

Using Hunt's text, Harris returned to the theme of the filibusterers and arguments for Manifest Destiny, the idea that white Americans had somehow been destined by God to take possession of the United States from sea to shining sea and (from the southern perspective at least) spread slavery south to the Caribbean and Central America. Hunt dismissed the "pro-slavery adventurer [who] may yet gain a footing Central America." He may indeed succeed, but "it will not be to establish slavery. Slavery once abolished, has never been re established [*sic*] in the same place, in America. . . . The vain effort to re-enslave St. Domingo cost the French forty thousand men." Hunt concluded, "To re-establish slavery permanently, where it has once been abolished, is to swim against the great moral current of the age."[21]

Hunt then went on to make a claim that became the central argument of Harris's essay. Hunt's argument, by discovering positive outcomes, followed in the tradition of seeking to understand how God tolerates evil. Hunt began by pointing out that Archbishop William Laud's persecution of the Puritans had the intent of policing religious conformity, while it actually "produced New England." As another example of this trope of unintended consequences, the obstinacy of King George III had as much to do with creating American independence as John Adams did. Then Hunt urged the reader to consider a third great question, perhaps the greatest evil of all, from a similar perspective. Harris foregrounded its importance with italics in his essay: "*If then, I were asked what was probably the final purpose of negro slavery, I should answer,—to furnish the basis of a free population for the tropics of America.*"[22]

Harris next argued, using Hunt, that prejudice against Africans would persist even in the northern United States, including among those who contended for the rights of all men. "In spite of themselves, they shrink from the thought of an amalgamation," where this last word was code for racial mixing and reproduction. From his familiarity with the Caribbean, however, he knew that where peoples of African blood had achieved "respected" class status, such prejudices faded away. The prejudice was a reaction to class, in other words, and not to race.[23]

Before continuing with the Anglo-African empire vision, Hunt paused to answer one argument against it that was prevalent among slaveholding Americans. This was the claim that mixed-race persons lacked vitality and would die out after three or four generations. Harris allowed that it might be correct in very cold climates, but in the tropics, nothing could be further from the truth. Here Hunt (and Harris quoting him) translated Médéric-Louis-Élie Moreau de Saint-Méry's words from his book on Haiti: "Of all the combinations of white and Black, the mulatto unites the most physical advantages. It is he who derives the strongest constitution from these crossings of race, and who is the best suited to the climate of St. Domingo." So not only did the mulatto exhibit robust health, but his vitality was better than either the "pure white" or the "pure negro." Moreau de Saint-Méry attributed this state of affairs to the mixing of traits. "To the strength and soberness of the negro, he [the mulatto] adds the grace of form and intelligence of the whites, and of all the human beings of St. Domingo he is the longest-lived."[24]

Harris then moved on to the ideas of Hermann Burmeister, professor of zoology at the University of Halle who studied mulattoes in Brazil. Again, following Hunt's summary of Burmeister's study, Harris noted that the mixed-race class was thriving and that mulattoes in villages assumed the roles of artisans of all sorts. "There is nothing," Harris concluded, "to indicate that the Brazilian mulatto is dying out." He lauded Burmeister as a man of science and impartial observation. "The Professor speaks elsewhere in high, but qualified terms of the moral and intellectual qualities of the mulatto, coming to conclusions similar to those of Moreau de Saint-Mery, except that he does not accuse them of indolence."[25]

To illustrate the leadership roles that "men of color" occupied in Haiti, Harris followed Hunt in listing their various occupations: merchants, lawyers, physicians, educators, artisans, and even editors. Although the rulers might be Black (and he was here distinguishing the "pure Negro" from the men of mixed race), most of the government functionaries were of the mulatto class. They were the authors of the literary, political, and historical works produced in the country and also made up the artistic contingent. Always with an eye to the degree of mixture, Harris agreed with Hunt that "as common laborers, also, if not too light-colored, the individuals of this class are equal to the Blacks in strength and endurance, and superior to them in skill and address." Altogether the conclusion was striking: this people "possesses within itself a combination of all the mental and physical qualities necessary to form a civilized and progressive population for the tropics, *and it is the only race yet found of which this can be said.*"[26] The italic emphasis is, again, the addition of Harris to Hunt's text.

It is worth pausing for a moment to consider why Harris found the Hunt pamphlet so very enlightening and spot-on. He himself was a "man of color" in this definition, with light brown skin indicative of race mixing. Harris may have grown up a "free man," albeit always hemmed in by laws that threatened and limited his rights. But there was a slave market in Fayetteville, and the reality of slavery was everywhere before him (as we saw in his poem). He was raised a Christian, and if he did not display his belief as freely as did his brothers the ministers, still it was likely an important part of his identity. Here in Hunt's words, he had found an explanation for how a just and loving God could have allowed the evil of slavery to exist: it was all to transform the heathen African into the religiously enlightened American and to blend the best biological traits of Black and white into a new race. *His race.* His very body manifested God's plan, and his destiny was to illuminate the path to an Anglo-African empire in the Caribbean. He saw in the mixture an improvement on either the pure white person or the pure Black person. He did not mean to undervalue Blacks, but "the Blacks form no exception to the well-known law, that culture and advancement in man are the result of a combination of races."[27]

Having quoted extensively from Hunt, Harris now turned to events of his own recent past. At a state convention held recently in Ohio, he heard debate on the question of whether the colored people of the state should pledge their "lives, property and honor" to "resist by force, the execution of the laws of the United States." The principal law in question was the Fugitive Slave Act, pursued vigorously by slave catchers from Kentucky and farther south. Feelings were running high after the crisis of the Wellington rescue and similar actions. Harris noted that William H. Watkins, John Mercer Langston, William Day, and others all spoke for the measure (that is, resistance) and few against it. "We trample the fugitive Slave Law and the dicta of the Dred Scott decision beneath our feet, as huge outrages, not only upon the Declaration of Independence and Constitution of the United States, but upon humanity itself," the resolution declared. The next day there was "whispering with white lips," and when the vote was taken, "and without any premeditation whatever, every mulatto voted for it, and every Black man against it." The printed proceedings of the convention recorded only that the resolution carried, but Harris was there, so his report is probably accurate.[28] I am not sure what Harris means here with his "whispering white lips," but somehow they turned the Blacks against the measure.

Harris, perhaps recognizing that he had gone too far, decided to desist and demur. "I have no desire to pursue this subject. I am not an amalgamationist, certainly not in the commonly accepted sense of that term. The whole subject of social intercourse is a matter which must be left to regulate itself ... subject only to the laws of nature." By "amalgamationist" he meant a proponent of mixed-race marriages, as a matter of principle. Still, he believed, "a combination of the two vital species is essential to produce a race possessing all the attributes necessary to raise the states and islands of the tropics up to what they should be—the centre of attraction for the civilized world."[29] Little could he know that eight years later he would, himself, marry a white woman from New Jersey.

Harris punctuated this point of African superiority with two examples of Black achievement. He described the fierceness of the French Zouaves, who were "fiendish, sable and irresistible," and the English reaction of enlisting Black men from the West Indies who with flashing teeth could "grin lightning as fiercely" as the French troops.[30] Echoing Phillips's text, Harris cinched the point: "Add to this the glory of the Haytian revolution, the only instance in the history of the world where a race of slaves has freed themselves without some outside assistance, and let the dunces who slander the colored race ponder."[31] Harris was switching back and forth here, at one point valorizing the mixed-race man over the "Black man" and at others including all persons with African blood into his roll of honor.

After extolling the fruitfulness, climate, and beauties of the Caribbean, Harris closed with a ringing call for his brethren to join him in creating a new civilization in these glorious lands. "I have only to add, how proudly will the colored race honor that day, when, abandoning the policy which make[s] them the tools and lickspittles of the whites, they shall set themselves zealously at work to create a position of their own." And not just a modest settlement, but "an Empire, which shall challenge the admiration of the world, and shall bloom with all the glory of its luxuriant clime, and live and flourish when our polar patrons shall have faded as these autumn leaves."[32]

Harris was not alone in calling for Black Americans to move to the Caribbean by rights of destiny. Elias P. Walker told the Ohio Colored Convention in 1858 that "the Cotton, Sugar, and Coffee growing regions of the world, belonged to the colored race, and that the nation or nations which produced those articles, must necessarily control the commerce of the world. Here then, was the path opened by Providence for our elevation. Let us concentrate upon the West Indies, upon Central America, where by our superior intelligence and energy, we would wield a wide influence, and many years would not pass away before we would have the world at our feet." Walker spoke here of "our superior intelligence," but how he defined "our" is unclear. A confidence in the superiority of Christianity, American education, and other traits is as likely as some aspect of skin tone, not to mention that he was talking to a convention of literate, free, and politically active African American men (and, actually, a few women as well).[33]

Thomas Hamilton, the editor of the *Anglo-African Magazine*, sought to temper Harris's racially divisive words as laid down in this article. Hamilton hurried to reassure readers that the magazine did not support the view that racially mixed people were superior to either the darker Black individual or the white person. This was not an official opinion of the magazine but rather presented because he valued every shade of opinion among the Black community. Hamilton spoke strongly against suppressing any ideas about our "condition," as such suppression would breed murk, gloom, and reticence. Still, he proclaimed, "no matter what complexion we bear, from milky white to jetty Black, so long as there can be traced in us one drop of negro blood, we are all in the same category of the oppressed." This was codified into law in the French and English West Indies (including Haiti), although he allowed that the Spanish were more "Catholic in their humanity" due to the "infusion of Moorish blood."[34]

Hamilton found that the rhetoric about mixed race had amusing implications. Familiar with the mathematics that calculated quadroons and octoroons as having one-quarter or one-eighth Black blood, he pointed to the power of African influence to dominate the whole. "The towering potency of the latter [Black blood] is fairly admitted when one-tenth or one-twentieth proportion of Black blood is admitted to overrule the other nine-tenths or nineteen-twentieths of white blood." Of course, this was not humorous at all to the many mixed-race persons in slavery; historian Joel Williamson estimated that by the 1850s some 25 percent of slaves in the newly opened regions of Missouri, Mississippi, Arkansas, and Texas were of mixed race, and 10.4 percent of slaves altogether were so. Yet the world where Harris lived, the free states of the Midwest, had by 1850 a predominance of mulatto citizens. More than half of the free African Americans in the midwestern states of Ohio,

Indiana, Illinois, Michigan, and Wisconsin were of mixed race. So the Harris conception of the "mulatto" was shaped by his own family and the educated men among whom he moved in the antislavery societies.[35]

Editor Hamilton's point was to illustrate the ludicrous nature of the whole calculation.[36] Although Harris probably would have known of the sort of mathematical formulas used by Moreau de Saint-Méry in the work on Haiti to calculate the exact percentages of "white" and "Black" blood in any given racial pairings, there is no indication that he divided people any more finely than "Negro" and "colored." In this he followed the usages of Haiti before the revolution, when the population was divided between slave, persons of color, and white. As Laurent Dubois points out, this was not an exact sorting of various shades, as fully Black men might end up free in the country. And the rights of men of color were contested and always at risk in pre-revolution Haiti.[37] Harris, however, seems to have had clear categories in mind.

The editor offered an explanation for the reality that Harris was trying to encompass. Of Harris, he wrote, "The writer ... does not state one fact which should be taken into the account in comparing the Blacks and mulattoes in the West Indies, and especially in Hayti. The reason why the mulattoes are the educated class in such localities, is not any special fondness or superior aptness on their part for learning." Rather, the sorting of skin color was due to opportunities inextricably tied to the conditions of slavery and treatment of mixed-race children. He argued that "whites, following that bent which the Catholic religion seems to foster in a larger degree than the Protestant, the bent of affection towards their half-breed offspring; educated their mulatto children with great care. And to this cause must be attributed the fact that this latter class have, in time, relatively to the Blacks—become the educated class." Given how this story had played out in the family histories of Harris and his friends the Langston brothers, Harris might have recognized the accuracy of this claim. Hamilton concluded, "This fact of course destroys the assumption of any relative superiority of one class from an admixture of white blood."[38]

Hamilton noted at the end of his comments that Harris was currently in "that part of Hayti held by those of Spanish descent" (at that point in time the government of Haiti claimed sovereignty over the Spanish-speaking Dominican Republic). If so, and if Harris wrote his essay when autumn leaves decorated his city, then it is likely that Harris fled the United States in the wake of the failed John Brown raid.[39] His name had been "outed" by several newspapers, and some people were arrested for even peripheral connections to the John Brown raid. John Brown Jr. had fled to Canada. There is conflicting evidence about when Harris made his first trip to the Caribbean. Editor

Harrison said that Harris was there at the time of the publication of the essay in March 1860. But in the opening pages of his travelogue, Harris said he departed New York on May 19, 1860.[40] One way of reconciling these dates is to imagine that the "March 1, 1860" issue of the journal actually appeared later than it was dated, and the editor added his note at the last minute. Erratic publication dates would not be inconsistent with the periodical's known financial difficulties of the time.

By the time of Harris's departure in May, he was the paid agent of James Redpath, a white man who had received $20,000 from the newly installed Haitian president Fabre Geffrard in 1859 for the promotion of Black immigration to the country. (While Harris and like-minded supporters of Black emigration had hoped to receive financial help from the US Congress, that did not materialize.) Redpath in turn paid agents, including Harris and John Brown Jr., to speak on his behalf in Ohio (Harris) and Chatham, Ontario (Brown) to drum up support for the plan, educate the people, and facilitate the move. The Harris trip and the subsequent travelogue were part of Redpath's campaign to make the Caribbean island familiar, approachable, and possible as a new home for Black Americans. Redpath worked for the Haitian government, but when he published his own *Guide to Hayti* in 1860, the map that was included as a frontispiece (and explicitly supplied by President Geffrard) labeled the whole island Haiti and then divided it into the eastern Spanish part and the western French part.[41] So although Harris visited "the Spanish side," he was indeed furthering Geffrard's ambitions.

LESSONS FROM THE HAITIAN REVOLUTION

The Harris monograph, *A Summer on the Borders of the Caribbean Sea* (1860), was divided into two sections. Each chapter was initially intended to be an article in the *Weekly Anglo-African*, but that foundered before the project was well begun. The first half of the book chronicled Harris's trip to the "Spanish" side of Haiti, which was a weak but independent country in 1860, albeit one claimed by the Haitian government. Spain reoccupied Haiti in that year, shutting down the possibility of African American settlement. That section will be discussed in the next chapter, because it focused principally on finding a good location for an American colony of resettled Blacks. First, though, it is worth exploring in detail the way Harris told the story of the founding of the Black Haitian Republic. In it he reveals the anger evident in his John Brown correspondence and the persistent antagonism to whites and joy in the success of Africans at arms, no matter how brutal.

In his first chapter written about Haiti, he characterized (Spanish) Dominica as "a garden of poetry and the home of legendary song," while (francophone) Haiti he saw as "a land of historical facts, and the field of unparalleled glory."[42] James Redpath had urged him to write a summary of the country's history, as that was essential for understanding its situation around this time. Harris did not visit Haiti on this first trip to the island and instead drew on historical accounts by Marcus Rainsford, on the Haiti sections on Santo Domingo; Bryan Edwards, on the British West Indies; and especially Thomas Coke, on the West Indies.[43] Harris proceeded with a thumbnail sketch of the area's occupation by first the Spanish and then the French. As Howard H. Bell points out in his introduction of the 1970 reprint of Harris's volume, there are multiple errors here, especially in chronology.[44] Nonetheless, the Harris summary of Haiti's revolutionary history is most valuable for this biography in what it tells us about the author himself.

In describing the town of Cap-Français (later named Cap-Haïtien), Harris noted some problems with the setting, but overall he found that the "air is temperate, though the days and nights are constantly cool. In short, it is another Eden." He did allow, however, that Port-au-Prince was low and marshy, "and the air is impregnated with noxious vapors, rendering it extremely unwholesome. To this day it is commonly regarded as the graveyard of American seamen." So obviously this Eden had more than one snake slithering in the grass. The town of St. Mark, which he noted already had a community nearby of "colored emigrants" from the United States, was situated in a healthier location.[45]

Harris sketched a varied picture of Haiti under the French occupation. On the one hand the land was incredibly productive, making more sugar than all of the British West Indies combined, as well as producing cotton, indigo, and other products. But it was also a land where "immorality and irreligion everywhere prevailed," for the white settlers indulged "guilty passions to their foul embrace" and seduced "the daughters of the swarthy race."[46] After this lyric, Harris announced that they had arrived at the "negro question," which was "the immortal question of the rights of man." He reminded his readers that by the final decade of the eighteenth century, the country was divided into three populations. "The whites conducted themselves as if born to command, and the blacks, awed into submission, yielded obedience to their imperious mandates, while the mulattos were despised by both parties."[47] One wonders how much personal experience was expressed in that final line. Harris detailed the injustices showered on the mulattoes—they could not take their father's name, they were forced to serve in a militia, they could not hold office, and if a colored man struck a white one, he could lose his right arm. "In fact, they were not much above the condition of the free blacks in the United States."[48] Yes, he was certainly talking about himself.

In the next letter Harris backed off on his claim of total degradation for the mulattoes. They could, he admitted, own land and slaves, "and many of them had actually acquired considerable estates. By these means the wealthiest had sent their children to France for education, just as many are now sent to Oberlin."[49] Harris knew Oberlin College well, given its proximity to Cleveland. It had been among the first American colleges to admit Blacks as well as whites and had become a focus of abolitionism and opposition to the Fugitive Slave Law. Mentioning it also recalled to the contemporary reader the story of the Wellington rescue, related here in chapter 4. As Harris continued his narration, describing the path of Vincent Ogé, a Haitian mulatto who studied in Paris, associated with the Marquis de Lafayette, and generally learned ideas about equality and revolution, did he continue to see parallels? Were free Blacks in the United States likewise learning to push for equality and contemplate revolution in the groves of northern Ohio academe? Certainly, Harris had been through a process of radicalization, including in his association with John Brown's revolutionaries, and perhaps he saw Ogé's unfortunate story as parallel to that experience.[50]

According to Harris's telling, Ogé came home from Paris convinced that "all the mulattoes of Hayti were actuated by the same high-minded principle," so he sacrificed his fortune and planned an uprising against the slavocracy. "What was Ogé's disappointment when, after evading the vigilance of the police and secretly succeeding in reaching these shores, he found no party prepared to receive him, or willing to take up arms in their own defence!"[51] And John Brown? He too thought the slaves would rise up and join the revolution. Ogé's revolution turned especially brutal, said Harris, as his men began to murder the mulattoes who would not join. One man, "who excused himself from joining them on account of his family, was murdered, together with his wife and six children." Harris too had canvassed the countryside seeking support for John Brown, to be told by one that family had to come first. So he had been there, but not to the next horrific steps. And Ogé himself was not just hanged, like John Brown, but broken on the wheel while yet alive.[52]

Harris drew another parallel between the American story and the Haitian one. When the French government heard of the uprising of 1793, it wanted to support the planter class but also to placate the mulattoes to avoid further unrest. So, it decreed that "every person of the age of twenty-five and upwards, possessing property or having resided two years in the colony and paid taxes, should be permitted to vote in the formation of the colonial assembly." Harris declared, "It was like the Dred Scott decision of the United States, for the question immediately arose whether the term 'every person' included the mulattoes." Again, he probed the deep wound of Justice Taney's words, that free Blacks could not be citizens and were not legal persons with rights. Meanwhile, in Haiti people of mixed Black-white heritage were increasingly treated as criminals by the whites, and they accordingly began to arm themselves for protection. As Harris wrote of the "far more awful mine, surcharged with combustibles, and destined to appall all parties, [that] was at that moment on the very eve of an explosion," were they words not just of history, but of hope for his own home front?[53]

Everything he writes here is autobiography. As he sat reading the history of the Haitian Revolution, he was simultaneously envisioning just such an uprising in his native land. Yet he also acknowledged the awfulness of war, calling the essay a "Chapter of Horrors" and giving the delicate reader the option of omitting it. He began by giving full agency to the revolting slaves, saying that they chose to "assert their freedom and legislate for themselves," as they recognized that "violence was necessary to prosperity. Such measures they adopted; and no sooner adopted than they were carried into effect."[54] The slaves had gone from plantation to plantation, massacring the white masters and adding liberated slaves to their new army.

The Harris narrative spared no details of atrocity. White women were violated "*on the mangled bodies of their dead husbands, friends, or brothers, to whom they had been clinging for protection.*"[55] The emphasis is in the original. Did Harris include such detail to titillate his readers? To feed fantasies of revenge? Or to warn southern plantation masters of the horrific alternative to peaceful abolition? Free your slaves, or else... Harris drew an object lesson from the story of one plantation, whose slaves "had been treated with such remarkable tenderness that their happiness had become proverbial." The master thought to raise the slaves to fight *against* the insurrection and found instead that they not only were in full rebellion "but had actually erected for their standard THE BODY OF A WHITE INFANT, *which they had impaled on a stake*" (italics and capitals in original). Harris drew the obvious moral to the tale: "So much for happy negroes and contented slaves!" White attempts to quell the rebellion failed, for the "slaves, as if impelled by one common instinct, seemed to catch the contagion without any visible communication."[56]

Harris admitted that the story he was telling was "too horrible for description," and he would not proceed, except there were so many who denied that such events had happened. In the parlance of the modern day, they claimed it was "fake news" that could not be substantiated. So, he felt bound to record the grisly details. He quoted extensively from Bryan Edwards's history of the Haitian Revolution, although as with his usage of the Hunt volume, his use of quotation marks was somewhat capricious. The preceding stories were taken verbatim from Edwards; now Harris begins to acknowledge his source overtly. One white policeman was nailed alive to a gate and dismembered one limb at a time. Another, a carpenter who had hidden from the rioters, was found, and "the negroes declared that he *should die in the way of his occupation*; accordingly, they laid him between two boards, and deliberately sawed him asunder."[57] Although Harris made some minor errors in transcription, one suspects one change in this sentence was deliberate: Edwards had "savages" making the declaration, whereas Harris changed that word to "negroes." It is easy to suspect that Harris was enjoying these stories, whatever his pious protestations. He was one angry man, getting revenge in fantasy if not yet in reality.

The horror continues in the next paragraph. "All the white and even the mulatto children whose fathers had not joined in the revolt were murdered without exception, frequently before their eyes, or while clinging to the bosoms of their mothers. Young women of all ranks were first violated by whole troops of barbarians, and then, generally, put to death."[58] Some unfortunates were forced into concubinage "for the gratification of the lust of the leaders," while others had their eyes cut out with a knife. Harris was writing revenge pornography on a vicious scale. And again, he changed a word—where Harris referenced lusty "leaders," Edwards again used the word "savages." But in the next paragraph Harris kept the label "savage," as he told the story of two beautiful daughters ravished in the presence of their father, and then all three were killed, the rioters' "passions being satisfied."[59] After recounting the story of two mulatto sons who killed their white father, he modified the atrocity chronicle by recording the story of a "*soft-hearted* slave [who] saved the lives of his master and family by sending them adrift on the river by moonlight." That hero was the "*Washington* of Hayti, Toussaint L'Ouverture."[60] Edwards told the story to illuminate the fact that some slaves were presumably well-treated and loved their masters.[61] Harris drew no moral from it except, perhaps, that a great man, destined for leadership, could behave with compassion.

Then there followed an interlude, when the free mulattoes joined with the whites to counter the Black slave insurrection. There had been a decree from France that allotted mulattoes increased civil rights, a decree the whites had resisted. Now the whites were willing to compromise in order to acquire free mulatto support. They passed an "act of oblivion" that supposedly erased from memory all the horrors that had passed and declared the infamous treatment of Ogé to be an act of "everlasting execration." Harris harrumphed, "So much for Ogé." Yet, said he, "the great lesson of the revolution was speedily to be learned. The hurricane of terror which was yet to overcome them was at that moment on the Atlantic, and hastening with fatal impetuosity towards these uncertain shores."[62] So much for détente with the white slavocracy. The mulattoes would soon learn to think differently. The French government repealed the decree, and the white Haitians crowed in conquest. The mulatto resentments simmered, Harris said, until finally "exploding in a frenzy which produced the most diabolical excesses yet on record."[63] Harris had lived through the frustrations of the 1850s, first in Iowa and later in Ohio, as measure after measure to ensure the equal rights of free Blacks before the law had failed to achieve legislative approval. He knew something of such simmering resentments.

He then told of the first battle in which mulattoes aligned with the revolutionary slaves, a battle that saw thousands of Black people killed or taken prisoner. One Black man was publicly tortured by white people, "to their everlasting infamy." They nailed him into a cart and paraded him through the streets. "He was then liberated from this partial crucifixion to suffer a new mode of torment. His bones were then broken in pieces, and finally he was cast alive into the fire, where he expired. So much for the whites." The mulattoes, "irritated to madness at the inhumanity with which one of their leaders had been treated," revenged themselves on a white couple. She was hugely pregnant. First they murdered him and then "ripped open her body, took out the infant and *gave it to the hogs*; after which they cut off her husband's head and entombed it in her bowels."[64] While Edwards called these men "monsters" and moaned that "my hand trembles while I write," Harris instead closed with a poem:

> A law there is of ancient fame,
> By nature's self in every land implanted,
> *Lex Talionis* is its Latin name;
> But if an English term be wanted,
> Give [y]our next neighbor but a pat,
> He'll give you back as good and tell you—*tit for tat!*[65]

Clearly, from his perspective, it served the white couple right.

The following chapter described the French army's invasion of Haiti, including the arrest of L'Ouverture under the guise of friendship and his death in a French prison. "Such was the fate of Toussaint L'Ouverture, the *Washington*, but not '*the Napoleon*,' of Hayti."[66] L'Ouverture may have led the revolution, but he did not complete it. That leader was Jean-Jacques Dessalines, who would succeed in casting out the French and establishing Haiti as an independent country. Sparked by indignation over L'Ouverture's treatment, Dessalines and his men resolved to throw off the French. This endeavor was aided by the diseases that decimated the European troops. Harris reported that the French treated captured troops with particular "barbarity." "Some [of the Black Haitian troops] perished on the spot; others were mutilated in their limbs, legs, and vital parts, and left in that horrible condition to disturb with their shrieks and groans the silence of the night." But Dessalines was not Toussaint, Harris reported. Not for him the motto "*never to retaliate.*" In contrast, Dessalines gibbeted the French officers and privates whom his men had captured, in a place "most exposed to the French army."[67] Dessalines knew well the philosophy of "tit for tat."

Dessalines and his army surrounded the French and drove them from Cap-Français, sending their ships into the waiting arms of the British fleet blockading the harbor. "Thus ended this visionary expedition through which Napoleon and Le Clerc flattered themselves and the country that the inhabitants of Hayti were to be again reduced to slavery," Harris wrote triumphantly. "And thus, by the unrelenting determination of Dessalines, were the fearful thunderbolts of war made to recoil on the heads of those who hurled them." So then, to the acclaim of his jubilant people, Dessalines was crowned first emperor of Haiti. The people followed the celebration with a church service, where they gave thanks to "Him who had guided them through this arduous struggle in defence of those rights with which He had originally endowed them."[68] Here we see the Methodist piety that Harris no doubt imbibed in his childhood finally able to assert itself after all the atrocity narratives had fed his vengeful soul.

Harris sketches the subsequent history of Haiti up to his present day of 1860. Unlike his detailed description of the Dominican Republic as a location for immigration, he has very little descriptive material about Haiti proper. Like James Redpath, Harris saw the current administration of President Fabre Geffrard as progressive and prosperous. The money was sound. And the educational system showed promise. "Under Protestant influences, also, several large schools, in which hundreds of young girls and boys are being educated, promise in due time to present to the world a virtuous female offspring of these heroic revolutionists" who were competent in both French and English. The boys, in turn, would be "skilled at once in commerce, and in the sciences of government, the sword, the anvil, and the plow." He reported that President Geffrard particularly invited immigrants capable of teaching in such schools.[69]

This brief consideration of immigration was followed by a summary paragraph that conveyed the main point of Harris's text on Haiti. "It is difficult to believe these fields of natural beauty, embellished with all the decorations of art, have at any time presented to earth and heaven such spectacles of horror," he began. Such events caused Europe "to stand aghast," but more importantly they "will serve Americans as a finger-board of terror so long as slavery there exists. The torch of conflagration and the sword of destruction have marched in fearful union through the land, and covered the hills and plains with desolation." With the tones of Jeremiah, he cried, "Tyranny, scorn, and retaliating vengeance have displayed their utmost rage, and in the end have given birth to an empire which has not only hurled its thunderbolts on its assailants, but at this moment bids defiance to the world."[70] As Julia Ward Howe would express it in the following year, "Mine eyes have seen the glory of the coming of the Lord," who would loose "the fateful lightning of His terrible swift sword."[71] The vengeance, horror, and joyous success of the Haitian Revolution was just a prelude to the coming conflagration threatening American slavocracy.

By the time Harris closed his Haitian section, his tone has shifted to promoting that country for immigration over the Dominican Republic. What is clear in these lines is that he still clings to his plan for an Afro-American empire: "Hayti may yet become the counterpart of England, head-quarters of a colored American nationality, and supreme mistress of the Caribbean Sea." His England reference draws on his recall that in the days of imperial Rome, the Brits were considered wretched barbarians, "just as Americans speak of Haytiens to-day."[72]

The book then shifts with no transition to a travelogue again, this time to other Caribbean islands. On his way to the Grand Turks and Caicos, he remarked, "It is usually no more to 'dangle around' this sea than it is to cross Lake Erie."[73] Such a crossing had an important place in the life of Cleveland—it was the route to Canada and a free society. Along the way he mentioned that Queen Victoria had recently conferred a knighthood on "Sir Edward Jordon, Mayor of the city of Kingston and Prime Minister of Jamaica—a degree of dignity never before attained by a colored man . . . since the British government began." Harris saw great portent in this fact. "The day of the Anglo-African in America has not yet clearly dawned, but it is dawning." He gloried in the experience of Black men in power. "A great many of the officers here, too, are colored. How strange it seems to stand before a large, fine-looking black or colored man, entitled Sir, Honorable, Esquire, and the like! To save me, I cannot realize it, although I see, hear, and shake hands with them every day."[74] Harris enjoyed hearing heroic stories of the times when former Jamaican slaves escaped to Haiti, "reminding one much of our Canadian friends. The history of the escape of slaves in our day is as full of heroism as any history in the world."[75] Britain had liberated her West Indian slaves twenty-two years earlier. Yes, many whites still held political posts, but the Blacks had begun "to tread on their political heels." While this was not popular with some whites, Harris advised "the easiest way for them is to allow themselves to be peacefully absorbed by the colored race in these regions, for their destiny is sealed."[76]

Harris noted that the vessel upon which he was traveling island to island had cleared "$1,400 on his trip out, with a cargo of lumber from the States." Harris then asked, "How much will our friend Wm. Whipper make in a year running his craft up a Canadian creek? The tenacity with which our leading colored men embrace that short-sighted policy which teaches them to confine their enterprises to certain proscribed, prejudice-cursed districts, is not only extraordinary—it is marvellous."[77] Harris here was railing against those who clung to poverty in Canada when the Caribbean offered such possibilities for both Black equality and prosperity. Commercial opportunities in the islands promised much greater returns.

On his way to British Honduras, Harris described being becalmed at sea and making friends with a heretofore unknown American. "For, my dear H., nobody ever knows what true friendship is until they have been shipwrecked, nor does anyone conceive how mutual are the sympathies of persons coming from the same country . . . until they have met away from home." He was beginning to yield a bit in his harsh anti-Americanism, the country whose Declaration of Independence had decreed that all men are created equal but whose Supreme Court had declared that no Black man could ever be a citizen. "Strange as it may seem, I have not met a colored American out this way but who actually celebrates the Fourth of July."[78] Remember that in his Iowa poem Harris had contrasted the Fourth of July speeches from white politicians with the ongoing slave auction in the next square. Even though Blacks in the United States had yet to see *their* independence day, those abroad had embraced it.

On the way, Harris was enchanted by the British colony island of Ruatan (aka Roatán), off the coast of Nicaragua. Fruits were its principal export, he noted. "Could a vessel be run between this and Baltimore, or any other respectable port of the United States, it would pay beyond a peradventure."[79]

He recognized the problem of fruit rotting in the process but argued that if the boats were regularly scheduled, it would work. Now, one could slice pineapples off the tree and drink nectar of the gods, while crops of oranges and limes were regularly tossed away with no one to consume them. He particularly liked the "cocoa-nuts." Ruatan had other estimable qualities—land was cheap, there were no export duties, and English was the common language. Harris was right to see great opportunities in the fruit trade, but it would take regular steam vessels, and the possibility of refrigeration, for fruit transport to the Northeast to become commonplace. Such circumstances would not appear until the 1880s, when the Boston Fruit Company first began importing bananas and other fruit.[80]

A further problem with settling Ruatan, or even Nicaragua itself, was the recent unpleasantness with "the pirate Walker," namely William Walker, the American filibusterer who sought to impose a new government on Nicaragua and resurrect slavery. Walker was ultimately hanged, but his legacy persisted in the destruction of the Nicaraguan route across the Central American isthmus and the ascendancy of the Panamanian route. This experience had turned the people of Ruatan against all intercourse with the United States. "This feeling has been heightened recently by the fact that a merchant, who dealt in fruits with certain parties in New Orleans, went over there on business," Harris reported. The merchant was a British magistrate, a citizen in good British standing, and colored. "Hardly had he reached the shore [in Louisiana] before he was arrested and taken to prison." The charge was being Black; he protested and showed his magistrate papers. "The New Orleans constable replied: 'If Queen Victoria were to come over here, and she were black, I'd put her in jail.'"[81] This event highlighted the grave risks that any Black person took in the southern states, in spite of the shiniest of documents. Harris argued that "there is no hope for the Central American States except by intervention on the part of some government capable of protecting them."[82] So despite his effusions about Ruatan, it could not be the new homeland, at least at present.

In the end, Harris concluded that it was in the Spanish-speaking area of the island of Haiti that an emigration scheme for Black Americans could best prosper. He reminded his readers of the opportunities for agriculture, mining, and commerce, particularly praising the deep harbor at Samana. Indeed, one mining enterprise was already at work. But then for the first time he alluded to governmental instability in Dominica. His proposed colony of emigrants would "not be interrupted by the present government, but the durability of that government is, I am sorry to say, a question which may be agitated, and even settled, *before I finish writing this book.*"[83]

In his last paragraph Harris offered a way out of this tangled situation. Gone here were his words about a colored empire. Rather, he turned to the "new administration" in the United States to facilitate the progressive change that he envisioned. By the time he wrote those words, Abraham Lincoln had been elected president, if not yet inaugurated. Here was hope that the United States could abandon "that policy which makes them the indiscriminate oppressors of the weak" and instead take up a position of promoting peace and prosperity in the islands. "Such a measure would in some degree recompense the colored race for the services they have rendered to the government, the fruits of which they have not been permitted to enjoy; would make this great nation less obnoxious to the weak; lay the foundation of a future empire; and cause those lovely regions to bloom with industry and skill as they now bloom with eternal verdure."[84] Historian Chris Dixon has described the many emotions that the possibility of immigration to Haiti elicited from free Black Americans. In this move Blacks were choosing between nationalism and race, and, as we shall see for Harris, angrily rejecting American citizenship could be one aspect of that choice. But for all they valorized Haiti, they also saw it as an *unfinished* revolution. The country needed educated Black Americans to bring modern agriculture and Protestant religion to the country, as was clear. Dixon observed, "The antebellum period was one of rapid change and uncertainty, but for Black Americans each moment in the increasingly bitter sectional conflict suggested that emancipation for the Southern slaves was becoming more distant, and that Northern Blacks' already marginal freedom was becoming ever more precarious."[85] There was, in other words, "push" as well as "pull" in the language of immigration historians. Harris echoed themes of other desperate Blacks who sought a country they could call their own, a purpose in the mission of helping their own people, and an escape from a country where free Blacks were kidnapped into slavery, were not allowed to vote, and "had no rights to be respected by a white man." Americans in the 1850s Midwest were surrounded by emigrants—Irish, German, Scandinavians—who had left one country for the opportunities in the United States. Why shouldn't they emigrate too, heading for their land of freedom and opportunity? If in the process Harris and others glossed over the insurmountable problems to be met in Haiti—the unstable government, the pervasive illnesses, and the difficulties in agriculture—one can forgive the blinders imposed by their own desperation. In the next chapter we will learn of his enthusiastic exploration of the Spanish-speaking side of the island and then of how he tried to put his ambitions into practice.

6

Colonizing the Caribbean

After laying out his bold plan for colonization and empire for the *Weekly Anglo-African* audience, Harris was finally able to visit the island of his dreams in the summer of 1860. He was disappointed by the backwardness he found but cheered by the vast field of work for skilled and hardworking Americans that the green land promised. Thrilled at the sight of Black men in all sorts of official jobs, such as harbormaster, policeman, and even president, he saw what might be if his expectations came to pass. Now, if those persons could only be replaced by educated Black Americans, what a wonderful world it would be! Finally, Black Americans would have a homeland where they could grow as full and welcome citizens. That summer he visited the island to survey opportunities for farming communities; two years later he would return with a shipload of Black Americans to found such a settlement.

Harris chronicled his first visit with letters and ultimately a book, *A Summer on the Borders of the Caribbean Sea*. This voyage did not take him to francophone Haiti at all; his firsthand description was of the Spanish-speaking side of the island. At the time of his travel, Haiti claimed political sovereignty over the entire island. Where did he get the money to pay for this travel? Probably from James Redpath, who was promoting immigration schemes to francophone Haiti. If he indeed funded the Harris trip, Redpath may have been hedging his bets by having Harris scope out not only Spanish Santo Domingo but also Honduras, as well as other Caribbean islands. Harris and like-minded men also had solicited funds for Caribbean colonization from the Honorable F. P. Blair of Missouri, and they considered memorializing Congress on the subject. But they knew that was a futile plan under the James Buchanan administration.[1] Whatever the reason, Harris went to the Spanish-speaking side of the island first and wrote as if he planned to settle there himself. The fact that he was studying the Spanish Creole language of the country was one marker of his intent. Once the Spanish government retook control of the land that would become the Dominican Republic in March 1861, that option was no longer possible.[2]

A third source of funding may have been his employment by the editor of the newspaper that published his letters. In one of the letters from the Dominican Republic, Harris spoke sentimentally of his experience with Thomas Hamilton, the editor of the *Weekly Anglo-African*. "Not a morning, my dear H., do I look upon these fields of living green but that I think of you and your daily routine of office duties," Harris wrote. "You are toiling away, arranging rude manuscripts, at times almost discouraged, but still toiling on in your close, hot rooms—and this for the good of your race."[3] Harris had definitely been in those rooms, to describe them so, and perhaps worked there. Given that his mother's family published the paper in Fayetteville and one of his sisters listed her occupation as "printer" in the 1860 census, it is certainly possible that Harris had acquired typesetting skills either in North Carolina or Ohio. The newspaper folded in the spring of 1861 for lack of sufficient funds, so it is very unlikely that it was a major sponsor of Harris's expedition, but it did support him by publishing the letters when it could.

SURVEYING THE DOMINICAN REPUBLIC

A Summer on the Borders of the Caribbean Sea is divided into eight letters from the Dominican Republic, five about Haiti (discussed in the previous chapter), one from Grand Turks and Caicos, and one from Honduras. After the concluding chapter the book ends with a slightly abridged version of the "Anglo-African Empire" essay analyzed in the last chapter. The chapters appear to have been destined for the *Weekly Anglo-African*, but after its demise Harris lost that venue. This is particularly regrettable because the first letter had more content in the *Weekly Anglo-African* version than the one published in the book; it would have been enlightening to know what else was edited out (and to speculate about why it was cut). Although the book's title page sports a publication date of 1860, a mid-March 1861 issue of the (newly revitalized) *Weekly Anglo-African* contained an ad for the volume with the words, "Just published."[4]

The book began with a preface by abolitionist George William Curtis, a well-known author, editor, and public speaker of New York. Curtis reported that "Mr. Harris thinks that the island of Hayti or San Domingo, in its eastern or Dominican portion, offers the most promising prospect for such an experiment," that is, planting a colony of Black Americans in the Caribbean.[5] The language is a bit confusing, but if read with the assumption that the words "Hayti" and "San Domingo" both refer to the whole island, then it is clear that Harris had told Curtis that the eastern/Spanish/Dominican end of the island was "the most promising prospect." The proposition that Harris had chosen the "Spanish side" of the island before he left as the site for his future colony is reinforced by the revelation in Letter 1 that he studied the "Dominican language" on board ship, the Creole language of the eastern island that was, he said, "a compound of Spanish, French, English, Congo, and Caribbean—but, of course, principally Spanish."[6] Harris said "we" and "our" in this opening chapter, but the identity of his companions was not listed, and he may have been using the plural as an authorial convention.

Harris was moved when the great island came into view and wrote about his anticipation of finally landing. Earlier in the chapter, he spoke of "the novelty of being at sea for the first time." Both comments refute the Hamilton claim that he was already there in March 1860. In Porto del Plata Harris was greeted by a Mr. Collins, "an American gentleman to whom I was addressed. He received me liberally, invited me to stop with him, promising to show me around the country." Collins was "decidedly un-American, but very gentlemanly indeed," reported Harris. This makes me suspect that his host was white, although this was not specified.[7]

He noted that there was a "non-progressive appearance of everything around him," indicated in part by the fact that the houses were but one story high. The harbor needed dredging, which would alleviate need to lighter goods from ships moored out in the deeper water up to the docks. He found the people were indolent, "excelling only in superstition, idleness, and profound stupidity." They were listless and apathetic, suggesting an enervation beyond just laziness. Even the military band (which accompanied a government official who was making a pronouncement) looked "all the world like a parcel of ragamuffin boys playing militia." The shores were lined with valuable trees such as mahogany, but no one seemed to be harvesting them. The dress of the men—cool, white linen with panama hats—was acceptable, but the women shocked him: "red-turbaned, often bare-stockinged, [and] loosely-dress[ed]." Not only that, but the men practiced polygamy. One told him he had two wives, as "one is not a plenty." This scanty development of the island's riches required an explanation, as it could not be grounded in the race of these happy-go-lucky people. Why had it remained, at least to American eyes, so lacking in progress? It was the prevalence, no doubt, of what he called an "apathy of stupidity."[8]

Then Harris turned to history, including works by James McCune Smith and W. S. Courtney, to explain the island and its appearance. Smith had argued that the island had declined from its ancient splendor because of the "effeminating [sic] influences attending all tropical climates," summarized Harris.[9] This theory countered arguments based on inherent racial deficiencies, to be sure, but introduced a new problem for Harris, who wanted to convince people to immigrate there. After all, some might think that "the climate [would be] hotter and less healthy than was desirable." So Harris denied that climate and disease had anything to do with the decline. "The country is as healthy as Virginia, and, except in its excessive beauty and fertility, resembles much the state of North Carolina."[10] Then he offered another explanation. The decline in the island's prosperity was entirely due to the cruelty of the Spanish and French in killing off the Indigenous peoples and enslaving Blacks under the worst possible conditions. He then proceeded to give a brief sketch of the island's history, including the rule of the two parts of the island by shifting governments.[11] The Spanish side of the island was particularly bereft, Harris believed, because many of the Spanish had abandoned it for greater opportunities in the home country, and after the Haitian Revolution many slaves escaped to the Spanish side for freedom from the French. The country was at times subjugated by, and at other times at war with, the French Haitians.

Harris had his own plan for the future of the two sides of the island. "The destiny of the island is union:—one in government, wants, and interest," he proclaimed. This happy state of affairs was to be "brought about by the introduction of the English language . . . such language, wants and interests to be introduced by the emigration hither of North Americans." These North Americans would be principally "colored" like himself, that is, mixed-race and light-skinned. And they would be Protestant like him, too, at least in the Harris vision. Only the Protestant religion could infuse "a tone of morality in the country."[12] Having imagined this new republic led by prosperous African American immigrants, Harris then crowed that England, France, and other countries would of course recognize it and form various treaties with the "weak little Republic." But Harris knew that this would not be forthcoming from the United States, a country that had yet to recognize Haiti sixty years after its revolution. "I hope you do not suppose the government of the United States could be *guilty* of anything that looks like generosity." And then his anger and despair boiled over into an anguished cry. "God grant that I may never die in the United States of America!"[13]

However much Harris sought to renounce his American birth, he still had to register as a visitor with the local authorities. "The meanest thing I have been obliged to do, and the greatest sin I have committed, has been registering my name as an American citizen," he confessed. "I presented myself to the United States consul." After noting that the man's clerk (who was also his son) was a mulatto, he continued, "The nice correspondence of Mr. Marcy was produced, not with any evil intent at all, but just to show what indefinable definitions there are between colored and black and white and negroes as American citizens." In Ohio, for example, if a person was "half white" they had all the privileges of white people, including access to the vote and schools.[14] "I should like to find out how a man *knows* he is an American citizen! There are members of Congress who can no more tell this than they can tell who are their fathers." Zing! He then cited a recent court case in Virginia that proclaimed that "an Octoroon is not a negro. Now, then, if an octoroon is not a *negro*, is an octoroon a citizen? And if an octoroon is not a negro, is a quadroon a negro?" Harris recognized the humor in this hairsplitting but also knew it was dead serious. If a person of the slightest darker skin tone could not prove citizenship, he or she might be "arrested as a fugitive slave."[15] The Black man in America had no rights.

The tirade against US institutions continued in his next chapter. Harris noted that the local gentry rode horses for transportation and always had a sword hanging by their side or had a knife in their belts. "It is an old, superannuated, hundred-years-behind-the-age custom," he admitted. But it kept the peace, as otherwise "the difficulty is generally settled at the sword's point, and there it ends." He contrasted "this rude mode of settling disputes" with the "one-sided, blaspheming, defrauding den of thieves called a court of justice in the States!" Harris lacked a sword and the knowledge to use one but instead made do with a pair of holsters for pistols. He felt this made a good enough show to convince evildoers to stay away.[16] We have no record of Harris being personally involved in a court case up to this time, although of course he was on the sidelines of the Wellington rescue. Discrimination against Black people was written into most state legal codes, with the words and rights of whites always privileged over those of African Americans. And in the enforcement of the Fugitive Slave Law, and especially the trial of his friend Charles Langston, he had seen such iniquities firsthand.

Harris was on an expedition out to the countryside to see the Pastorisa Place, which he called "a perfect Arcadia." Señor Pastorisa had offered his large plat of land as a possible site for African American settlers. After the long journey by horseback, often on narrow trails and rocky paths over the mountains, Harris came to an enchanting scene that marked one of the "'gilt letter' chapters of my life." Feted with a succulent meal of fried plantains, pineapple syrup, and scorched sweet milk, he rested content. Such a day and such food would soon cure "a dyspeptic Northerner," for sure. It was an idyllic valley, five miles wide, bounded by mountains and watered by a central stream. Señor Pastorisa was a genial host, but it was his wife who particularly entranced Harris. She was "'a little tinged'—the handsomest woman in the world." Was he thinking of Belle, the beautiful octoroon of his poem? Then Harris added, "Her complexion is that of a clear ripe orange." Despite his admiration, Harris saw much that could be done to improve the plantation. His host had a new plow but lacked the knowledge and gear to link oxen to it. Harris might have shown him how to make the yoke, but there were no tools suitable for its construction. Above all else the valley needed a wagon path to the outside world or a river route that could carry a flatboat. Through his American eyes Harris saw a bountiful farm, worked by able American emigrants using farming technology imported from home, a farm that would ship luscious produce to the world.[17] What a wonderful world it could become!

Particularly attentive to the island women he met in his travels, Harris was at least a bit aroused by their less-than-modest clothing. "The women are frequently good-looking, but seldom spirited. The prevailing question seems to be, How low in the neck can their dresses be worn? and the answer is, Very low indeed!" One supposes that mother Charlotte Harris did not dress her girls in such a fashion. Even more exciting, he noted, "white Swiss is worn as [a] dress, and when seen on a handsome woman is like Balm of Gilead to the wounded eye."[18] "White Swiss" meant "white dotted Swiss," a thin cotton fabric used for summer garments. I suspect that in the Harris household this fabric would have been worn as an undergarment such as a petticoat but not all alone. Clearly, he found the sheer fabric an alluring article on the island women.

He was more condemnatory of another custom. In the Pastorisa household he learned that it was usual for women to eat "second table." In other words, the men ate first and the women waited on them as servants before having their own turn to dine. "She sees that his baths are ready, and at times even that his horse is fed" before taking her own plate. This was not, he explained, from lack of respect. Rather, "it is their stupid custom." Americans were more inclined to respect women, especially in public encounters. The Dominican males would learn this soon enough if the Americans moved in. If an American stagecoach company ever ran a coach up this valley, he mused, "and two or three of these fellows have to climb on top for the sake of giving one lady an inside seat, they will comprehend somewhat better for whose convenience the world was made."[19] Although this was acutely true for nonwhites, this custom was described here as a gendered behavior, not a racial one.

On June 14 he was still at the Pastorisa household. As Señor Pastorisa was ill with a fever, Harris had more time to write. In this section he lauded the many wonderful details of the customs and country. He was particularly impressed with the comforts of a hammock, which he described to his American readers as if it would be unfamiliar to them. Similarly, the exotic palm tree was described; it had "berries" used for fattening pork and a bark that could be turned into a variety of items. It was "the most useful tree in the world, its usefulness is excelled by its own beauty." His point here was to reinforce the natural riches of the landscape.[20]

There was no truth to the reports that the country was full of snakes, he wrote: "The world does not contain another thing so brazenly destitute of the least common sense." He had not seen one, not even a "dead garter-snake!" He did watch a sailor catch a young shark, as "wicked a little thing as I ever saw, and strong as a new-born giant." The sailor proceeded to prepare the shark for eating, which repulsed Harris. But he tried some, saying it was coarse and that "the idea that its mother might some day eat me, made the thing disgusting." But he drew a lesson from the story, applicable to the immigrant experience. The Irish, he reported, were afraid to go to America "on account of its frogs," whereas a "Frenchman makes a dish of them."[21] Other people ate cats or rats. He did not draw a summary conclusion but seemed to be preaching that humans could find a broad range of foods palatable and should be willing to learn new tastes in a new land.

Harris went on to express his desire to see the local reptiles while he had a chance. Was this a segue from what could be eaten? Or just a continuation of ideas about interesting local fauna and flora? At any rate, he mused, "I should be sorry to miss seeing some lazy old crocodile sunning in the sand." Then he made a surprising claim: "Should it have seven heads, however, I shall very likely catch it, and send it straight to Barnum; but if not, why, as Banks would the Union, let the snaky thing slide."[22] Harris referenced a quotation from Nathaniel P. Banks, Speaker of the US House of Representatives in 1855. Banks said, at a campaign meeting supporting John C. Frémont in his battle against James Buchanan for the presidency, "Although I am not one of that class of men who cry for the perpetuation of the Union, though I am willing in a certain state of circumstances *to let it slide,* . . . if the chief object of the people of this country be to maintain and propagate chattel property in man, in other words, human slavery, *this Union cannot stand, and ought not to stand.*"[23] Harris's thoughts were never far from the fraught politics of his homeland.

He continued this free association on reptiles in the next paragraph, with a reference to a southern folk song. "Your 'Allergater in de brake' song may do for the Southern States, with their rhythmetical-and-stolen-from-the-African-coast slaves; but to apply it to this country would disgrace the most idiotic 'What-is-it' ever imported."[24] The song he referred to is probably similar to "O, Get Along Home, My Yaller Gals," said to be "An Ethiopian Lyric" in an 1851 collection of slave folk songs. The singer began by saying that he was playing his banjo at the end of day and calling "my yaller gals" to come on home. After reporting on the possum and the bullfrog, he continued,

> De alligator in de brake
> Plays fast asleep when wide awake
> He wants to suck some n—— in
> As massa do a glass ob gin
> Oh, git along home, my yaller gals,
> De ebening sun is declining.[25]

In the second part of this sentence Harris called up a display from P. T. Barnum, the "What Is It?" exhibited three months after the publication of Darwin's *On the Origin of Species* in 1859. The "What Is It?" was a New Jersey–born African American man named William Henry Johnson.[26] Barnum dressed him up in furs and said he was some sort of half monkey, half man who proved Darwin's theory. It is likely that Harris was not the only observer to find this claim "idiotic," not to mention racist.

So what was Harris's point in this perplexing paragraph? The folk song spoke to the alligator eating the unsuspecting human, sucking him in like the master gulped gin. Nonsense, said Harris. Just as idiotic as the "what is it"! There were not any fearsome beasts here on the island. Not even so much as a squirrel. Birds without number, yes, but no alligators and no snakes. Be not afraid![27] To put it another way, the United States has fearsome beasts, like snakes, alligators—and white men who enslave our race. The islands are much, much safer.

Finally, his host, Stanley, was well again. (Presumably Stanley and Señor Pastorisa were one and the same.) They traveled down the Isabela River to the town of the same name, the first landing site for Columbus. Harris saw mahogany logs on the shore and ships in the harbor ready to take them away, but otherwise Columbus would find the town without "a particle more of improvement" than on his original sighting. (Although of course the Indigenous people were absent.) The modern traveler to the Dominican Republic would discover that the neighborhood of La Isabela on the north coast is commemorated as the landing site for Columbus; the river reaching it is the Río Bajabonico. There is a Río Isabela that flows to the sea on the south side of the island, but the Harris description more clearly matches the former. "To get a better view, you must cross the promontory (the northernmost point of the island) to where Columbus first landed." Columbus had abandoned La Isabela by 1496, so it is not surprising that the site was "unimproved" when Harris visited it. But it was all part of his object lesson: there was great potential for development of the land, even though the harbor was too shallow for vessels of "a hundred tons burthen." He wondered why "a man of Columbus' sense ever stopped there at all."[28]

His companion led Harris in a scramble over the cliffs and arrived at the Columbus landing beach. Like any tourist, Harris sought a memoir of the site. He fed his "zeal to commemorate the landing of Columbus by gathering a few tiny tinted shells," which was tolerated by his host, who got to sit in the shade for a while. "But I have no doubt he had rather see me as expert at gathering peas or picking up potatoes." Indeed, Pastorisa laughed at his friend. "Ah! H.,' says he, 'leave off writing books and gathering shells; get married, and come to farming.'" Harris agreed it was a good plan, all except for the marriage proposal.[29]

On the way back, Harris and Pastorisa paused for a meal with local people. They were having fresh roasted goat, along with winter squash and plantains stewed together. The woman of the house washed her hands by taking a ladle full of water in her mouth and then spraying her hands with it. Harris found this mode of washing quite remarkable. As to the children, well: "The four, and even six year old, running about the place, were as innocent of even a shirt as any son of Adam at his coming into the world." Old and young sat around on the dirt floor of the open-sided kitchen to enjoy the meal. Harris seems to be presenting the scene as a marker of primitive life, but he also expressed something like envy for their carefree ways. "Our dinner is over; we bid these folks good-bye, and pronounce them the happiest set of miserably contented mortals the sun ever shone upon. Man needs excitement; he prays for ease."

They made their way back to Pastorisa's farm and, after a couple of days of rest, returned to Porto Cabello. "So ends the week," he wrote in conclusion. "One at least in my life for which it was worth the trouble to have lived."[30]

In the next letter, Harris was back on the theme of how healthy the island was for its inhabitants. The people wore a white head kerchief to express mourning, but it was rarely seen as the population mostly died of old age. There was an eighty-year-old man in sight whose father died only last year. Harris then went on to tell of the abundant food, frequently offered: great coffee, alligator pears (avocados), pineapples, mangoes, oranges, bananas, and sticks of sugar cane. Such tropical fruits, luxuries in the United States, abounded there. And he taught the concurrent lesson that the people were so generous, they were constantly offering more food and drink. The temperature was mild and sunstroke rare. The hottest day there, in late June, was eighty-eight degrees Fahrenheit. It was a paradise.[31]

The Dominican Republic had a great potential for development, Harris believed. It was "ripening for immigration," especially now that the "Pike's Peak fever will ere long be exhausted." All that was needed was to build some good roads and bring in plows, cotton gins, sawmills, and practical American workers. He acknowledged that the Dominican people had a "lingering prejudice against white Americans," but what really mattered was this: "Are colored men in America competent to infuse the spirit of enterprise which the country demands? *Let the common-sense working-men answer!*"[32] Not only that, but the local government supported the plan. It promoted immigration schemes that would welcome farmers or other useful professions and at least laid open the possibility of giving immigrants travel and establishment funds. (Harris could not know that this agreement, signed in 1860, would become null after the Spanish retook control of its former colony in 1861. Harris may have preferred the Dominican Republic over Haiti, but within a few months of his trip that destination was no longer open.)

By early July Harris was back in a place he called Porto Cabello, a Dominican Republic port about sixteen miles west from Puerto Plata (per Harris), where he had initially landed.[33] His companion remarked that "a man that could find fault with this climate would find fault with Paradise." Yet now Harris was not so quick to agree. For the first time illness clouded his view of its beauty. "Whether the day and night trips along the coast have been too much for me or not, I have certainly got the chill-fever."[34] He said no more about this illness, which might have been any number of diseases, such as malaria or dengue. Either it was mild, perhaps abbreviated by quinine, or he chose to pass lightly over it as his purpose was to extol the paradise, not condemn it.

The Dominican Republic had only a quarter million inhabitants, leaving it very sparsely cultivated by the metric Harris employed. If the valley that led to the port of Cabello was developed with American technology and the harbor readied for shipping, then a prosperous community was guaranteed. They had only to see his vision and not be put off by the current primitive state of affairs.[35] Like John Adams, he was filled with "reverence and awe" at the dream land that lay before him.[36] The emotions evident in Adams's famous letter to his wife, Abigail, are relevant here, as depicting a future undaunted by military disaster and colony discord. "Yet through all the Gloom I can see the Rays of ravishing Light and Glory. I can see that the End is more than worth all the Means. And that Posterity will triumph," proclaimed Adams in a famous passage.[37] Harris too, writing less eloquently but nonetheless from the heart, saw a new land where his people would prosper in safety, respect, and happiness.

As if to build on a "Garden of Eden" trope, in the next section Harris described the agricultural abundance just waiting to be exploited in the Dominican Republic. He used W. S. Courtney's *Gold Fields of St. Domingo* (1860) as his main source. Mahogany trees were a major source of wood for export and still plentiful in the hinterland. Tobacco was grown as well, although Harris believed the quantity produced could be much increased and would rival in quality the output of Cuba. Likewise, beeswax was a local product extracted from the numerous bees and flowers but was harvested only as a small craft industry, whereas there was great opportunity for increased production. The locals did not bother to harvest honey, except in small batches—again, a lost opportunity. There was ample prospect in the production of hides and subsequently leather—the occupation of his friends the Learys in Fayetteville. He noted that sugar was produced in a small way—locals found cane growing wild and "have nothing whatever to do but cut and grind it in wooden mills and boil day after day." They lacked the sugar mills used elsewhere. "It is easy to conceive what a source of incalculable wealth the culture of this staple there would become, if in the hands of a skillful and enterprising population."[38]

Here Harris failed to realize that the mass production of sugar, on an order that prevailed before the Haitian Revolution, was impossible without the concomitant use of slaves forced into the grueling labor of sugar harvesting and syrup production. As historian Laurent Dubois describes for the situation in Haiti, the freed Black families chose subsistence agriculture on their own land over the riches of plantation-style production.[39] Harris did not understand this aspect of mass production necessary to produce major cash crops like tobacco and sugar on the order of the Cuban output. Cuba, after all, still had slaves in 1860.

Harris was particularly annoyed that the locals failed to harvest and ship their profusion of fruits and coffee. The fruits included coconuts, oranges, lemons, and limes—all high-value items on the US market. He found these crops both "cultivated and grow[ing] wild in vast abundance on the island." But, he lamented, "the labor necessary to collect them, prepare them for shipment, and carry them to the ports is not there. From this cause, indeed, the whole Spanish end of the island languishes in sloth, and its transcendent wealth goes year after year incontinently to waste." Similarly, the capacity for coffee production remained to be fully exploited since "the abandonment of the coffee plantations"—that is, the end of slavery.[40] All told, "the labor of cultivating coffee and sugar in Dominica, with all the modern appliances of civilization, would be absolutely insignificant compared with the rich returns it would bring the planter."[41] So under this vision, technology would replace the slave system. To him, it seemed so obvious! Harris was naive and uninformed here, but no more so than the many leaders of the island who sought and failed to achieve reforms.[42]

In the spring of 1861 the Dominican Republic government of Pedro Santana, impoverished and weak, had asked the Spanish government to again annex the country. He feared repeat invasion by the Haitian army and encroachments by the United States. Yet the monetary system was in such shambles that he could not mount an army or preserve the economy. The Spanish offered the financial support needed for prosperity and military might, although Santana did not realize that his abdication was the price for Spanish intervention. By the fall of 1861 it had become clear that the island would be ruled by leadership directly from Spain and that dark-skinned inhabitants would have few rights.[43] In his book, Harris followed his gloomy prediction of the demise of Santana's government with the conclusion, "And now I have struck the key note of all I have to say. The most beautiful countries in the world are the most lamentably ill-governed." The white people might have some protection from such vicissitudes, but the free colored people of America "have no protection anywhere. Now this is a shame and a disgrace to the civilized world." Only if a significant number of free Blacks did immigrate could they protect themselves, and even then, it would be "a matter of great risk."[44]

THE HAITIAN COLONY

By March 1861 Harris was back in Ohio, recruiting new emigrants for Caribbean settlement under James Redpath's colonization scheme. Together they sought African American families who were ready to move to francophone Haiti. (John Brown Jr. was serving a similar role in Windsor, Canada, where many escaped slaves had settled after traveling through Cleveland on the Underground Railroad.) Harris may have come home earlier in the year. One January 1861 correspondent from Cleveland ("W. E. A."), writing to the *Weekly Anglo-African*, took issue with an earlier letter writer with the initials J. P. S., who had claimed that there were "but three leading colored men in Cleveland—viz: Charles H. Langston, J. D. Harris, and B. K. Sampson." W. E. A. disagreed, saying that C. H. Langston no longer lived in Cleveland, and "Mr. Harris had not been here for better than a year until last fall, and is only here occasionally."[45] In February 1861 Harris was in Toledo, speaking at an emigration meeting.[46] And by March 1861, James Redpath had bought the *Weekly Anglo-African* and installed George Lawrence, an African American newspaperman, as its editor.[47]

This purchase did not please many in the northeastern literate Black community. Thomas Hamilton's paper had been open to multiple points of view, which he presented with limited censorship. He had published essays, stories, and poetry by Black authors and overall, according to one historical account, "create[d] a unified black press that allowed black readers and writers of all stripes to speak and collective[ly] participate in creating a black print community," one that spread far beyond New York City.[48] Under new editorial leadership—that of James Redpath himself—the paper was primarily dedicated to promoting Haitian emigration. Critics said that Redpath had appointed a Black man (Lawrence) only "as a figure head of a ship," in the words of an editorial in the *Christian Recorder*.[49] The paper's new focus became even more evident when Redpath changed the name of the weekly newspaper to the *Pine and Palm*, connecting the pinelands of the South with the palm trees of the islands.

Amid the rising political tensions of early 1861, Harris did not always speak unmolested about the immigration of free Blacks to the Caribbean. In late March the opponents of emigration in Cincinnati managed to lock him out of a speaking venue, but the next night he was able to talk and found many attentive listeners. He particularly sought farmers who could move with their skills and equipment to Haiti, but even when such men were interested, they deferred emigration until after the next harvest.[50] The March issues of the *Weekly Anglo-African* were full of statements pro and con about the Haitian emigration movement. By April, however, its comments had become one-sided. On April 13, for example, an editorial proclaimed, "The Haytian fever is spreading far and wide." The paper reported that John Brown Jr. (surely a name to conjure with) was up in Chatham, Ontario, lecturing on Haiti and recruiting more emigrants from the escaped slave population there.[51]

In March 1861 James Redpath listed J. D. Harris as the local emigration agent for Ohio.[52] Seven months later Harris had become even more closely associated with Redpath's enterprise for Haiti. A hostile letter about him appeared in the *Christian Recorder* that October. Parker T. Smith wrote from Dresden, Canada, to describe an emigration meeting headed by William Wells Brown and J. D. Harris. Smith found Brown "arrogant and condescending," while "Harris appeared as agent for the *Pine and Palm*," there to tout subscriptions. According to the irritated Smith, Harris said the main reason to subscribe was that "it is the only living newspaper published by colored people in the United States." Smith was indignant. He "asked if the *Christian Recorder* is not a living paper, but he [Harris] would not answer the question." "Who publishes the *Pine and Palm*?" Smith ranted. James Redpath, that was who, a white man, not a colored person at all.[53] If this account is true, it sounds like Harris had become a thorough acolyte of the Redpath vision. Certainly, he and Redpath agreed on the concept of the African American Caribbean empire that Harris had espoused in the previous year.[54] And on October 6, 1861, Harris sailed at the head of an Ohio cohort of settlers bound for their new homeland in Haiti.[55]

What we know about the history of the Harris-led settlement is filtered through the *Pine and Palm*, the Redpath newspaper with the principal goal of recruiting settlers for Haiti. So bad news was no doubt abridged and good news overemphasized in order to keep the people coming. Redpath's agents, including Harris, were paid twenty dollars a week to serve the Haitian Emigration Bureau, and they got an extra two dollars per emigrant landed in Haiti.[56] A further problem with using the *Pine and Palm* as a source, and particularly as a source of Harris's thoughts, is that the paper's articles could be months out of date. Events that happened in January might only be reported in June, and then again repeated a couple of months later. A letter dated January 24, 1862, was printed in September of that year. Mails from the island were erratic, and it is also possible that the delay served some political purpose for Redpath.[57]

Writing under his pseudonym Peregrine Cope, Harris described his trip to the capital of Haiti, Port-au-Prince, in an undated letter whose contents suggest it was written in late January 1862. In the capital Harris was taken by multiple incongruities that he saw. A well-attended Protestant church sat close by "a place where a singular kind of dance is carried on, which is but little in advance of downright African heathenism." A neat classroom with all in order had a naked boy in one corner. He found a painting of Sabès Pétion, one of the heroes of the Revolution, disturbing, for his forehead sloped back, an indicator (according to cranial theory) of low intelligence. Harris wondered, "How did Pétion gain such a name as posterity accords him?" It must have been that he had greater intellects around him who facilitated his greatness, he reasoned.[58] Here Harris showed familiarity with the concepts of Samuel Morton, whose influential book *Crania Americana* appeared in 1839. Morton, like others of his time, sorted human skulls by race and intelligence and claimed differences in mental capacity based on those classifications. The forehead that sloped backward was supposedly a sign of primitive, low intelligence.

After describing the magnificence of a high mass celebrated to honor President Geffrard's patron saint, Harris turned to the situation of Drouillard, the colony of emigrants begun by Theodore Holly, which was near the capital.[59] Apparently, Harris had heard of much misfortune afflicting the colony but found Holly full of good cheer: the situation was improving and the sick were on the mend. Early on, this was the persistent theme of his reports. He would supply a verse about hardship or tragedy but then a chorus of reassuring improvement.

Multiple earlier cadres of migrants had arrived at St. Mark and headed for the fertile Artibonite River valley—eleven shiploads and 1,166 persons, per a list Harris published in January 1862.[60] And the news of their many disappointments had already filtered back to the United States by that time. Their fates were entangled with issues of cooperation with the Haitian government and peoples, Redpath's inability to raise and manage funds, and a deep underestimation of the challenges faced by those living and farming in Haiti.[61] Some problems may have improved over the spring months, but overall, the enterprise was ill-conceived and unlikely to succeed. Some 4,000 African American immigrants moved to Haiti under Redpath's auspices, before Redpath resigned in September 1864 and abandoned the colonists. In 1864, when one investigator inquired of their numbers, he could find only about 200 were still in the country.[62] What happened?

Harris traveled with 280 aspiring colonists on the ship *Flight*, and it became the custom to name new settlements of migrants by the ship name. So, his group was called Flight I, and when the ship later brought another cadre, it was labeled Flight II. The Flight I group left on October 6, 1861, and arrived on November 2.[63] The location of his settlement was the Artibonite River valley, which drained into the port of St. Mark, the most popular of American settlement areas. The river itself was not then suitable for flatboat travel, so

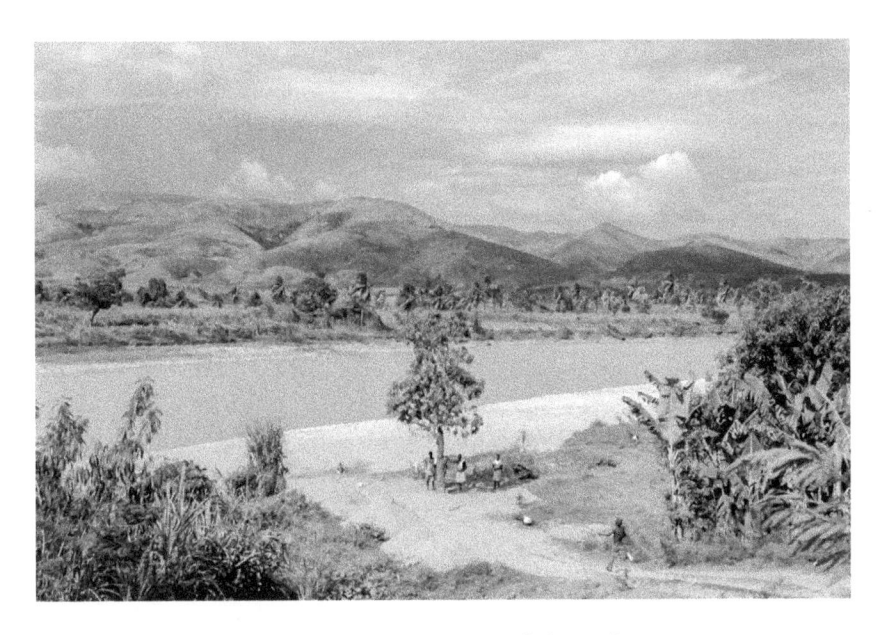

Artibonite River valley, Haiti. Courtesy of Library of Congress.

one of the first tasks was to build a canal along its length to create a wider passage. Settlers received sixteen acres of land per married man (six acres for a single one), and if they arrived with the means to purchase food and farming implements, they started clearing the land right away. The Haitian government provided food and shelter for their first eight days, but afterward the American emigrants were expected to be self-sustaining. Redpath's agents had advised settlers to purchase equipment before leaving the United States, as it was apparently much cheaper there. But if they arrived impoverished (as many of the former slaves recruited for the task did), they could work on the canal for a salary, purchase food and rent a space, and save until they had the means to buy farming equipment and till their designated land parcel.[64]

Harris wrote an account of the first *Flight*'s arrival and the migrants' travel to their settlement lands that appeared on January 2, 1862, in the *Pine and Palm*.[65] It was bundled with a group of letters from other emigrants that were dated November and December 1861, but his missive had no date. In the harbor of St. Mark, he admired the natural beauty of the place and reported the need for renovation of many houses and the presence of a barque that, having deposited immigrants, was now sailing back to New York with 50,000 pounds of cotton and lumber. He marveled at the thousands of people milling about an active market offering produce, meats, manufactured goods, and animals.[66]

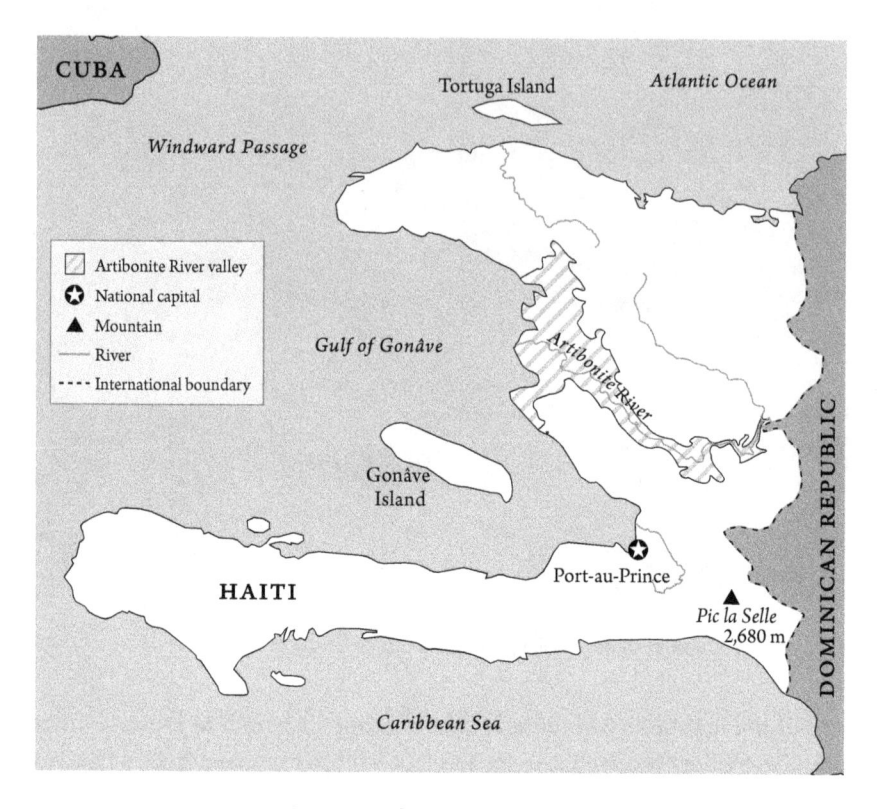

Haiti. Adapted from Freeworldmaps.net.

As soon as the migrants on the *Flight* had disembarked, they received money from the government for eight days of support, as promised. Harris was startled to see others who had come months before but had still not settled on their own land. They could not get to work until the government had surveyed the land and divided it up. Apparently, the river had flooded, impairing movement to their new colony. And the government was still supporting them while they waited, with half pay (which shows the generosity of the government, Harris pointed out). He set out to inspect the settlement lands, in the company of Auguste Élie, the Haitian director general for emigration. The Artibonite valley, which stretches almost 200 miles across the inland of Haiti, was a vision of fertility and had room for 10,000 homesteads (said Harris).[67]

As he and Élie traveled up the valley they talked to various migrants. From these conversations one hears Harris answering the charges brought against the wholesomeness of the enterprise. One person was sick and complained that the French-speaking doctor did not understand him. Harris had "the satisfaction of informing him that the said doctor has been removed, and an English physician appointed." After talking to other immigrants about their problems, Harris concluded, "There is no fundamental reason why the immigration should not succeed." The government was financing the canal, which would eventually carry their produce and lumber to port. The lands would be surveyed—a backhanded way of admitting the truth that one impediment to settlement was the fact that the lots had not been marked off yet, and thus promised acres were yet to be assigned. So, all was well![68] Another agent, P. Hall, noted further problems in the St. Mark area, unmentioned by Harris. There was not enough lodging for the arrivals in the city. Too few of their number had money on hand, so the settlement began impoverished. Hall begged that migrants arrive with provisions. And he noted that (in December) the mornings and evenings were pleasant, but "in the middle of the day the weather is very warm."[69]

In late January Harris wrote another letter to the *Pine and Palm*, continuing the report on Port-au-Prince. He was writing as Peregrine Cope, but the text was supposedly edited by J. D. Harris. He began by extolling the weather: sunny in the daytime, and the nights, well, the nights were "cloudless, cool, and delicious." To further entice those at home, he remarked on the "lately arrived passengers from Canada [who] remind us of the freezing and thawing ... of the variable, mud-generating, and consumption-giving latitudes." Certainly, one might catch a cold here in Haiti, but take "a sea bath the next morning, and the cold will pass away like money in New York—one never remembers how." So, he answered those critics who spoke of the wretched heat and humidity of Haiti, finishing with a quip that was likely better remembered than the weather report itself.[70]

Harris was flush with enthusiasm for the prospects of the coming spring. Already many had built houses and cleared their land of brush. And then, in just a couple of months, the spring rains would fall, "at which time the corn, cotton, and rice crops, the sugar-cane and coffee plant will spring from the earth, [and] a change will be wrought in the prospect of affairs, as if following the sweep of a magician's wand!" This paradise was the dream of his life made real. "When I settle down, for good and all, in Hayti,—with the nice little wife in the neat little cottage, surrounded by a grove of orange trees ... it will be up this valley, about four miles from the city on the slope of a mountain, overlooking the sea." He had already given a name to his own homestead in his envisioned community in the Artibonite River valley. "This miniature Eden," he proclaimed, "shall be *Doucé-Amère*." The phrase means "bittersweet"—the name of a particular plant but also, most likely, a name expressive of both happiness and regret that he could not make such a home in his native land.[71]

Here the supposed essay by Peregrine Cope ended, and a letter by J. D. Harris to Élie, dated St. Mark, January 29, 1862, began. He was making a formal report to Élie as the director general for immigration in Haiti. For the moment, things were a bit rough in his imagined Eden. It took at least seven weeks for the migrants, mostly from Canada, to receive their land and get to work. Many of these people were old men, he noted without explaining why that mattered. Many would have been slaves who had escaped across the border to freedom in Ontario. Harris cheerily reported that their produce would soon "swell the markets of St. Marks." He continued to travel up the valley, visiting communities made up of settlers from various ships, such as the *Truxillo* and the *Pearl*. Of the *Pearl*'s community he admitted, "It is true they have had some sickness, and they were kept a long time without their lands."[72] But, he said jovially, the sick were now recuperating, and those who were now so disposed would soon have their lands. Another colony was very little developed because the settlers had been flooded out in the spring by the Artibonite overflow; there had been sickness there too, and some lacked the proper dedication to hard work.

After completing his report, Harris, in a backhanded way telling certain groups to stay home, confessed to the difficulties that migrants continued to face. The government here wanted laborers and farmers. "What can inexperienced young men, brought up in the city, or unprotected females, do here? Nothing—worse than nothing. Nine chances to one, if compelled to expose themselves, by undertaking to clear land, they will take the fever." Not only that, but emigrants needed to have at least some capital when they set out. "If a man comes to a strange country, to work, without tools, without money, even a cent, without anything to eat, without medicine, with a large family ... and does not suffer, he will be lucky." The island government wanted men of "small capital" and "sturdy" farmers.[73] So here was another answer to why the immigrant communities were not thriving: they were populated by the wrong sort of people.

THE TROUBLED DREAM

Harris provided continued warnings about the settlements under his purview and their many needs. But there was a filter on his words, both psychological and actual. Between December 1861 and the summer of 1862, Redpath was desperately trying to salvage his operation. And positive reports from agents of successful colonies were just the thing to buoy continued emigration. While Redpath did send one of his closest associates in March 1862 to investigate complaints, the results were downplayed in the *Pine and Palm*, often under the rubric of "well, this was a problem, but now it's on the mend." Harris was the constant companion of this inspector, Henry Melrose, and through the accounts in *Pine and Palm* it gradually becomes clear that Harris was the only Redpath agent (Melrose included) who spoke French and who was thus able to communicate directly with the Haitian government spokesmen. Harris became perforce part of the inner circle; he was not just an employee but a management spokesman. On the other hand, he was an honest, ethical man, and his comments became less rosy as the weeks went on, until finally he resigned. We cannot know whether he deliberately deceived potential emigrants on the orders of his boss, or perhaps the small part of the enterprise under his direct observation really was as promising as he reported.

More detail existed in Melrose's report back to Redpath. He found things in the St. Mark area not at all as dire as returning colonists had claimed. Everyone who wanted land had acquired it, and most were living in houses they had constructed. He interviewed Reverend Robert Tripp, a settler who could not understand why any colonist would be disappointed. "If every man would only do his best, it would be better for every one of us. For my own part I like the country very much." Melrose generalized from multiple conversations like this one to claim that "the majority of the emigrants are on the high road to success."[74]

Henry Melrose held a public meeting in "the temporary chapel in the Flight Valley" to hear from the people of the settlement. Multiple calumnies were being spread in the United States about excessive sickness, hostility of the locals, lack of help from the government, and general broken promises from Redpath's Haitian Emigration Bureau. The various people quoted in the subsequent report in the *Pine and Palm* all talked about how well they were doing. Yes, there was sickness and some had died, but they were through that now. Even if the settlers were negative, Redpath could have censored their words. The reports about this meeting and subsequent investigations were not published until July.[75]

Soon Melrose came to the Flight I colony, which he called "the crack colony of the whole settlement, and by far the most prosperous." And then Melrose explained why. "This is owing chiefly to the exertions of Mr. J. D. Harris ... who came out as its leader. During the voyage he impressed upon the emigrants the necessity of casting aside all sectional prejudices, of being united one body." Helping each other was the fundamental attitude for success, and Melrose cited this behavior as key to the speed in which the settlement had matured. Both sides of the road were fenced, and row after row of log cabins sat at intervals. The only drawback was the absence of fresh water, as the first attempt to sink a well had failed. But they were digging a new one and expected to hit water any day. All around, Melrose praised these colonists for their common sense, energy, and general "go-aheadedness." An observer credited the fact that they arrived very impoverished, with no cash for cheap rum or fruit. So, the joys of town did not appeal, and they headed straight to their land and got to work. Some of the other settlers who arrived with money "thought themselves too fine gentlemen to go to work so long as it lasted, and loafed around and spent it in dissipation." Those are the ones who invited fever and disease, said this anonymous settler.[76]

On the way back to St. Mark, Melrose was hailed by a woman and invited into her cottage for tea. The husband reported that his health had been very poor, but he was better. And, "We have lost our children." But the government officials took good care of him. All told, "This is the country for a poor man. . . . I like the place first rate." The farmer spoke of great prospects in regard to the cotton crop. Melrose broke in with a caveat: "In spite of the loss of their children,—which both appeared to deeply regret,—they yet seemed *very* happy."[77] This conversation reflects in micro the message that Redpath's agents wanted to broadcast—horrible things had happened, but despite it all, the people were happy.

Melrose then began a summary of the "hard facts." He reported that 1,214 emigrants had been sponsored to Haiti since the enterprise began. (His count differs slightly from that of Harris, above.) Of that number, 900 were at work on their farms, 120 had died, and 194 had left. That is 10 percent mortality in two years, hardly an acceptable record. But Melrose just went on, documenting in turn the construction of settlements and clearing of farms. He did admit, "That there has been much sickness among the emigrants at St. Mark is true; but there is very little now. Fever is rapidly disappearing." Melrose offered several explanations, which were remarkable in that they could with some validity be assigned to the past but not to the future. These included heavy spring rains, arrival of smallpox from New York, orphans without caregivers, gross imprudence of some colonists in eating and drinking and working in the heat of the day, and drinking impure water from streams. Finally, as the American consul at Port-au-Prince noted, large population movements always produce higher mortality. Therefore, Melrose could conclude, not only was the fever gone, but the principal etiological agents were gone as well.[78]

Melrose then consulted a local physician, Dr. Relman, giving him a long survey of questions regarding the emigrants' health. Relman believed the colonists were unclean in body and refused to learn how to eat in the tropics. "They would not bathe . . . [and took] no advice, but only gratif[ied] their amazing Northern appetites." The migrants might be drunk all day, sometimes lying "under a burning sun." Their fellow settlers were so callow as to refuse to care for their neighbors. Relman concluded, "There is nothing about the climate of Hayti to alarm or discourage" the emigrant.[79]

Melrose then addressed the reasons that so many emigrants had returned to the United States and complained so loudly about Haiti. "A great many persons have come to Hayti, who were totally unfit to be pioneers in such a great Movement as this." They were afraid of work and lacked perseverance, and "when they encountered any obstacles, instead of doing as live Yankees do under such circumstances—put forth all their energy and overcome them—they made up their minds" that Haiti was not the country for them. Melrose noted that he had generally seen it true that when incompetent persons were unsuccessful, they blame everyone but themselves.[80]

Melrose was particularly piqued that the emigrants would not help each other. The exception was Harris's Flight I group, who had been taught to do so by his lectures on ship. Harris was Melrose's guide around the Haiti settlements and likely shared this attitude toward laziness. Melrose reported one story that he told in illustration: "Mr. Harris told me that one day when visiting the settlements, he saw one of the emigrants building his house. He was tugging away at a log, with all his might and main, endeavoring to get it into its proper position in the house, while just across the road were half a dozen men talking and laughing among themselves." This was not the Flight settlement, but another. "'Why don't you ask those men to come and help you?' asked Mr. Harris. 'Because they won't,' was the reply. 'Why don't you assist that man to build his house?' inquired he of the emigrants across the road. 'Because it's none of our business.'"[81] Melrose drew on the knowledge that Harris had accumulated in the local culture in other ways. For instance, it was said by returning emigrants in the United States that the native Haitians were opposed to the movement. "'Have you observed any ill-feeling between the emigrants and the Natives?' I [Melrose] asked Mr. J. D. Harris one day, as we were talking about matters connected with the Movement. 'No, not a bit,' was the reply."[82]

In the next installment of Melrose's report, the unique position of Harris became clearer. One of Melrose's recommendations to Redpath was modeled on Harris and his work with the Flight I colony. "It would have been decidedly for the advantage of both the Government and the emigrants, had you sent an agent with the first colony, to be subordinate to, yet to coöperate with, the Government officials at St. Mark, as Mr. Harris now does." As Melrose put it in his list of suggestions, "I would strongly recommend you, whenever a new settlement is to be formed, to send an agent along with the emigrants to assist and cooperate with the Haytian officials, and officiate as interpreter between them." This last phrase elucidates an aspect of the situation not very clear until now. Harris could speak French, as could the members of the government and other educated men in Haiti. Harris likely translated not only emigrant to government official, but even Mr. Melrose to government officials. No wonder he accompanied Melrose on his path of investigation![83]

Melrose had further recommendations for Redpath if the enterprise was to continue. The first was to send no further colonies until the fall, avoiding the summer fevers. Another step to alleviate the fever problem was to settle the colonies in the highlands instead of on the floor of the river valley. The soil there was less fertile but the living much healthier. The agent should interview each emigrant beforehand, to determine his or her suitability for the island's work environment. And finally, mail for the migrant colonies should be sent in a locked bag in care of Mr. Harris. That should improve the problem of lost letters and papers.[84]

Haiti became increasingly unstable in 1862. Just as the migrants began to arrive in late 1861, President Fabre Geffrard faced an internal revolt; he fought off two more in 1862, including one in September. Spain had reoccupied the Spanish-speaking half of the island in 1861, and there were fears in 1862 of a war between Haiti and Santo Domingo. Indeed, one fear of the potential colonists was not just that war would disrupt their homestead but that they themselves would be drafted into combat.[85] Little of this situation was evident in the positive settler recruitment literature that continued to appear in the *Pine and Palm*.

Our knowledge of what happened at the Flight I colony is scanty. The records go from reports that everything was fine and growing to the sudden end of the project a few months later. James Redpath announced on September 4, 1862, that the Haitian government had suspended the *Pine and Palm*, which had been "one of the semi-official organs" of that government.[86] He was shrinking the American operation to one office in New York and no field agents. He listed Mr. Harris of Ohio as among those who were "retir[ing] from the Movement with him."[87] Redpath reviewed in his essay the many problems of the emigration scheme, including poor leadership and organization on the ground in Haiti, poor government cooperation, and, perhaps in some cases, the fact that the lighter mulatto Americans were prone to dismiss darker-skinned people as "darkies" and inferiors. Redpath did still believe that Haiti was a good target for African American emigration, but he himself was giving up the fight.[88]

The record reveals only one further comment from Harris since the Melrose visit in the spring. Redpath said of him, in September 1862, that Harris "agreed to raise [further] colonies only on condition that I should revisit Hayti and that the reforms which I had so often advised, and the necessity of which they also urged, were immediately adopted."[89] Here Redpath was both acknowledging that Harris's critiques were valid and claiming them as his own. Some time that fall, Harris sailed back to the United States and then traveled to Cleveland. There he began or continued medical studies with his mentor at the US Marine Hospital. Given the death rate in the Haitian colonies, there is no doubt that he had learned, as he said later, something of the diseases of the islands. He may well have learned something, too, about working under a boss with whom one disagrees. It would serve him in good stead when he took jobs in the Union army and Freedmen's Bureau hospitals. His dream of an African American Caribbean empire was gone; his fantasy of settling with a wife in a cabin on the hillside of Haiti was likewise squashed. He went home to the United States in the fall of 1862, a country at war and already transformed from the one he had left. There he would find new challenges, new opportunities, and, sadly, new disappointments.

7

The Great Transition, 1862-1864

In the fall of 1862, Joseph Dennis Harris came home from Haiti. He had left the Caribbean with his dreams in tatters but returned to a country radically transformed. While he was gone, the southern states had seceded from the United States, Fort Sumter had fallen, and the first great battles of the Civil War had been waged. Although the impact of the war on slavery and on the civil rights of free Blacks was still in the balance, these were exciting times to be Black in the militarized North. J. D. Harris moved back to Cleveland, rejoining his mother and youngest siblings. By the fall of 1863 J. D. was attending medical school in Cleveland, and in the following summer the Union army recognized his new skills by hiring him as a contract surgeon for its hospital in Portsmouth, Virginia. This remarkable transition is the story of this chapter.

Most of the African American physicians who served in the last years of the war were stationed in Washington, DC, or in nearby Baltimore. As far as can be discovered, Harris was the only African American MD working in southern Virginia, which may have contributed to his historical obscurity. In his review of the early history of trained Black physicians in the United States, Herbert Morais found Charles Purvis and John Rapier (who served in Washington hospitals for the US Colored Troops) but did not mention Harris.[1] Of note, Harris's very first medical contract, in late June 1864, was for Dr. J. D. Harris of Portsmouth, Virginia. He had already moved there after completing his medical education. His mother and younger siblings were still in Cleveland. What was he doing in the South, even if it was the occupied South? The answer lies in two aspects key to his choices at this time. First, he wanted to serve the freedpeople and the Black troops. Second, he joined a family cluster that had already formed in that neighborhood. His move to Virginia opened a new and exciting phase of his life.

The war years offered free African Americans, as well as newly freed slaves, untold opportunities that could not have been imagined a few years earlier. In 1858, an escaped slave could be captured in the North and returned to slavery, all with the support of the US government. In 1863, that same government began facilitating emancipation and forming Black regiments to fight the South. African Americans suddenly found themselves in a very unfamiliar country. Gone was the rhetoric about no place for free Blacks in the United States. Now exciting new opportunities were opening. Harris, his brothers, and even his nephews sought new roles sanctioned by the Union, including medical training and, in his brothers' cases, openly teaching freedpeople to read and write. Two of his nephews (sister Sarah's sons) joined the 54th Massachusetts Regiment (of later cinematic fame in *Glory*). His friend John Mercer Langston had already made inroads in the field of law; now Harris dared to believe that he himself could become a doctor.

So did two other free African Americans who intersected Harris's path in medicine—John H. Rapier and Charles B. Purvis, mentioned above. Purvis overlapped with Harris at Western Reserve Medical School in 1863–64. A member of a noted abolitionist family in Philadelphia, Purvis came to Western Reserve because no East Coast school would admit him. He spent 1863–64 and 1864–65 there, becoming its first African American medical student to receive a diploma. (Harris graduated in 1864, but not from Western Reserve.)[2]

Rapier has even more similarities to Harris. He was born to a prosperous free Black family in Alabama that could support Rapier's ambitions, first to be a revolutionary and later to become a professional. While Harris condemned William Walker's attempt to colonize Central America, young Rapier found it exciting, especially since his uncle knew Walker. Rapier joined Walker's colony in Nicaragua in 1856 but became disillusioned by the leader's dictatorial methods, his persistent racism, and the poverty of the colonists. Like Harris, Rapier gave life on the northern frontier a try, in his case in Minnesota. There he was disappointed again, as the federal government was not honoring Black homestead applications. Rapier then began writing articles for five Minnesota newspapers. Like Harris, disgust with the *Dred Scott* decision led him to abandon the persistent racism of the United States for the possibility of a new life in the Caribbean. He went first to Haiti and then to Jamaica. As his biographer noted, "A black American, he felt that he had a better chance of finding social and professional opportunities in the West Indies than in either Europe or his homeland."[3] In Jamaica, Rapier decided to establish himself as a dentist but then sought the higher social standing that medical training would bring.

Rapier dreamed of attending Canadian medical schools, followed by a year in Scotland, but could not raise the money for such an ambitious plan from his family.[4] So he began "reading" medicine with a preceptor in Jamaica. As was typical in such student posts, his work included bandaging wounds, mixing medications, visiting patients, and whatever else the doctor asked him to do. It was the usual exchange—he learned the elements of medicine, and the mentor acquired free labor. In order to practice in Jamaica, Rapier thought he needed a degree from an English, Scottish, or Irish school. Since he could not afford foreign study, he enrolled at the University of Michigan as the first Black man to attend its medical school. Rapier himself attributed his success at Michigan to the fact that he acted the part of a Caribbean native, not an American; the students had previously rioted over the prospect of an American Black man in attendance. Like Harris, Rapier enrolled in didactic lectures from 1863 to 1864 (at Michigan) and then acquired the MD from the same Iowa school, Keokuk, that would also give Harris a diploma. He moved quickly to join the army as an acting assistant surgeon and was stationed at the Freedmen's Hospital in Washington, DC, until his death the following year.[5]

So, while Harris was not unique, he was certainly among a very small cluster of successful African American medical graduates. At this point we need to move forward to 1865, when Harris applied for a three-year appointment as a regular army physician (in contrast to his tenuous status as a temporary surgeon with a month-to-month contract). When Harris presented himself to the army examiners to apply for the three-year position, he was required to write a brief summary of his medical training and experience, labeled his "autobiography" in the government files, and take a written exam. This process will come back into the story in its own time, but for now let us listen to Harris describing his motivation for medical study. He first explained how he became interested in medicine. "In the West Indies it is necessary to know something of fever. I made it a study."[6] As there were no medical schools in the islands, he chose to return to Cleveland and study there. (Of note, he said nothing of this decision in his writings on Haiti.) Given the cost of boarding on his own, it seems likely that he moved in with his family on Fourteenth Street in Cleveland. The first challenge was to find a preceptor who could teach him the elements of medical practice at the bedside; medical schools required such experiences *before* admission to medical lectures. He was a Black man seeking medical training in an era when most white physicians would not dream of taking such a hued assistant into patient homes.

MEDICAL TRAINING IN CLEVELAND

Harris was lucky to be in Cleveland, where abolitionist spirit ran high among whites and Blacks. And he was especially lucky to find Dr. Martin Luther Brooks as a preceptor. At the age of six Brooks had moved from Connecticut when his family took up farming in the wilderness of northern Ohio. At sixteen, Brooks broke his leg while cutting lumber, a misfortune that left him unfit for manual labor, so his father sent him to school instead. He caught the fire of abolitionism from a lecture by William Lloyd Garrison, and he himself gave the first pro-abolition lecture heard at his chosen college, Oberlin. After completing college, he traveled to Gallipolis, Ohio, a Virginia border town with many Black families. There Brooks put his politics into action, teaching a large school for "colored students." His home also became a safe house on the Underground Railroad, which helped escaping slaves reach the freedom of Canada. Such blatant radicalism aroused the antipathy of the locals, some of whom expressed their dismay in violence. Undeterred, Brooks had the ruffians arrested and jailed.[7] He was on record delivering a wagonload of escaped slaves to Oberlin in 1837, where the students raucously welcomed their guests with a great feast. After some time for rest, the students sent them off to Canada with huzzahs.[8]

To further his career, Brooks attended the Medical College of Ohio in Cincinnati. As he lacked enough money to complete the course, he found a business position in Kaskaskia, Illinois, where he reportedly met Abraham Lincoln. Cash in hand, Brooks returned to Ohio and finished his medical training in 1843. He tried to make a go of it in Patriot, Indiana, and returned for a brief time to the Gallipolis area. What both of these small towns had in common was their location on the Ohio River, which suggests he continued Underground Railroad work. In any event, he soon returned to Cleveland

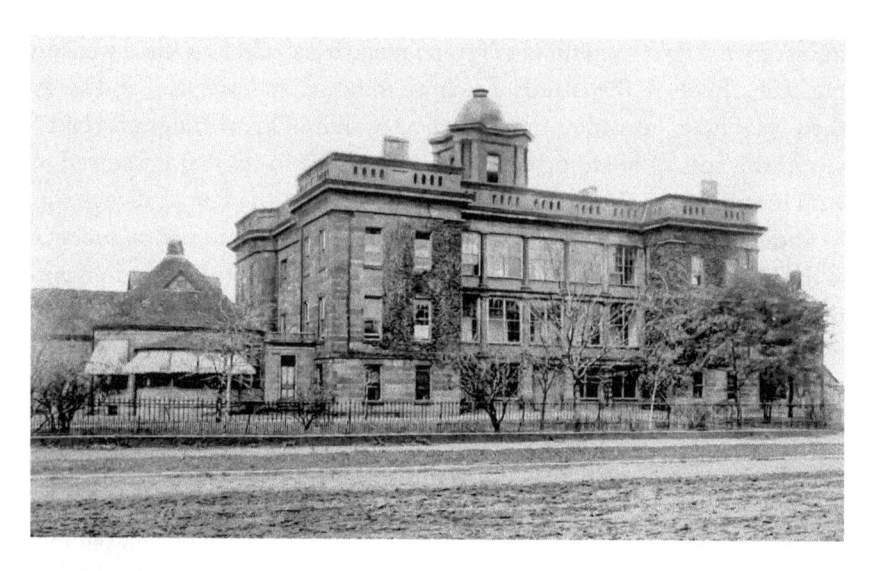

US Marine Hospital, Cleveland, Ohio. US Public Health Service, *Annual Report of 1896*.

and private practice.[9] Following sixteen years of such work, he received the appointment as physician to the US Marine Hospital in Cleveland.[10]

What was a marine hospital, and why was there one more than 400 miles from the nearest ocean? The Marine Hospital Service had first been created by Congress in 1798, to provide hospital insurance for sailors in maritime ports.[11] Its financial basis came from the federal government, ship owners, and the sailors themselves. In 1837 Congress extended the system to care for sailors on the inland waterways, including the Great Lakes.[12] The US Marine Hospital in Cleveland opened in 1852, in a newly built structure that contained fifty beds and a portico that faced Lake Erie. Doctors from Western Reserve Medical School held weekly clinics there during the school term, so Harris the student would have been very familiar with the place from his time as Brooks's apprentice. The hospital faced Lake (now Lakeside) Avenue and stretched between the corners of Erie and Muirson Streets, now East Ninth and East Twelfth Streets, conveniently located near the medical school.[13] It was just over a mile from Harris's mother's house.

Thus, Martin Brooks emerged almost magically as the perfect mentor for J. D. Harris. His abolitionist sentiments ran deep, and there is a direct line between teaching those Black children in Gallipolis in his youth and taking Harris as a student in 1862 or 1863. He had trained at one of the best available orthodox medical schools in the Midwest and had almost two decades of medical experience. Finally, his position at the US Marine Hospital meant that his patients were all male, so the negotiation over a Black man examining a white woman did not have to be made. The sick and wounded sailors may not have been thrilled to see a Black man assisting the doctor, but at least he was essentially there in a servant role—just where the Black man belonged, said some, whether in slavery or freedom. Brooks may also have been tolerant of Harris's peculiar situation in other ways. Perhaps he waived or reduced the usual fee of a $100 per year.[14] And Brooks may have certified Harris as educated enough in medicine to enter formal schooling before Harris had completed the expected two to three years of apprentice experience. In any event, we know that Harris could not have returned stateside any sooner than the fall of 1862. He started medical school in Cleveland in the fall of 1863. In the pressure of wartime, Brooks may have urged Western Reserve to take Harris with only a year of preceptor training, rather than the usual three years. It was wartime and the army needed doctors; this path of accelerated medical education was likely common.

In the fall of 1863 Harris matriculated at the medical school he called the "Medical Department of the Western Reserve College, or the Cleveland College." Others referred to the school as the Cleveland Medical College. As Frederick Waite pointed out in his chapter on the Western Reserve Medical School, it was common in the mid-nineteenth century for a school to have both an official name (which might be a mouthful) and a secondary nickname. Hence this medical school was known not only by the names already listed but also as the Erie Street Medical College.[15] This location was very convenient for Harris, as he could walk there from his mother's house. Again, he was lucky—he had no extra transportation or lodging costs when he started medical school. We do not know where he found the money for tuition. Perhaps from his mother—with money left over from selling the North Carolina property—or from his several siblings who were employed. It is even possible that in a burst of wartime fervor, Western Reserve reduced his fees. No records exist to answer this question.

Western Reserve had something of a progressive spirit, having admitted women for medical training in the 1850s, including Emily Blackwell and Marie Zakrzewska.[16] In 1865 it would graduate another African American physician, Charles B. Purvis, as mentioned above. Such progressiveness did not flow unchallenged by the Western Reserve medical faculty, however; after graduating six women in the 1850s, the conservative bloc triumphed in barring women from the school. Still, school leaders Drs. John J. DeLamater and Jared Potter Kirtland were both pro–female students as well as staunch abolitionists.[17] Although Kirtland was emeritus by the time Harris and Purvis applied, it seems possible that the pendulum had swung toward Black admissions in 1863 due to wartime influences, including the Emancipation Proclamation of January 1, 1863, and the enlistment of thousands of Blacks into the US Colored Troops.

In describing the Western Reserve experience in his 1865 application for a commission as a surgeon in the US Army, Harris reported that he studied chemistry with Professor (John Long) Cassells, who was also the school's first dean. From Dr. (Jared) Kirtland, professor emeritus of theory and practice of medicine, he learned disease causation, process, and treatment. Dr. (Henry K.) Cushing was his professor of surgery.[18] (Cushing's brother Harvey, trained on the East Coast, went on to pioneer the field of neurosurgery, with appointments at Yale, Harvard, and Johns Hopkins.) Harris offered letters of support from all three professors, letters that unfortunately did not survive in his file.[19] The University Archives at Case Western Reserve do list him as a medical student in the 1863–64 school year, and at the time these professors did teach the courses attributed to them.[20] He was not, at least, inflating this aspect of his medical school experience.

So, by the spring of 1864, Harris's medical training amounted to a preceptor year with Brooks at the US Marine Hospital and one solid year of didactic medical education at Western Reserve. The usual fees for this instruction would have been $100 per year with his preceptor and $60 per year for the lectures.[21] A "year" at Western Reserve was fifteen weeks; in specific terms of 1863–64, the lectures began on November 4 and ended with commencement on February 21.[22] Not surprisingly, the curriculum now included a new course not taught in the 1850s: a survey of military medicine. One school historian, Frederick Waite, reported, "The content of this course included military hygiene, army diseases, military surgery, and the routine duties of an army surgeon in the field."[23] The professor for this course was able to pair the lectures with appropriate cases of army patients at the US Marine Hospital in Cleveland, which had been partially taken over by the army for military patients. This continued the tradition begun in 1852. "One medical and one surgical clinic had been held each week at the medical college since its origin in 1843," wrote historian Waite. Once the marine hospital opened in 1852, it became a valuable location for clinical learning and demonstration.[24]

Western Reserve Medical School went through hard times in the 1860s. Enrollment had dropped after a second medical school opened in Cleveland in 1857, and with young men off to war, attendance fell off dramatically by mid-decade. The school stopped keeping minutes for six years (1862–68), which makes it hard for the historian to say with certainty that the admission of Black students was discussed and planned or in fact not even recognized as such, and no programs or catalogs were printed. Enrollment dropped to sixty-one students in the year Harris and Purvis were admitted and to twenty in 1864–65. Historian Waite did not note Harris or Purvis as the first African Americans at the school, although he did chronicle the first women. Did Harris and Purvis "pass"? Did the faculty "look the other way" in their desperate need for tuition as the school tried to stay afloat? It was an era of heavy facial hair, and they were both light-skinned. Certainly, there does not seem to have been an antagonistic white student reaction.

THE IOWA CONNECTION

A few months after finishing at Western Reserve, the Union army hired Harris as a contract surgeon (with an MD after his name) on June 23, 1864. (He may have been working with the Black troops earlier, either without a contract or on a monthly contract now lost. He referred to diseases seen in the field above, and what may have been new was his appointment at Portsmouth, not his appointment at all.) How did he acquire the MD in such a short time? He had completed only one out of two years at Western Reserve. He says simply, in his autobiography, "I went to Iowa. While there I attended the Lectures of the Professors at 'The Medical Department of the Iowa University.'"[25] He does not name these professors (as he did for Western Reserve) or give the dates of attendance. If he is referring to Keokuk, then the term likewise lasted from November through February. So, for the 1863–64 school year, the Iowa lectures overlapped the Ohio ones.[26] His explanation for going there? These professors were ones "whose ideas of Medicine are more modern than those of the Western Reserve College and consequently more correct." So, he concluded, "I took my Diploma there."[27]

The first challenge is finding this school. What was the "Medical Department of the Iowa University"? The current University of Iowa Medical School (in Iowa City) opened in 1870.[28] However, there was a school in Keokuk, Iowa, that was associated, at least initially, with the State University of Iowa (not to be confused with the current Iowa State University, which graduated its first class in 1869). Initially called the College of Physicians and Surgeons, Keokuk, Medical Department of the State University, it opened in 1850.[29] In 1857 a new state constitution in Iowa said that all segments of the state university must be located in Iowa City, but the Keokuk school appealed to the state legislature for exemption. This makes it clear that the medical school was associated with the University of Iowa (in Iowa City), and not the Iowa

State University (in Ames). The Keokuk school remained the state medical school until 1870, when the medical school in Iowa City opened. The Keokuk school's official requirements for graduation were these: (1) the candidate must be at least twenty-one; (2) he must have attended two courses of medical lectures; (3) he must have had two years of study with a preceptor; (4) he must write a medical thesis; (5) he must pass an examination; and (6) he must pay the graduation fee. The cost of a diploma was twenty dollars; what the school charged a candidate from another school is unknown.[30] It seems likely that Harris meant this medical school in Keokuk when he listed it in his autobiographical statement. But he certainly had not completed the two years of lectures there.

Was it just a "diploma mill" that would sell students a piece of official paper in return for cash? I suspect the situation was more complicated. The school's initial dean was John Sanborn, a high-minded physician dedicated to elevating the status of medicine and medical training in Iowa, as is evident in such dramatic remarks as "Every young physician who passes forth from the halls of medical instruction, goes as an apostle of medical science." He led the faculty at the Keokuk school, was instrumental in founding the first state medical society, and participated in publishing the first medical journals in the state. The initial Keokuk professors were all well qualified for their day, and the school got off to a good start. So, all around it was, initially at least, a school that taught orthodox medicine (by nineteenth-century standards) and had typical requirements (two years of lecture and at least one year of apprenticeship). It was allied to the new University of Iowa in Iowa City and had some state support. Sanborn had high hopes of it being the "best western medical school." As historian Susan Lawrence noted, "With a hospital, large lecture theaters, growing collections of materia medical specimens and anatomical models, a library, and considerable civic support, the Keokuk College seemed to be headed for a long and successful place in Iowa medical education."[31]

School records are scanty for 1864, the year that Harris supposedly studied there and received his diploma. The University of Iowa alumni register does list Harris and Rapier as graduates of the medical college in Keokuk in that year.[32] The last available copy of the medical journal sponsored by the school was published in 1858 and did not resume until 1867. The midwestern states were particularly hard-hit by the Panic of 1857, and this recession may well have influenced the ability of students to pay enrollment fees. The school lost state support in the 1870s, especially when the legislature discovered that despite the $15,000 the state had loaned the school for a new building in

1858, the school was still totally in arrears in 1879.[33] And of course the Civil War would have drained the pool of young men eager to learn medicine, as happened at Western Reserve. A further influence of the war was the great demand for doctors, particularly after the creation of the US Colored Troops regiments in 1863.[34] The USCT would come to make up 10 percent of the Union army and yet never had anywhere near the expected enrollment of surgeons for its regiments. It would not be surprising that patriotic northern medical schools *might* have been more inclined to admit African American students in these years.

So, we have three free Black men from the Midwest—Harris, Purvis, and Rapier—who all decided to go to medical school in 1863 with the ambition of serving "their people" in the army. One, Purvis, continued at Western Reserve for the usual two years, graduating in 1865. His acquisition of a medical degree from an orthodox medical school put him in rare company, as one of the pioneering Black medical doctors in the United States. But it also meant that, as he was a student, he was unable to act as a physician during the war. The other two, Harris and Rapier, had graduated from Keokuk by the fall of 1864. Until very recently neither has been recognized as an early African American medical graduate in the United States. Yet the medical school in Keokuk was an undeniable regular school—that is, neither homeopathic or Eclectic.

How can we explain these oddities? Each had a medical diploma from a respectable school, but one that Harris and Rapier did not have the time to attend before we see them accepted by the Union government as MDs and practitioners of medicine. In an era when students often raised a ruckus about Black classmates, there is no record of this response in Iowa. In a photograph of Iowa medical students from 1860, there are no apparent Black students.[35] And the population of African Americans in 1860 Iowa was vanishingly small. One solution that fits the evidence is that both Harris and Rapier received their degrees by mail. Harris perhaps submitted the same evidence that he produced when applying for a regular army appointment in 1865—letters from his Cleveland preceptor and professors at Western Reserve. Rapier likely had similar testimonials from Michigan. In the heat of war and in desperate need of doctors, the medical college at Keokuk may have issued them diplomas upon evidence of work completed. All that the school asked was that the student write a thesis. For Harris, a thesis title was listed in the graduation program: "The Fevers of the South." If this scenario indeed happened, the Keokuk school never knew Harris and Rapier's race, but they did see men capable of serving the troops and gave them the ticket that would put them where doctors were so urgently needed. Western Reserve and Michigan would not take this step, but perhaps the Iowa school did so. There is no further evidence, and if this speculation is correct, then Harris lied in his autobiography: "While there [Iowa] I attended the lectures of the Professors."[36] Of course, he could have attended only one or two lectures for this sentence to be technically true. If he actually attended a year's worth of lectures, I am at a loss as to how he did so.

HARRIS AS A PHYSICIAN

The question next arises: If Harris cut corners in acquiring his medical degree, was that reflected by inadequate medical knowledge and practice? We have none of the modern data typically used to assess a physician in the United States. First, the medical examination he conducted on patients was limited to the five senses, without support from X-ray or laboratory blood work. The urine might be inspected and even tasted, but only researchers would go further, trying to elucidate its chemical components or visualize red blood cells. The stethoscope was in common use, which allowed the physician to recognize the sounds of cardiac irregularities, pneumonia, fluid overload, and pneumothorax. But we have no way of knowing whether Harris missed the diagnosis in many cases or was a wizard at figuring out what the patient had.

How well did he treat his patients? On the formal therapeutic front, we have some evidence that he followed the most progressive ideas of the day. In the exam he had to pass for his regular army physician appointment, he said he believed bloodletting was overused, for example, and instead he treated pneumonia "expectantly."[37] Thus, he revealed familiarity with "the healing power of nature" or, in Latin, the "*vis medicatrix naturae*." Bloodletting for pneumonia was the standard of care earlier in the century, but from the 1820s physicians at the medical centers in France began questioning its usefulness. One, P. C. A. Louis, even divided his patients and treated one batch with bloodletting and the other with supportive care. The supportive care group had better outcomes.[38] Such ideas were increasingly taken up in elite medical schools on the East Coast, while the West and South were slower to give up the practice so representative of the orthodox medical man that the field's premier journal in England was named *The Lancet*.

The Harris exam was not marked and no answer sheet was included. So, we cannot know what the examiners thought of his performance. Still, comparison of his answers to the more popular and common medical handbooks available to the Union army surgeon reveals his understanding to be mainstream. And he was confident writing this exam. After explaining the "use of bile," he noted, "*It is a subject upon which a vast deal has been written—which is the best sign that it was not well understood*" (emphasis in the original). Harris was also a conventional "regular" doctor when it came to medical treatments. He closed his test with "PS Homeopathy is folly. What could infinitesimal doses do with the enormous Diarrhea we have in the field? Possibly however the agitation of this question did good by calling attention to the abuses of Mercurous Blistering."[39] Condemnation of excessive use of calomel was another tenet of those who believed in the healing power of nature, and one famously promoted by the army's surgeon general, William A. Hammond.[40]

In my eagerness to lay this information from the exam before you, I have muddled our time line. Let me straighten that out now. Once Harris finished his formal medical training and had degree in hand, he applied to the army to serve as a contract surgeon. There is no evidence of a contract before June 23, 1864, but he could have spent the previous month or two with the US Colored Troops in the field in Virginia. In late June 1864, he was posted to the coastal Virginia city of Portsmouth. The area of coastal and peninsular Virginia, including Fort Monroe, was a staging point for the USCT fighting to take Petersburg and Richmond, as well as for slaves escaping to Union-occupied Virginia soil. Harris had been there for seven months when he applied for a commission as a regular (not contract) physician in the army. Under such an appointment he would agree to serve for three years, rather than the three months with option for renewal that came with the contract job. The papers quoted from above—the autobiography, the letter, the exam questions and answers—are from his application to become a commissioned surgeon and were written in February 1865.

Now, let us proceed. Do we have any information from his patients or their relatives about his reputation as a physician? His medical superiors at his first documented post as a contract surgeon, Balfour Hospital in Portsmouth, Virginia, apparently respected him. When he began his contract (dated June 23, 1864), he was assigned to a ward with about a hundred patients. Then another ward was added, and finally a third. In fact, Harris proudly reported in his autobiography, "in testimonial of my services the patients and attendants have purchased Gross Surgery to be presented me as you will see in my accompanying pages."[41] Such tributes were usually presented when a doctor or officer left a post. And in his autobiography Harris said, "I quit there [Balfour Hospital] to come here [to the place of the examining body]."

By "quit" he did not necessarily mean that he resigned but rather that he left Portsmouth to come to DC. The "Gross Surgery" to which Harris referred was probably Samuel D. Gross's *Manual of Military Surgery*, a well-known, widely distributed, and respected handbook on surgery during the war. Or, it could have been the massive textbook *A System of Surgery*. The former seems more likely, given its portability as a short handbook designed for saddlebag storage.

A further encomium came in the pages of the *Christian Recorder*, a newspaper published by the African Methodist Episcopal Church. An anonymous correspondent (pseudonym "LOOK IN"), writing on July 2, 1864, reported on a visit to Portsmouth, Virginia, where the Union was now in command and a local hotel had been converted into a "colored" hospital for USCT men and freedmen from the area. With joy the writer reported on the local reaction among the native southerners. "The Union-hating, rebel-loving, good men provoking and gallows deserving Portsmouthians were terribly startled, and with eyes extended, mouth opened, hair on end and hands in pockets, they could be seen in groups, talking very low. A Union man approached one of the groups, and inquired what was the matter," the author reported. "Why, says one of the F.F.V.'s, "*There's a n—— doctor in Portsmouth*, in the capacity of a U.S. Surgeon." It was too much: A Black MD upon the sacred soil? Those claiming status in the First Families of Virginia were prone to make saints out of George Washington, Thomas Jefferson, the Lee family, and such and to see Virginia as the birthplace of America, the sacred ground. "They could not stand it," the reporter noted with glee. "Some of them tried to die, others went in search of the last ditch, while Surgeon Harris, with an ability that is second to no surgeon in this department, is rendering invaluable service to the sick and wounded soldiers."[42]

The timing of this letter is interesting and somewhat diminishes its value as an actual measure of Harris's therapeutic skill. His contract began June 23, 1864, and according to this periodical source he already had a reputation of being "second to no surgeon in this department" nine days later. Of course, it is possible that he had been practicing there earlier and the association went unrecorded. Those other surgeons were, as far as I have been able to discover, all white. So, one suspects a bit of exaggeration was modifying the pride the letter writer felt in seeing a man of color holding such an educated and authoritative position. Harris practiced in the Portsmouth hospital until early fall 1865; he next moved to a Freedmen's Bureau assignment at Howard's Grove Hospital outside of Richmond. It had first been the Confederate smallpox hospital and following the occupation was converted to a hospital

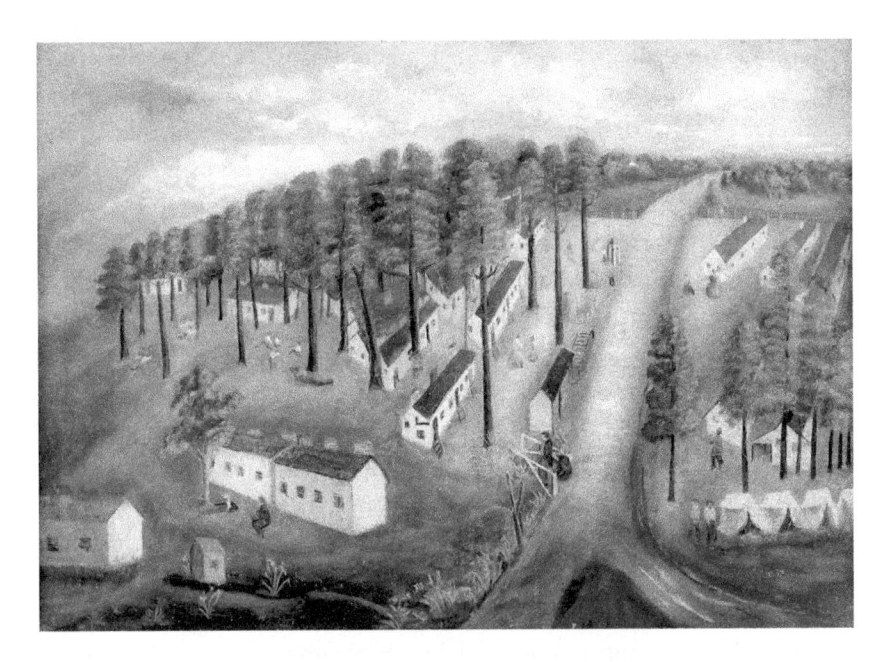

Drawing of Howard's Grove Military Hospital, Richmond, Virginia, during the Civil War, artist unknown.
Courtesy of Chicago Historical Society.

for the USCT and freedmen. Another *Christian Recorder* letter brought news of a local church service in November 1865 and mentioned "Miss Colton, from the dear A.M.A., who is matron at Howard Grove Hospital, where J. D. Harris, M.D., is surgeon in charge."[43] What pride that singular last sentence portrayed!

Given the manifest barbarity of Civil War medicine (as some might argue), what difference did it make if a physician was excellent or mediocre? As I argue in my book *Marrow of Tragedy*, the key aspects of survival in Civil War hospitals were all related to what might today be more broadly described as nursing. Someone to keep the patient clean, or to be sure he was fed, or to call the doctor's attention to a poorly healing wound—all of these interventions were probably more important than specific medicines (with the exceptions of quinine, chloroform, and opiates). One key difference between hospitals north and south was the inadequacy of food in the South. Union troops received lemonade and oranges; Confederates were lucky to have peas and biscuits. Malnourished men could not fight infection or heal wounds.[44]

It is likely that a dedicated Black physician who was "serving his own people" would be more attentive than at least some white physicians. In my volume on Black troops and their medical care in the war, the cruelties and indifference of some white physicians toward Black patients was documented. Also described in that book was an experiment that Union surgeon (in charge) Ira Russell carried out in one St. Louis hospital with several Black wards. He found that the patients in one ward, tended by Dr. James M. Martin, thrived and mostly recovered. In other wards the Black patients had much worse outcomes. The doctors complained that Martin got the healthier patients to start with, so Russell called their bluff. He moved Martin to the ward with the highest mortality, while sending one of the other complaining doctors to the healthy ward. That doctor was known to say, "It was useless to doctor a sick negro, for he was sure to die, do what you will." But under Martin's care, the malignant ward became in time one of the best in the hospital.[45] The point here is that a concerned surgeon who saw that his patients were well cared for could make a difference—and the patients could see that as well.

Russell called Martin a man who "entered, heart and soul, upon the duties of his ward." And, continued Russell, he "thoroughly understood the negro characteristics and, in addition to the care and skill he bestowed upon his patients, he knew exactly what psychological influences to bring upon them as remedial agents."[46] We know next to nothing about what the wards were like that J. D. Harris controlled. But his expressions of zeal toward his fellow Black men and the influence of friends and family around him made it likely that he tried his best. He may also have been able to recruit volunteer nurses from both the local Black community and from the white women who came south with the US Sanitary Commission or the American Missionary Association.

Union surgeon Ira Russell met J. D. Harris in the fall of 1865, as noted in the introduction. By this point Harris was working for the Freedmen's Bureau in Richmond. Here my point is to emphasize the opinion of one thoughtful northern physician of the demeanor and learning of our protagonist. At the behest of the US Sanitary Commission, Russell was touring the hospitals on the East Coast that cared for the Black troops and freedmen, assessing their quality, cleanliness, and care. He was also quite interested in the questions of whether health and disease appeared differently in Blacks and whites and whether people of mixed African and European ancestry had suffered from a decrease in vitality. As he inspected such hospitals in Richmond, he "visited the Howard Grove Hospital in charge of Dr. Harris, a very intelligent colored gentleman from Cleveland Ohio. This hospital is managed by the Freedman Bureau and is neat, orderly and well located. Dr. Harris has seen a good deal of service, is familiar with the peculiarities of his race, and deeply interested in its elevation and welfare." Russell was a Massachusetts native and supporter of the Black soldier, having overseen a hospital in St. Louis that cared for Black troops. As noted above, he was well aware that compassionate medical care made a life-or-death difference to these men and likewise recognized that an able and interested Black surgeon could be the best possible physician for the Black soldiers and freedmen now resident at Howard's Grove.[47]

Russell put his research questions to Harris and conveyed his replies. Harris, he said, "scoffs at the idea that blacks have lower vital force and says when he hears the remark as he often does,—'A sick negro will die, do what you will,' coming from the lips of Surgeons and men who ought to know better, he regards it as a sure sign of laziness, indifference or ignorance and looks upon such allegations as an excuse to cover up the results of bad practice." When quizzed about the prevalence of tuberculosis among his Black patients, Harris said the disease was no more common among Blacks than whites and indeed was actually more prevalent among poor northerners. Pneumonia, on the other hand, was much more common among the colored troops and freedmen.[48]

Russell found Harris adamant on the issue of mixed-race healthiness. "The doctor has given a great deal of attention to the influence of the admixture of the races upon health, physical endurance and fecundity and is convinced that such admixture does not tend towards deterioration or extinction."[49] Later Russell reported in general on medical opinion regarding mixed-race heath, endurance, and fecundity and again summarized Harris's conclusions. "Dr. Harris, the colored Surgeon ... was very emphatic and decided in his opinion that the admixture of the races, does not impair physical endurance or fecundity, but on the contrary, promotes both."[50] Harris must have told Russell about his Caribbean book, as later Russell quoted from it on this very question.[51]

Historian Leslie Schwalm likewise focuses on Russell's interest in the physiological differences between Black and white bodies. While she acknowledges that he paid "insistent attention to the material impact of slavery, racism and discrimination on the health and survival of Black troops, Russell was nonetheless willing to seek out and accept the common argument that race was embodied, a biological fact, rather than an ideological justification for race-based slavery."[52] Here it should be noted that Harris shared many of these ideas. While he recognized the many social determinants of health (to use the modern phrase) that created differences among the races, Harris was also open to the possibility of differential disease susceptibility that depended on race. Still, he knew the borders between Black and white were porous and fungible; his humor over the degree of racial mixing and the question of when a child became white or Black indicates the omnipresence of these concepts in his own mixed-race experience.

This encounter is remarkable. In just a few lines Russell limns the great transition that has happened in the life of J. D. Harris over a few years. Five years earlier he had fled the United States, in despair of ever rising to the status of citizen, voter, or gentleman. By mid-decade that same government that had believed a few years earlier, in the words of Charles Langston at the Oberlin trial following the Wellington rescue, that "colored men have no rights in the United States which white men are bound to respect" had now accepted J. D.'s credentials as a learned man deserving of hire by his country. A white man, albeit admittedly one strongly supportive of Black freedom, found him "a very intelligent colored gentleman." He was accepted into the professional classes, no longer a blacksmith, a plasterer, or a farmer. He was a published author, with two books to his name. And he signed his name on government reports: J. D. Harris, acting assistant surgeon in charge, Howard's Grove Hospital, USA. Where would he go from here? The move to Virginia had opened a new and exciting phase of his life.

8

Family Ties in Reconstruction, 1864-1869

This chapter explores the social network that surrounded Dr. Harris on the Virginia Peninsula and environs during Reconstruction. His brothers William and Robert are prominent here, as are the ladies sent by the American Missionary Association (AMA) to serve freedpeople in Virginia. It would be grand to find dialog between these important players and the good doctor, but here we must make do with conversations held with other people, particularly those in the home office of the AMA. The protagonists here—William Harris, Robert Harris, Cicero Harris, and Elizabeth Worthington—all worked under the auspices of the AMA as teachers and preachers to freedpeople. Their correspondence survives in the archives of the AMA, where letters sketch a picture of their aspirations, personalities, and emotions. To some extent, they shaped J. D. Harris's world, and it is worthwhile to imagine their conversations with and about him in the strange context of the postwar South. From them we glean the important family values that were key to his own principles and actions as he transitioned from rebellious youth into respectable middle-aged professional and citizen.

It was no accident that of all the locations in the southern states, the Union first occupied and defended the tip of the lower Virginia Peninsula and nearby areas. Protected by Fort Monroe, a strategic structure that had guarded three rivers since the colonial era, it never fell to the Confederate government. Fort Monroe and an ever-expanding swath of land around it became the Union staging ground for major, unsuccessful expeditions toward Richmond in 1862, as well as for later invasions of Virginia. But more important for our story, it was the first place that a Union army commander announced that escaped slaves would be protected by Union guns. In May 1861 General Benjamin Butler declared such people "contraband of war," refused to hand them over when angry Confederate "owners" came calling, and instead gave them safe lodging and rations in return for heavy labor. As the war went on and more and more enslaved people found safe harbor in and near Fort Monroe, their label changed to "freedmen," and it was here that the first steps toward education and medical care for these needy people began.[1]

The largest antislavery organization in the northern United States, the American Missionary Association, responded to this confluence of freedpeople in Virginia (and in Port Royal, South Carolina) by organizing schools and churches for these new citizens. The AMA began when a group of Congregationalists joined together to defend the escaped slaves who had captured the ship *Amistad* from its white slaver owners and sailed the ship to Connecticut. Before the war the organization's influence had first exploded in the northern United States, where it birthed 115 antislavery churches in Illinois alone. It was more than ready to venture south as soon as there was an accessible population of southern freedpeople to serve. Altogether the AMA planted 500 schools and 200 Congregational churches in the South, churches now part of the United Churches of Christ. While most of its schools were at the elementary level, it also founded colleges for Black students, including Fisk, Hampton Institute, Dillard, Tougaloo, and, in coordination with the Freedmen's Bureau, Howard University in Washington, DC.[2] W. E. B. Du Bois described this movement, peopled by thousands of intrepid volunteer teachers and preachers, as "that finest thing in American History.... The teachers in these institutions came not to keep the Negroes in their place, but to raise them out of their places where the filth of slavery had wallowed them."[3]

One official estimate in 1866 counted half a million freedpeople in Virginia. The US government's Freedmen's Bureau had ten hospitals in the state for this population, with around a thousand beds and an occupancy of 659 patients at the end of 1866. At Howard's Grove Hospital in Richmond there was a ward for insane colored patients, then numbering 31, as well as "a home for the aged and infirm." J. D. Harris was surgeon in charge of this hospital in late 1865. Overall, 16,559 Black patients (males, females, and children) had been admitted to Virginia Freedmen's Bureau hospitals in 1866, with a mortality rate of 5.3 percent, an admirable figure for the day, especially given the crowded and unhygienic state of the freedmen's camps, as well as the prevalence of smallpox. The chief physician of the Virginia freedmen's hospitals estimated that about this many people again had been treated as outpatients. Fifteen doctors were at work in the department.[4]

A local woman named Mary Peake opened the first school for freedpeople on September 17, 1861. It was located on the James River near Fort Monroe and the "contraband camps" that formed around the security of the Union encampment. Before her death a few months later she wrote to the AMA describing the many needs of the freedpeople and urging the organization to take up her education work.[5] The process of setting up schools did not take off until 1864, when more real estate had been secured by Union troops and the military presence could protect the northern teachers who sought to bring education to the freedpeople. Multiple philanthropic groups sent such teachers, but our cluster all came under the auspices of the AMA. The first of these among the Harris relatives was William.

WILLIAM D. HARRIS

William D. Harris was born on June 6, 1827, the third child and first son of Jacob and Charlotte Harris.[6] William learned the plastering trade, presumably from his father. In 1850 he married Kate "Kitty" Stanley in New Bern. Kitty was the granddaughter of John C. Stanly, one of the richest men of color in antebellum North Carolina.[7] The fact that twenty-three-year-old William had made the acquaintance of Kitty to the point of marriage suggests that he spent considerable time in that city, perhaps expanding his skills within the circle of connected families that had initially nurtured his father.[8] Or, he could have gone to New Bern after his father died in 1847 to continue his education or find work.

William traveled with his new wife to Ohio, where he settled on a farm in Delaware, Ohio, by 1856. William was a recording secretary at the Ohio Colored Convention in that year and listed as representing Delaware. In the 1860 census he was recorded as thirty-two years old, his wife, Kitty, was thirty-three, and they had four children, aged two through nine. William had $1,300 worth of real estate, probably a farm, and also worked as a plasterer.[9]

In 1864 William asked the American Missionary Association to appoint him as a teacher in eastern Virginia or North Carolina, saying that he had been a plasterer for seventeen years but in addition had taught school for two years in North Carolina before going to Ohio. Also, he had taught a "Sabbath school" for five years and witnessed many hopeful conversions. The AMA accepted him, and he traveled to Portsmouth, Virginia, to teach in March 1864. He was likely the first family member on the scene, although J. D. would join him soon.[10] These were difficult times. The war continued, but Federal troops controlled (and patrolled) Portsmouth and environs. Still, angry whites attacked William's pupils. "Soon after I commenced here we were troubled somewhat by white boys gathering at a certain point, where my scholars had to pass, on their way to school, they would knock shake them and throw brickbats & stones at them," he reported to the AMA. William soon had the white boys sorted, however. "I handed 8 of their names to the A. Provost Marshal and he very promptly detached a squad of Col'd Soldiers with me to arrest them. We accordingly brought them before the Marshal, who sentenced them all to imprisonment in the guard house. I am happy to report that all has been quiet since."[11]

The other threat to the families of his schoolchildren was smallpox, which was ravaging the freedpeople in his vicinity. "The first part of the month, the small pox prevailed in our school worse than ever," he wrote at the end of May 1864. "The contraband Doctor, informs me that now only 7 or 8 cases are reported per day, at the first of the Mo. 18 or 20, and there are now only 130 at the Hospital. Only one of my pupils has died by this dreaded and loathsome disease. I feel thankful that I have escaped thus far, as I have been much exposed to it by visiting my pupils and others in its first stages." The "contraband doctor" was his brother J. D., who cared for local freed Blacks before he received his appointment at the Portsmouth hospital for contraband and Black troops at the end of June 1864.[12] William likely collaborated with his brother in the care and succor of men at the hospital, acting as a visitor and reading the Bible to them. In July 1864 William opened a school for the convalescents and told the AMA, "As a large number of wounded soldiers have been brought in our midst, we felt constrained to do what we could for these noble, and brave sufferers. One thing was to open a school for the benefit of the convalescents or slightly wounded of the Hospital opposite the Mission House."[13]

William was just as focused on conversions as teaching, something that the AMA no doubt encouraged. He proudly told one AMA official, "I have been doing what I could for the salvation of souls, I have witnessed several hopeful conversions, one was an Old man of seventy years."[14] William frequently referenced the Lord and his religious beliefs in his letters, but it is clear that his style of worship was one of comparative restraint. He found the religious enthusiasm displayed by some colored troops and other freedpeople distasteful. "The meetings are generally, demonstrative, and often boisterous, as they seem to worship on the principle, that the kingdom of Heaven suffereth violence and the violent take it by force."[15] (The word "suffer" here is used in its archaic meaning of "allow," as in Jesus saying, "Suffer little children ... to come unto me.")[16]

Two years later he recalled the Portsmouth excesses to another AMA correspondent, W. S. Bell, with whom he had worked on the peninsula, and compared his calmer Richmond experiences with them. "I mean you would find very little of that wild excitement, shrieks, & boisterous demonstrations, rolling on the floor and dancing around the altar which you, and I, will always remember with a shudder."[17] Perhaps William was actually comparing the Black congregants to little children, who are of course prone to shrieks, dancing, wild excitement, and chaotic dancing.

While William felt proud of his accomplishments after one season in Virginia, the financial demands of supporting a family of six back at home in Ohio overwhelmed the salary that the AMA could offer. Even by the "strictest economy" he found that "family expenses at home exceed my entire salary to the amount of 64 48/100 [$64.48]." William was torn.

> I am making some sacrifice for our Holy cause, and while I believe it to be my duty to do all I can for the elevation and salvation of my people, in this auspicious and momentous hour as they have just begun to struggle up from chattelism, to manhood, from bruised, and mangled slaves, to good citizens; [yet] ... while I feel the heavy responsibilities and self-sacrificing duties of the hour, I also feel that it is my duty, in view of my limited means and in justice to my family to ask the Society to increase my salary.

He sought to go back into the field "to a place where I am *most needed* or where I can be most useful, most successful in *winning souls to Christ*, [e]ither as a Preacher or School teacher or both." But he advised them not to forget "that we cannot do anything, anywhere, in the south without military protection."[18]

The next day, July 27, 1865, William heard remarkable news. Reverend Daniel Payne of the African Methodist Episcopal Church had invited him to take a church in Richmond with 500 parishioners. Although William had no formal schooling, in August the Central Ohio Yearly Conference of the Wesleyan Methodist Convention recognized his considerable skills as a preacher and teacher of the Bible. They ordained William Harris and made him an elder. He then communicated with the AMA to try to work out an agreement under which he would both take the church in Richmond and continue as a salaried AMA teacher, which was made possible in part by the fact that an AMA school met on the church property.[19] The church position was a high honor but not a financially viable one. The relationship between his two paymasters, the AMA and the AME Church, did not remain cordial, and the church in Richmond was too poor to sustain his salary.[20] He did find the time to preach at Howard's Grove Hospital in 1866, where his brother J. D. had doctored sick men from the colored regiments as well as local freedmen.[21] And Miss Marcia Colton, whom he knew through the AMA, was now there acting as matron. William mentioned his brother specifically only once, telling W. S. Bell of the AMA in the summer of 1866, "The Dr. is well."[22]

William was a temperance man and tried to lead his congregation in that direction. "Seeing the already innumerable drinking saloons increasing almost every day—The rapid encroachment of the Monster Intemperance in all grades of society—even to some extent in the churches, although it seems like a hopeless undertaking against this monstrous though popular iniquity—although I believe it will render me unpopular—I have preached one sermon and had two regular Temperance meetings." He reported that 112 people had taken the temperance pledge: "I hereby sacredly promise to abstain from the use of all intoxicating liquors as a beverage, and to do my best to persuade others to the same."[23]

Only one sign of unpopularity filters through the William Harris correspondence, and there is no way to know if his temperance stand had anything to do with it. A man had him arrested for supposedly encouraging that man's daughter to marry against her father's wishes. The charges were false, as was quickly proved by testimony of witnesses. Still, the local newspaper reporters were "greedy at first to report something bad against the 'Yankee N——Teacher,'" but in the end they had to "put on their overcoats and leave the room." In the company of the letter to the AMA about these events is a December 13, [1866,] newspaper clipping that described Harris as "a gentleman and minister of the gospel who stands very high in the estimation of his entire congregation and the masses of the colored people of this city for more than a year, and all the whites who have had any acquaintance with him regard him with the utmost respect and confidence on account of his gentlemanly and Christian deportment." The name of the paper is unknown, but it presumably was not one of the rabidly pro-Confederate papers such as the *Examiner*, which would have such negative things to say about J. D. in years to come.[24]

In May 1867, Bishop Payne sent William to Georgetown, DC. By the end of his service in Richmond, William was supervising ten churches with 1,041 members. His parishioners there were in a bad way—destitute and suffering in the winter and afflicted with cholera during the summer. William was sorry to leave them but obedient to his new orders. He wrote the AMA with hopes of continuing his sideline of teaching them.[25] He again contacted George Whipple at the AMA in September 1867, from Georgetown. He sought a teaching position for his seventeen-year-old daughter, Lottie, then studying at Wilberforce University in Ohio, an institution founded by the AME Church with Bishop Payne as its first president, but "my limited means will not allow me to continue her there." He said he would be happy to have her nearby in DC or "under Miss Daffin or Miss Worthington." (Miss Worthington, as will soon be evident, would be his sister-in-law before the next year was out.) Or he would be glad to place her with brothers Robert or Cicero in Fayetteville.[26] By November 1868 William was in Charleston, South Carolina, where he was a minister and teaching in a freedmen's school. Lottie was with him.[27] This family did what it could to group and regroup, valuing the creation of new family clusters.

Bishop Payne moved him again in the new year. In February 1869 William wrote the AMA, "Having been assigned to duty in Columbia by our Bishop & Conference I find a large field of missionary work. My daughter who has been teaching successfully in Charleston since May (as I desire to have her with me), is now out of employment." So again, he tried to get the AMA to hire her and to renew his own commission. He said of the Howard School in Columbia, South Carolina, that it was supported by several different associations, but none of them AMA.[28] Still, his letter describes a substantial northern presence in the schools of the town. A month later he reiterated the need in Columbia. "Columbia needs Missionary labors more than any which I have yet seen. Intemperance is especially fearfully increasing among both white and colored, boys & women are seen in the streets staggering from intoxication and many members of the General Assembly indulge to an alarming extent. There is a great want of principle & rectitude in other directions."[29] By now Dr. and Mrs. J. D. Harris were in Columbia as well. The

1870 census found William Harris in Columbia, where Kitty and their four children now lived. William died four years later of "typhoid dysentery."[30]

ROBERT W. HARRIS

Robert Harris, called Robbie by his family, was seven when his father died and ten when the family traveled to Ohio. In 1860 he was living with his mother, brother Cicero (b. 1844), brother Jarvis (b. 1841), and sister Catharine (aka Kate, b. 1836, m. 1869). During the summer of 1864, Robert decided to follow William's footsteps and applied to the AMA for a post. "Desirous of assisting in the noble work of elevating and evangelizing our oppressed and long abused race, and of promoting the interests of Christ's spiritual kingdom on earth, I make this application to you for an appointment as a Teacher of the Freedmen of the South," he began. "I am nearly 25 years of age, in general good health, and of strong powers of endurance. A Plasterer by trade, but during the past year engaged in Rail-Roading." Although he had completed high school in Cleveland, along with his brother Cicero, Robert did not mention that credential here.[31]

Robert's letter illuminated the continued network of support provided by Harris family members and those affiliated with them. His mother had planned that the younger boys would get a high school education, and she must have mustered support from other family members to help support her household while the boys were not engaged in remunerative tasks. Robert in turn took care of his mother and the children remaining at home. He was too young to have learned plastering and bricklaying from his father, but through the people Jacob had trained—William, George, brother-in-law Cicero—he learned the crafts at one remove. The social capital built by his parents in Fayetteville continued to pay into the next generation. Cicero Richardson, once his father's apprentice, now had a prosperous construction company in Cleveland. Robert continued, in his application letter, "I am unmarried but have the care of a small family consisting of a widowed mother and a younger brother and sister who are dependent on me for support." His twenty-year-old brother Cicero was likely already earning a living, but Kate and his impaired brother Jarvis would have still been at home and dependent. "I respectfully ask you to be as liberal as you can afford in the matter of salary," Robbie added. And he asked to be stationed near his brother William in Portsmouth. In closing, he admitted, "I have had no experience in teaching except in privately teaching slaves, in the South, where I lived in my youth."[32]

If indeed he taught slaves in the South, he was doing so by the age of ten, when the family migrated.

Robert arrived in Portsmouth in November 1864, accompanied by a "large number of ladies," he reported in a letter to the AMA. One of these was Elizabeth Worthington, a white woman from New Jersey who would later marry his brother J. D. The AMA had apparently assembled a group of female teachers in Baltimore, where they took ship for Portsmouth. It sounds as if Robbie was providing male chaperone and support. Remember, the war was still on, and traveling by sea along the rebel landmass had persistent dangers. Robbie's first work was in helping the "lady Teachers" get settled, including fitting out their schoolrooms and "gathering in" the available freed children who were not yet attending school. The children were poorly clothed and shod, and Robbie feared that they would suffer much in the coming winter. Robert also commented, "I have had ample opportunities for visiting the various Hospitals for sick and wounded soldiers located in this place. The soldiers manifest much pleasure at our visits and desire us to come frequently."[33] Access to these hospitals would have been facilitated by his brother J. D., who had charge of three wards of Black troops in the Portsmouth hospital.

Robert's school for the freedpeople was located at a community called Providence Church, about four miles southeast of Norfolk. He found the people desperately poor and barely surviving on the government ration as they tried to raise a crop. "They are like children just beginning to walk and must be assisted till they can walk *alone*," he reported in late December 1864. Robert faced multiple challenges in setting up his school, including making a decrepit building habitable, acquiring adequate benches and books for it, and distributing donations of clothing from friends in the North so that children could be clothed sufficiently to travel to school during winter weather. The children of soldiers were worst off; Robbie tried to help them by writing letters to the Black soldiers who should be supporting them, only to find that those soldiers had not yet been paid and had nothing to send. Robert himself lodged with a family of freedpeople, as there was no other boarding situation nearby.[34]

By April 1, 1865, Robert could report that his school was finally in good order, and his pupils were learning quickly. He and his students did meet hostility from disgruntled whites, however. "Some rowdies in the neighborhood have attempted to break it up by way-laying and abusing some of the pupils. By threatening to send for a guard of soldiers, they have been induced to cease their annoyance, and I hope we shall have no more of it. They have a wholesome dread of soldiers, especially colored soldiers."[35] These comments, which echo those of his brother William, are a reminder of the physical dangers that these teachers faced, perhaps all the more so when the teachers were themselves African Americans. Even after Robert E. Lee's surrender a week after Robert's letter was written, racial hostilities did not just melt away, and every trip on a lonely road presented the possibility of violence.

As was typical for AMA schools, Robert's assignment ended in June and did not commence again until the fall, when he returned to Providence Church. They continued to be harassed by nearby whites. He mentions that "poor white trash" had threatened to burn the school as a New Year's Day frolic, but he had the building guarded and nothing came of it. Nearby white neighbors would not sell them wood or allow it to be cut on their land, so wood had to be transported from quite a distance.[36] Otherwise, the school prospered. In April 1866, Robert fell ill of a fever that left him with laryngitis, and "my doctor thinks that rest and change of scene will be beneficial." One suspects he consulted his brother J. D. in this regard.[37] Robert headed back home to Cleveland for the summer.

The following fall of 1866 found Robert at a school in his old hometown of Fayetteville, North Carolina. He went there under AMA auspices but his role soon grew larger. In 1867 a group of Fayetteville African American citizens raised money to buy the land to build a schoolhouse for children of color.[38] Among them was Matthew Leary, friend of Jacob Harris and executor of his will, and Andrew J. Chesnutt, Harris family friend whose son Charles would study with both Robert and Cicero.[39] As Charles Chesnutt's biographer Richard Brodhead noted, "The $136 they [the citizens] paid, like the labor they lost when their children attended the school, represented the sacrifice they were willing to incur to gain the good of literate education."[40] Robert Harris said in December 1868 that the Freedmen's Bureau paid to put up the building, now named the Howard School after General O. O. Howard of the bureau, but that the students could not use it as there was no furniture. "The people are not able to do it, and in consequence the house stands idle and useless for the lack of a few hundred dollars." He asked his AMA contact to see whether he could use his influence with the bureau. Or perhaps, "Can you not advise me what course to pursue in order to get a further loan from Uncle Sam?"[41]

The Howard School was both remarkable and typical—typical because it came into being as a school for freed slaves under the auspices of a northern philanthropic association. But such schools were always meant to be temporary; the hope was that southern state governments would see the value of freedpeople's education and take over the costs of running the schools and paying the teachers. This might have been feasible under the early Radical Republican governments, but as Reconstruction faded and leaders who favored slavery and the "old ways" of southern life returned to power, there was little interest in supporting Black schools—not to mention the fact that such governments were generally impoverished. So the Howard School in Fayetteville, led by Robert Harris until 1880, was remarkable for its persistence.

A new entrant on the philanthropic scene helped the Howard School weather its first storms. In 1867 the will of George Peabody created the Peabody Education Fund to help areas ravaged by the Civil War return to prosperity. The initial trustees, led by Burnas Sears of Brown University, decided the fund would be best spent shoring up education in the states of the former Confederacy. As historian Earle West has noted, "In his earliest observations of conditions in the South, Sears frequently remarked that in terms of need, at least, white children deserved more help than Negro children."[42] This was because the Freedmen's Bureau and multiple northern charities were on site helping freedpeople, including with education, but not poor white people. Of course, this Reconstruction funding and attention was temporary. Later, when the Peabody Education Fund dictated that communities had to contribute the requisite two-thirds of support to receive one-third and the school had to be free, there were few Black communities that could meet that standard. When the inadequacy of the Peabody disbursement to Black schools was publicized—a southern paper called the Peabody Education Fund "an important adjunct to the cause of education among the white people"—the trustees in embarrassment began to direct their funds through the Freedmen's Bureau to give more aid to Black schools.[43]

In any event, things at the Howard School were better by April 1869, perhaps because the school had finally acquired additional support from the Peabody Education Fund.[44] Robert reported to the AMA that the new schoolhouse was occupied and the students divided into two grades, primary and grammar. Most of the students were either just beginning to read, write, and do arithmetic or at the next higher stage of knowledge. He had borrowed chairs and otherwise gotten the necessary furniture. "The expense for grading, setting out trees, digging well, &tc. we have defrayed by a subscription among the citizens. The colored people came from far and near to attend the 'dedication' of the first school-house built for colored children in this county. The whites are a little jealous, as it surpasses all of theirs. This school will be the means under Providence of aiding immensely in the elevation of our race in this district." He said that promised support from the State of

North Carolina had not come through, but the state had no money anyway. He asked the AMA to send books, which were desperately needed. Other schools nearby were eager to hire his graduates, foreshadowing the school's future purpose as a training institute for teachers.[45]

It seems likely that the Harris name and the family's persistent networks were important in garnering such widespread support from the Black community. Both Jacob and Charlotte had friends and relations from their prior time living in the area, connections that spanned half a century. Included would be many who had been in slavery but now were free. Additionally, those merchants who raised the money to build the school would themselves have commercial connections. Robert Harris had multiple dimensions. He was the AMA man on the spot, able to communicate with the home office and bring in some funds. He had already created a school worthy of Peabody support and planned on staying. He was not a white humanitarian destined to leave in a few years; Robert was a local and able to speak the local dialect. In more ways than catching the words, he understood the situation locally in ways no outsider could. The Howard School was never rich, but the original school survived because it could call on the social capital that surrounded it in Fayetteville.

As the school grew, the AMA supported more teachers to help in educating the children. One of them, Mary Ellen Green, was hired in 1869 and sometime thereafter married Robert.[46] In the 1870 census, eighteen-year-old Mary Green boarded with a Mr. and Mrs. Turner in Cumberland County, North Carolina. Also boarding there were Robert and Cicero Harris.[47] In the 1880 census they were married; she was twelve years his junior and had no children by him.[48] Aside from beginning married life, Robert created a "Band of Hope" at the Howard School, whose members swore to abstain from alcohol, tobacco, and profane language. While sixty-nine pupils took the pledge, he reported that their parents were indifferent and that the use of tobacco was almost universal among them.[49] Temperance was an important plank in the acquisition of gentility, according to many who sought to "elevate the status" of Black people.

In 1877 North Carolina finally acted to create state-supported normal schools. A normal school was a vocational entity devoted to training teachers. The Howard School became the State Colored Normal School of Fayetteville and evolved into modern-day Fayetteville State University over the course of the twentieth century. One legend has it that the creation of normal schools for whites as well as Blacks was spurred by the success of the Howard School. In a court case, six Black and five white boys were asked to give testimony and sign their names as witnesses. The Black boys all signed, but the whites could only make their marks, that is, sign with an X. This shamed the local Fayetteville whites to set up a school for their race at least as good as the institution presided over by Robert Harris.[50] The State Colored Normal School offered a three-year course of study that certified its teachers with the equivalent of at least a high school education. Students learned not only literature but also science, algebra, geography, bookkeeping, and oratory—quite a metamorphosis from Robert's first school in 1864, whose students were mostly functioning at what would now be called an elementary school level. That he orchestrated and oversaw this transition speaks volumes about his leadership abilities, not to mention intellect.

Literary historian Richard Brodhead gives Robert and Cicero (see below) full credit for the education of Charles Chesnutt as a man of letters and educator himself. Chesnutt became Robert Harris's assistant at the normal school when it was established in 1877, and after some time spent with Cicero in Charlotte, Chesnutt returned to take over the normal school in 1880.[51] Chesnutt's diary affords us glimpses of Robert Harris as a man and the difficult days of his final illness. In May 1880 Chesnutt recorded, "Mr. Harris is still in a critical condition, which I am afraid will never be less critical than it now is. He has almost lost the use of his legs, which are swollen, the effect, he says, of a torpid liver. He goes on crutches, and still cherishes the delusion, which a merciful Providence leaves to us as long as we have any life left, that he will get well. I truly hope he may, but it is extremely improbable.... He was in great pain."[52] The 1880 census listed him as ill with dysentery.[53] The swelling sounds like ascites or a mass in the abdomen or both. Chesnutt did not say he was yellow, however. Robert could well have had amoebic dysentery with liver abscess and gross hepatic enlargement. Dysentery—that is, prolonged and bloody diarrhea—would be consistent with that infection. Amoebic dysentery does not cause jaundice. With a large liver abscess the compression of the vena cava could lead to lower extremity edema. The disease is spread through contaminated water supplies and was still common in the American South thirty years later.[54] At the time of Robert's illness the causative agent of this sort of dysentery had not yet been identified, so the absence of specificity in his diagnosis is unremarkable.

CICERO HARRIS

Cicero Harris, the youngest child of Jacob and Charlotte, was also on the Virginia Peninsula in the years that J. D. was living in the state. Born in 1844 and educated at Cleveland's Central High School, Cicero first appears in the American Missionary Association records in July 1866. Like his brother Robert, he wanted to serve the freed slaves. "Having an earnest desire to go among the Freedmen as Teacher, I have decided to apply to the Am. Miss. Society for position. I have had no experience as school teacher, but I hope by constant application and zeal to counterbalance my inexperience."[55] The principal of Cleveland Central High School, a white man, wrote him a letter of recommendation. "This is to certify that Cicero Harris was a pupil of the Central Cleveland High School for two years. He was not surpassed in scholarship by any of his class and his conduct was in all respects unexceptionable. I have often met him since he left school and I believe him to be in all respects worthy of confidence."[56] In another letter of recommendation, his brother William praised "his moral character, education, piety, and devotion to the cause of Christ, and humanity," noting that "he is a member of the Wesleyan Church and I think has an eye or mind towards the ministry eventually."[57] The pastor of that Wesleyan congregation compared him favorably to his brothers William and Robert, saying, "The brother I recommend partakes with them of a comparable zeal for the improvement and elevation of his long-oppressed brethren."[58] He gives us yet another attestation to this Harris family value.

Cicero got the job and joined his brother Robert in Virginia and then in Fayetteville by November 1866. Cicero was put in charge of the younger children, a group Robert labeled the "infant school."[59] Cicero was still there in Fayetteville at least until January 1869.[60] In the first half of the 1870s, Cicero moved to Charlotte to take over the Peabody Education Fund school for training Black teachers. This was the second normal school in the state for creating Black schoolteachers. There Charles W. Chesnutt worked under him for three years, teaching in rural schools around Charlotte. After Robert Harris died in 1880, Charles Chesnutt took over the running of the school back in Fayetteville. Cicero had achieved his plan of becoming a minister in the 1870s, being ordained by the African Methodist Episcopal Zion Church in 1872. Under the auspices of the AMEZ Church, he opened a seminary in Concord, North Carolina, in 1874 to train preachers for that faith. The school moved from Concord to Salisbury, North Carolina, where it changed its name to Livingstone College. There Cicero became "professor of Mathematics, Natural Science and Homiletics," and his wife, Meriah, served as matron. He was also secretary-treasurer of the school and vice president until he was elected a bishop in the AMEZ Church in 1889. In his role as bishop, Cicero presided over churches in the Blue Ridge, Western New York, and

South Florida Conferences of the church. In honor of his service and accomplishments, Howard University awarded him an honorary doctor of divinity degree in 1891. The youngest Harris boy, who crossed the Appalachians in a covered wagon at age six, had risen high indeed.[61]

ELIZABETH WORTHINGTON HARRIS

Elizabeth Worthington was born in 1840, the daughter of a Presbyterian minister then serving in Milford, Michigan, a small town forty-five miles northwest of Detroit. Her father was Albert Worthington (1804–93); her mother was Ruth Parker (1808–71). They married in Ypsilanti in 1836. Albert had studied at Hamilton College in New Jersey and then Princeton Theological Seminary, from which he graduated in 1830. Elizabeth had an older sister named Clara (1837–72), who before her early death gave birth to two daughters, Clara (b. 1868) and Florence (b. 1869, lived only one month). Elizabeth's brother, Albert Payson, was born in 1842.[62] Brother Albert was Phi Beta Kappa at Harvard, from which he graduated in 1867.[63] He attended theological seminary but had to withdraw due to illness. He died of tuberculosis in 1868, after repeated pulmonary hemorrhages and a trip to Iowa for his health.[64]

When she applied for a post as missionary teacher in 1864, Elizabeth described her education: "I am now twenty four years of age, of good health, and unmarried. I have been for three years a student of the Western Fem. Seminary, located in Oxford, Butler Co. Ohio. It is on Mt. Holyoke plan. I am completing the Scientific Course at Homer."[65] The Western Female Seminary was founded by teachers from Mount Holyoke College in Massachusetts. The "Scientific Course at Homer" was held at the Cortland Academy in Homer, New York, where Elizabeth's education was focused on learning to teach according to a "normal school" curriculum. One of her teachers there wrote, "Miss Lizzie P. Worthington having been under my instruction, I most heartily recommend her as a faithful student, an earnest Christian and as one who in my estimation is eminently qualified & adapted to the work of a teacher."[66] When the AMA asked her for a reference from her minister, she sent a letter from her father. He wrote,

> This certifies that my daughter Elizabeth is well qualified for the department of a teacher, both religiously and intellectually. She has enjoyed a thorough course of training in some of the best literary Institutions in our country. As a Christian, she is very much devoted

to the interests of her dear Redeemer's cause, taking an active part in Sabbath schools and Bible classes. I can confidently recommend her not only in these respects as a teacher, but also as a proficient in music. She is an excellent singer and can play well on any instrument. She is a member in good standing of the Presbyterian church.[67]

Elizabeth expressed in her letters to the AMA her ardent hope that she could teach the freedpeople. "I have been desirous for some time of teaching the African race, but not until now has it seemed advisable. It will be to me a great pleasure if I can do them any good."[68] In another letter she uses the word "expedient." Several factors determined the change in situation that allowed her to consider going. First, she finished her normal school course in June 1864, so she was ready for the next stage in her life. Second, she was unmarried with no apparent prospects in that line. The war continued, and many of the men of eligible age were in the army. So she was at loose ends. And as the war continued, there was the possible threat that areas now occupied by former slaves would be overrun. This indeed happened in Plymouth, North Carolina, the destination for one AMA teacher who then had to be reassigned to Virginia. Virginia seemed safe but was not entirely so until the war ended ten months later. Thus, there was both dedication and excitement in venturing into the South.

In the fall of 1864 she set out for her new post in Portsmouth, escorted, as we have seen, by Robert Harris. Once in Virginia, she initially earned $10 a month, plus her traveling expenses. In February 1865 she asked for a raise. She reminded Mr. W. E. Whiting of the AMA that she initially signed on to work for $10 a month and then returned $1 of that to the AMA (as she was, apparently, tithing). Now she wanted to increase her monthly pay to $15, and again return 10 percent, or $1.50. "I would like the money as soon as you can send it," she wrote, as expenses in Virginia were higher than expected.[69] On the last day of March and again in April she requested that her monthly salary be sent as soon as possible. Clearly Miss Worthington needed both her salary and to maintain a reputation for sanctity and charity.[70]

Elizabeth taught with William D. Harris in Portsmouth, Virginia, in the spring of 1865, at the same time J. D. Harris was employed at the hospital there. In April Elizabeth reported that she was quite pleased with her school and with the fact that "the children seem the better to appreciate their education privileges, and understand better their relation as moral beings." She told an anecdote that illustrated her sympathy with and enjoyment of the teaching style of Reverend Harris. In the mornings they would lock the doors at the start of the school day and conduct prayers. If children were tardy, they had to wait until such devotional exercises were complete. "The other morning at prayers he was reading 'Knock, and it shall be opened unto you,' when heavy knocks by tardy children drew my attention to the door," she said. "I was almost sorry that the knocks came just then, but my fears were all dispelled by the happy turn Mr. Harris gave to the matter." He asked the children if they heard the knocks, and the children answered yes. But they cannot come in just yet, and must wait, right? Right, they said. Elizabeth continued, "Just so Mr. Harris said is it with knocking on heavens gate. Do not delay. If you would be children of God, you must seek early, and you shall find." That same day the school learned of the capture of Richmond. The children told her "Tis nothing strange." When she asked them why, they said, "God helps us." Elizabeth closed her letter with the conclusion, "I felt the weight and beauty of their reasoning."[71]

The mission schools broke up for summer vacation, as the pupils went to work in the fields and the missionary teachers escaped the insalubrious climate of the peninsula near the James River. In August 1865, Elizabeth wrote to the AMA asking to have a new commission. She wanted to return to Virginia but preferred Richmond, as one Dr. Green in Portsmouth told her that the climate closer to the ocean "was not adapted to my constitution." Still, "My experience in Portsmouth the last year has taught me that teaching may not only seem a duty but may be a real pleasure heightened as it must be when the hearts of the children keep pace with the intellect and are grateful [illegible] Christ." She remembered William Harris, her supervisor, with especial fondness. "I first taught with Rev. W. D. Harris, whose fervent piety did much toward making this school a pleasant one." In the same letter she put forward her sister Clara's offer to accompany her as a teacher. Clara had studied at Mount Holyoke and later at the same Western Female Seminary in Oxford, Ohio, as her sister. Written at the bottom of the letter in a different hand is the phrase "decline giving a commission."[72]

It is not clear whether this phrase applied to one sister or to both. Clara never took a commission with the AMA, but Elizabeth was also rejected, initially. Apparently, the complaint against her was that she "lacked the force and nerve to maintain the needful discipline of a successful school."[73] Elizabeth fired off indignant letters in reply to this assessment. "Did anyone make the criticism of which you speak who is more qualified to judge the matter than Rev. W. D. Harris, with whom I was associated in teaching, seven months out of the eight that I spent there [in Portsmouth]? Has not my school sustained a creditable appearance?" She asked to know who had made the criticism so she could explain the circumstances that might have inspired his low opinion. In the meantime she enclosed a letter from W. D. Harris that endorsed her work (albeit "not wishing to be egotistical"). She fervently hoped she could return to Virginia.[74] In a later letter she attested to "the cherished purpose of my heart, to labor for the intellectual and moral good of the Freedmen."[75]

In a follow-up letter to an AMA officer, she was more adamant. "Let me explain some things, and I think you will say at once, that the *criticism was unjust*. I was well aware that I was no favorite with Mr. Bell." Bell had the supervision of several AMA schools near Fort Monroe in federally occupied Virginia. She described how scarce rooms were in Gosport, where she was teaching, so that she and W. D. Harris ended up teaching in the same room, and he had "the government" of them. They kept the large number of children in order and discipline. Later, Bell asked her to take over another school as the teacher had to leave. "Mr. Bell never came to my school for the purpose of ascertaining its progress, or my mode of discipline. How *could* he judge? How *could* he criticize? I was conscious that the school was well disciplined. I never allowed disobedience. I never suffered a falsehood to pass unnoticed. I knew that the children improved and were happy. I know that I am not deficient in force and nerve, or strength of character." She closed by saying that she would be willing to be a missionary if there were no teacher slots available.[76] She did not appear to have returned south under AMA auspices until January 1867, when she was assigned to Morehead City, North Carolina.

Elizabeth Worthington very likely made the acquaintance of J. D. Harris during the fall of 1864 and the spring of 1865. In December 1864 she lived in a boardinghouse with thirteen other AMA teachers, including W. D. Harris and his younger brother Robert Harris.[77] J. D. was in Portsmouth at that time, as a contract surgeon at the Portsmouth Hospital. W. D. talked about visiting the colored troops in the hospital as part of his duties, and perhaps Elizabeth accompanied him. If she read to the hospitalized men or wrote letters for them, she would be acting in just the same way that thousands of female hospital volunteers did in the North. The likelihood that J. D. should have visited his brothers in their lodging is likewise high, and he could have met her there. Her fondness for William D. and his returned fondness for her are evident in their letters.

January 1867 found her in Morehead City under the supervision of Mr. H. S. Beals. There she taught ninety-one students with the help of Mr. Jenkins, her assistant. Most of her pupils were at the very beginning of learning to read and write.[78] Her letters describe a destitute population of freedpeople whose children needed clothes so they could decently attend school. In her letters she criticized the clothing that arrived, saying that dresses for girls over ten were badly needed, as well as shoes and more pants. The blackboard was "soft and chalk hard and gritty and can only be cleaned by washing and hard scrubbing." The cook stove was burning the floor, but Mr. Beals told her there was none better to be had. She lacked sufficient books. And on and on. The situation had multiple difficulties.[79]

She apparently got on no better with Mr. Beals than with Mr. Bell in Portsmouth. One bone of contention was the design of a chimney for the stove that heated the schoolroom. He wanted to build a fireplace chimney, but she was sure that a stovepipe would be better (and outlined three reasons that it would be so). She had grown up on the Michigan frontier and probably felt she knew more about heating a room than the hapless Mr. Beals. She also requested that the schoolroom be properly boarded off in winter to keep out the winds. And "nothing has yet been done to keep the rain out of the School room or my room. I sit up late nights dreading to retire to my room that has been damp ever since one week ago last Thursday." She suspected Mr. Beals was too busy, but if so she wanted someone else appointed in his place. She apologized for writing in criticism of him, "but I could not endanger my life & the life of my school."[80] The man could not even buy the right food, in her eyes. In April he delivered a half barrel of flour to them that cost eleven dollars, but it was not as good as some that had been sent. "Thus you see southern prices."[81] Another time she bewailed the absence of potatoes from the Morehead City markets. She comes across as cranky, demanding, and hard to please, although in her defense she had more serious grief to deal with after bewailing the potato shortage and Mr. Beals's stubbornness about the chimney: she reported the news that her younger brother had died of tuberculosis during that same difficult spring.[82]

In the fall her problems with the schoolroom continued. She wrote to her AMA contact in despair: "Is it asking too much to have our School room boarded off from the garret part and plastered *at once*? Many of our pupils are thinly clad without shoes or stockings & must be so through the winter. They need a comfortable school room." She asked to go to Hampton, Virginia, to teach in a normal school there, "where I can have charge of more advanced pupils! My education has been with special reference to teaching & I would like a normal school."[83] She was tired of Mr. Beals, tired of that drafty schoolhouse, and tired of teaching primary school pupils. In February 1868 she was still in Morehead City, although there the record of her AMA teaching ends in the archives.[84]

MARRIAGE

Without any prologue in her AMA letters, Elizabeth Worthington married J. D. Harris three months later. The Reverend William D. Harris officiated at the ceremony on May 15, 1868, in Wayne County, North Carolina.[85] The choice of marriage site is peculiar. From his files we know that W. D. was in Richmond in 1868, heading a large church. Robert and Cicero Harris were in Fayetteville, North Carolina, which is close to Wayne County. The rest of the Harris clan was back in Ohio. Elizabeth's father and sister were in Vineland, New Jersey. Although Cicero Richardson (sister Sarah's husband) had lived briefly in Wayne County before the move to Ohio around 1850, no one in the Harris family lived there in May 1868. Even more peculiar are two letters from Elizabeth to the AMA in June 1868, a month after her wedding: she signed them "Miss Worthington," and they were mailed from her father's house in Vineland.[86] This persistence of apparent single status a month after her marriage, coupled with the odd choice of Wayne County, may be an indication that the marriage was a secret one. The marriage of white and Black was not a casual event in Reconstruction society.

Such "miscegenation" was illegal in both North Carolina and Virginia in the 1860s. So horrible was it that in the election of 1864, Lincoln's opposition published a book, complete with lascivious sketches, claiming Republicans' sponsorship of such couplings.[87] However, North Carolina allowed a clergyman to notify the county registrar of nuptials by mail. So W. D. Harris may have done just that, leaving the registrar to assume both were the default (white) race. Or, since he had spent part of his career in Wayne County, he may have made friends with the registrar, who accordingly did him a favor. Neither state would legalize mixed-race marriages until 1967, when the Supreme Court ruled, in *Loving v. State of Virginia*, that state laws prohibiting "racially mixed" marriages were unconstitutional.[88]

Beginning at least by April 1869, the former Elizabeth Worthington signed herself "Mrs. Dr. Harris." They were living in Hampton, Virginia, where she reported, "My home is the third house on the right-hand side from the Hampton Bridge—as one enters Hampton."[89] She was writing the AMA to secure copies of its magazine but made a point to invite guests to visit her at home. A few months later she wrote to her former AMA contact E. P. Smith to offer advice on the Hampton Institute, then growing around her. "I have watched the progress of Hampton *Agricultural* Institute with much interest," she began. Then she offered him advice. "If it is to be Normal School the standard is *too low*. *Every* teacher should understand *Physiology* both for his own wellbeing and for the welfare of his School. Every teacher fitted at a *Normal* School should understand *Algebra* in order the better to master the more difficult parts of Arithmetic." She recommended that the long-suffering Mr. Beals be brought in as a spiritual leader of the school and offered a character reference for his wife as being "lady-like," a woman who would make "a most excellent matron." She particularly praised their daughter Sara, who had much to offer at Hampton. "Miss Sara is a thorough scholar. Her labor in Beaufort (where I knew her) did not cease when she left the School room. She taught the older girls Palm-leaf hat-making and tatting *out of school hours* that they might be able to help themselves. I hope that these suggestions may not be impertinent." She closed with "Should you visit Hampton do not fail to call on Mrs. Dr. Harris."[90] She did love to use that title.

We have little direct testimony of J. D.'s opinions of events in this time frame. From his brothers' letters we get a sense of what it was like to be a free Black man during Reconstruction, working against violent threats from southern whites and odds of incredible poverty and need among the freedpeople. The prospects for "elevating our people" were never more immediate, and right at hand. This was a core Harris family value, one repeated in the job applications of J. D., Robert, William, and Cicero. There was no hint of tolerance for mixed-race marriage, though, before J. D. married, and there is no indication of how the Harris family reacted to the addition of Elizabeth Worthington. W. D.'s prior favorable impression of her must have helped and may explain why he was willing to officiate at the wedding. Still, the possibility that a Black gentleman could marry a white gentlewoman, in public, was astonishing. When J. D. ran for office in 1869, the press noted the oddity as a nasty fact but did not give it the attention that one might expect. It may be that it was so shocking that newspapers were loath to publish it when delicate white females might read about the scandal.

Medicine and Politics, 1864-1869

During the last half of the 1860s, J. D. Harris emerged as an accomplished professional man with a good salary and respect in his community. The US government appointed him first as surgeon to the Black wards of a Union army hospital and later as surgical director of various Freedmen's Bureau hospitals. He had a horse and carriage, suitable clothes, and the appellation of doctor. Like other single young men with an income, he soon found himself in need of a wife, and indeed marriage found him in 1868 (as noted in the previous chapter). As if that was not remarkable enough, he then became a candidate for the lieutenant governor of Virginia. It was not all easy going, but who would have thought it even possible, looking at the Black teenager on the edge of slavery in 1840s Fayetteville?

CONTRACT SURGEON FOR THE US ARMY

When J. D. Harris began as a surgeon for a US Army hospital in Portsmouth, Virginia, in June 1864, his appointment was by contract as an acting assistant surgeon, USA. As the war came to an end during the following spring, the army began closing hospitals and laying off contract surgeons. If he was to continue medical practice in the US government's pay, Harris needed a new job. First, he tried for a regular army appointment, with the US Colored Troops, but that did not materialize. Then he applied to the Freedmen's Bureau and worked in its Virginia hospitals until 1869. It was a turbulent time for Black men in Virginia. Harris found severe health problems among the newly freed slaves and a federal government that soon lost interest in supplying the medical needs of this desperate population.[1]

On June 23, 1864, Harris signed on with the Union army to work as an acting assistant surgeon. This category of appointment meant that his job was guaranteed only as long as the contract dictated, which was typically for three months at a time. His contract was ultimately extended through August 1865. Harris began work at the Portsmouth, Virginia, hospital in June 1864, where his practice was so lauded by the *Christian Recorder* letter quoted in chapter 7. Ultimately, he oversaw three wards of 100 patients each, patients who had come from the US Colored Troops regiments. Throughout his medical career, Harris cared mostly for Black patients, as doctor and patients were segregated together. That the hospital wards at Portsmouth could be overloaded and chaotic is seen in a complaint filed by Harris's superior Dr. J. H. Franz, who wrote to Brigadier General George F. Shepley of the District of East Virginia in October 1864. Franz complained, "Without any Notification of their arrival, one hundred & fifty (150) wounded men are here awaiting admission into Hospital. I can think of no other place than the Basement of the Baptist Church to put them, and with your consent will reoccupy that room."[2] The word "reoccupy" indicated that this was not the first time such a flood of injured men arrived without warning. The siege of Petersburg, including the disastrous Battle of the Crater (July 30, 1864), left nearly 2,000 Union men wounded, many of them from the USCT. Such "colored men" were likely patients for the young Dr. Harris.

With the ebb and flow of patients, hospital space expanded and contracted, as the Franz letter indicated. The major Civil War battles of the fall of 1864 were elsewhere, in Tennessee and Georgia. Not until April 1865 would the war again be centered in Virginia, when Richmond fell and Grant and Lee met at Appomattox to end it all. One bit of evidence that Dr. Harris's assignment shifted according to necessity in that time comes from a patient census report from November 18, 1864. His address is Freedmen's Hospital, Hampton, Virginia, where he was noted as surgeon in charge. Hampton is across the bay from Portsmouth, a distance of twenty-five miles that required a ferry ride. By February 1865 Harris was back in Portsmouth, at the Balfour

Hospital. In other words, he was moved as needed. Overall, his contract with the army lasted from June 23, 1864, to August 25, 1865.[3]

In February 1865, Harris applied to join the regular army to serve the US Colored Troops as a surgeon; doing so would gain him a commission, not just a temporary contract as a surgeon. But the situation with the rebellion was rapidly changing. General W. T. Sherman had marched across Georgia from Atlanta to Savannah in the fall of 1864. In perhaps the most famous telegram of the war, on December 22 Sherman sent Lincoln a jubilant message: "I beg to *present* you as a *Christmas gift* the city of *Savannah* with 150 heavy guns and plenty of ammunition and also about 25,000 bales of cotton."[4] The newly freed slaves descended on Savannah (or were there to start with), and the city was garrisoned in part by the USCT. While many of the slaves on the Virginia Peninsula had been free for three years or more, these newly freedpeople were fresh to liberty and often in acute need of medical attention.

In his application letter to Secretary of War E. M. Stanton, Harris asked to be made a commissioned surgeon-officer, either at the assistant or associate level. He wanted to go to Savannah and help with the new citizens there as they adapted to freedom. "I would now be glad to serve, as Surgeon and Physician, the freed people in and near Savannah, wish to grow up with them and help them to obtain the honorable position which I am sure they will speedily secure for themselves."[5] Even as Robert E. Lee held on, hoping to make a final stand in conjunction with the ragtag army under Joseph Johnston, it was clear to the Union army leadership that the war was near an end. Soon there would be no need for extra contract surgeons such as Harris to treat wounded and sick soldiers. Harris no doubt knew this and was trying to cement a permanent position before the layoffs began. Army physicians, like other recruits, signed on for a three-year commitment. Many of the Black regiments had formed in 1863 or 1864, and so their term of duty would last into 1866 or 1867. Harris wanted to serve with them in Savannah, but by the late spring of 1865 many army physicians were no longer needed, and most of the remaining Black regiments were sent to Texas.

Alexander Augusta was also drawn to Georgia, where he became surgeon-in-chief of Lincoln Hospital, the Freedmen's Bureau hospital in Savannah. Augusta was a famous figure—the first Black man appointed as a full surgeon in the US Army, and one who stayed in the news by challenging public segregation on streetcars and other entities when they barred his path. My first hypothesis was that Harris applied for the transfer south in order to join Augusta in Savannah. But that timeline does not work. Harris sent his letter in February 1865. At that point Augusta was still working as a recruiting surgeon for the USCT in Baltimore, "detached" from his appointed regiment, the 7th US Colored Infantry. He only resigned from this service in April 1865 and was then sent south to work with General Rufus Saxton in Beaufort, South Carolina. He arrived in Beaufort on May 3 and reported to Savannah on July 3, 1865. So, Harris acted independently of Augusta's possible leadership.[6]

It is worth pausing for a moment to consider similarities between Drs. Harris and Augusta. Both were fortunate to gain experience and income from working for the federal government, first as surgeons to Union army troops and later as surgeons in Freedmen's Bureau hospitals. The career of Alexander Augusta, the most prominent African American physician in the war, illustrates the sort of structural societal problems that the first Black physicians met. They had some markers of gentility, such as clothing, that spoke to their class, but their race overwhelmed these indicators as far as the white public was concerned. Augusta, who was born to a free Black woman in the South, chose to study at the University of Toronto, as no American medical school would admit him in the 1850s. With his medical degree in hand, Augusta wrote to Abraham Lincoln in early 1863, asking whether he could serve in the newly forming Black regiments, or else in areas like the Virginia Peninsula or the District of Columbia where freedpeople were congregating under the protection of Union troops. Cognizant of the quality of his degree and experience, the army appointed him as a major and full surgeon to the 7th US Colored Infantry Regiment, then forming in Bryantown, Maryland, a small town about twenty miles south of modern-day Joint Base Andrews. Maryland was still a slave state—it did not secede, so the Emancipation Proclamation freeing slaves in the states that would "then be in rebellion" did not apply to it.[7]

Augusta immediately ran into issues of hierarchy in the Union army medical corps. As a major and full surgeon, he had seniority over all assistant and associate surgeons. It was a matter of who saluted whom. As the more junior physicians appointed to the regiment were white men, this set up an intolerable situation in their eyes. "When we made applications for positions in the Colored Service, the understanding was universal that all Commissioned Officers were to be white men," they complained to Lincoln in early 1864. "Judge our Surprise and disappointment, when upon joining our respective regiments we found that the *Senior Surgeon* of the command was a Negro." The doctors proclaimed that they could not serve in such a subordinate position without losing all self-respect.[8] Another wrote his senator that the "amalgamation or miscegenation in the appointment of officers" was intolerable. He found this deep challenge to his honor to be "*grave, unjust,* and *humiliating*."[9] In response the army sent Augusta to Baltimore, where he worked examining African American recruits at an induction center. He remained "on leave" from his regiment throughout the war. And Harris? None of his appointments included the supervision of white male doctors. The army medical hierarchy would not make that mistake again.

There were similar problems finding a place for African American doctors to practice. Harris, like Augusta, cared for patients who were freed slaves, colored troops, or, later, indigent Black people in Washington, DC. But just because both men had respectable MDs and experience with patients did not mean that white patients would willingly be doctored by them. Breaking through this societal barrier would be a long time coming. Harris did follow along with his preceptor seeing white patients at the US Marine Hospital in Cleveland, but he worked in a servant or assistant mode, something quite acceptable for Black men. While it was unthinkable for many that a Black doctor should treat white women, this gender mixing apparently caused no alarm when Harris treated Black freedwomen at Fredericksburg. However, when Harris moved to the South Carolina state asylum to practice (see next chapter), a different outcome would disrupt his course. Segregation of doctors and patients by color became the rule. This was a major limitation for the training of Black physicians, then and later.

While Harris was disappointed in his goal of serving in Savannah, the US Army did find a place for him that satisfied the restraints of "only Black patients" and "no white men under his command." The army was mostly cutting regular medical staff, not adding to them as the war drew to its close. But the ranks of needy freedmen and freedwomen were growing all around Virginia military bases. Harris's letter to Secretary Stanton was forwarded to Major George Luckley, medical director of the Army of the James, an army that included the 25th "African Corps" of the USCT. Luckley ordered Harris to report to one W. A. Conover until the time that "you [Conover] may see fit to order him before the board." At the bottom of the letter, he added, "Maybe General Birney would like him?" General William Birney was in command of the Third Division of the X Corps of the Army of the James, which would soon split into the XXIV (white) and XXV (Black) Corps.[10]

In any event, on May 4, 1865, a medical board convened at the headquarters of the XXV Corps "to examine applicants for promotion to surgeon and assistant surgeon of colored troops." On the board were surgeons E. M. Pease, Norton Folsom, and P. G. Barrett. All had appointments to the USCT. They were all white. A sheet wrapped around the outside of the papers read, "Examination papers in the case of actg asst surg J. D. Harris." Handwritten in pencil on the outside was "25 a.c." This packet contained the autobiography and examination described in an earlier chapter. Included as well was the patient census report sent from the Freedmen's Hospital in Hampton, perhaps a sample showing that he knew how to prepare such reports.[11]

The XXV Corps would shortly be on its way to Texas, leaving Virginia in late May 1865. Its assignment was to protect Texas from invasion by French-occupied Mexico. So, if Harris received an offer to go with these troops, it would have come in the three weeks intervening between exam and corps embarkation. The arid area of south Texas had few freedpeople, and perhaps therefore little attraction to Harris. It certainly was not Savannah. It is also possible that he was turned down due to lack of available positions or the desire that all of the medical officers be white. E. M. Pease had been one of the surgeons to complain when Alexander Augusta was appointed at the rank of major, a sign that he had little inclination for mingling with Black doctors.[12]

CONTRACT SURGEON TO THE FREEDMEN'S BUREAU

Harris ended his contract with the US Army in August 1865 and then signed on with the Freedmen's Bureau in October. It is worth a pause here to consider employment opportunities open to him, a thirty-two-year-old Black man barely a year out of medical school. There were some affluent Blacks in his region, but probably not enough to support a medical practice. The freedpeople had a vast need of medical care, but they were mostly destitute. So, the fact that he was a salaried physician for the federal government over the next several years was a lucky opportunity and a logical choice. Salaried positions were uncommon for physicians at that time—except of course for the war years, when both the Confederate and Union armies paid for thousands of salaried doctors. Still, those men would mostly return to private practice at war's end. Harris lacked a clear path to make that possible—but he had a community on the Virginia Peninsula that welcomed him, among both freed Black people and the white charitable and missionary workers who had come to aid the former slaves.

So, Harris took a job with the Freedmen's Bureau. The bureau, formally known as the Bureau of Refugees, Freedmen, and Abandoned Lands, was created by Congress in 1865 as an entity of the War Department. Originally intended to last one year, its goals included setting up schools, providing temporary health care, adjudicating legal disputes between whites and Blacks, and generally smoothing the path to citizenship for the formerly enslaved southerners. For Harris, the bureau's hospital duties would have been familiar. Doctors used the same forms as in the army, just crossing out references to the military and replacing with the Freedmen's Bureau information across the top. The history of the bureau is a vast and evolving topic, as the National Archives continues to organize, microfilm, and release the documents of the "regional field offices." As an example of the size of this document cache, the records for the local Virginia field offices occupy 203 rolls (microfilm collection M1913) with images per roll of anywhere from 800 to 1,100 or more. There is no way to search specifically for an individual, so while I found many references to Dr. Harris, I make no claims to have exhausted this archive.[13]

Harris left his army position as a contract surgeon, stationed in Portsmouth, on August 25, 1865.[14] The letter sent to inform the surgeon general of this fact says that the army contract was annulled and he was transferred to the Freedmen's Bureau. Harris contracted with the bureau on October 1, 1865, so perhaps he had a few weeks' leave and some relocation time. Or he may have started work without a contract. His contract was not for a particular hospital but to work in the Henrico District of Virginia, which had several hospitals. The Freedmen's Bureau had divided each state into administrative districts, with Henrico close to Richmond but not included in it. The salary was the same as what he earned in his physician post with the army—$100 per month.[15] Taking the Freedmen's Bureau post may have been sweetened by the fact that the bureau surgeon-in-chief for the District of Virginia was Dr. J. J. De Lamater (sometimes spelled Delamater). De Lamater had been one of the organizers of the Cleveland Medical College in the 1840s, the same medical college that Harris had attended in 1863. De Lamater's colleagues from the early days, Drs. John L. Cassells and Jared P. Kirtland, were still teaching when Harris went through. De Lamater might have been more comfortable working with Harris, given their educational connection.[16]

CONDITIONS IN THE VIRGINIA FREEDMEN'S BUREAU HOSPITALS, 1865–1868

Dr. Harris was first assigned to Howard's Grove Hospital, where Ira Russell found him in the fall of 1865. Howard's Grove had been a Confederate hospital until early April 1865, when all Confederate hospitals were surrendered to Union management.[17] It was a large facility, built in the countryside with some sixty-two buildings nestled under shady trees. As many as 2,000 Confederate patients were housed there by 1865, although the Confederate army moved as many patients out of Union hands as possible before the surrender.

As the hospital grounds were bound by the Mechanicsville Turnpike, Redd Street, Coalter Street, and Q Street, it was only a mile and a half to two miles from the fortifications around Richmond.[18]

If Harris was initially the only surgeon at Howard's Grove, what of the attendants, the nurses? We learn about one by happenstance, an American Missionary Association nurse who volunteered at the hospital. A November 7, 1865, letter by "W. D. S.," published in the *Christian Recorder*, reported on a program at the Third Street AME Church of Richmond and mentioned "Miss Colton, from the dear A.M.A., who is matron at Howard Grove Hospital, where J. D. Harris, M.D., is surgeon in charge."[19] W. D. Harris was the reverend of this church; it is possible that the printer misread the handwritten *H* in his initials as an *S* when noting the author of the letter. Miss Colton was white but apparently had no problem working with the Harris brothers; members of the AMA were notoriously liberal in their tolerance of integration. It is quite possible that there were other Black workers in the hospital—perhaps even relatives of the patients whose only pay was food—but if so, that is not recorded.

So who was Miss Colton, and what was her opinion of Dr. Harris? Miss Colton was Marcia Colton, a Minnesota woman in her sixties who had worked with the Choctaw Mission prior to the Civil War. After being accepted by the AMA for work among the freedpeople in Virginia, she was first assigned to Craney Island, near Hampton Roads, Virginia. There the Union army housed freedwomen accused of being prostitutes, with the goal of education and redemption. Then in October 1865 the AMA asked her to take over the role of matron at Howard's Grove Hospital, with special assignment to the section that served as a home for the aged men and women recently freed from slavery. Over time this population grew to more than 900 men and women, many of them poorly clad and shod, in a hospital that sometimes could not be kept warm in winter. Miss Colton reported on October 16, 1865, that "Dr. Harris[,] a brother of D. W. [sic] Harris, [is] the surgeon in charge here which will make it pleasanter for me no doubt."[20] She noted the hospital was about nine miles from the Richmond City center. W. D. Harris's church was on Third Street in downtown Richmond. Colton may have been misinformed when she wrote the October letter, or it may be that it really took nine miles to get to the gap in the fortifications that would admit them to the city.

Unfortunately, Miss Colton says nothing more directly about J. D. Harris and his hospital management. Freedmen's Bureau records say that he was reassigned to Fredericksburg later on in the fall. Colton mentioned new doctors in the spring of 1866—Browne and Rayfield—so perhaps with hospital growth more doctors were needed. Both of the new doctors were white. As noted earlier, a Black doctor could not supervise a white one, so perhaps De Lamater thought it best to move Harris to a smaller, one-doctor hospital. In late May 1866 Colton wrote, "It is said by visitors and Inspectors alike that this is the best Hospital for Freedmen that there is in operation."[21] This letter followed another to Whipple from two months earlier, when she said that "there are some things needed in the medical practice here which the government does not furnish the Bureau and these physicians wish to have.... Mustard, C[h]amomile flowers. And Tinc[ture] of Valerian." She had spent some of her AMA stipend to make up the pharmacy shortfall, but that did not seem right, and the AMA should supply it directly, if possible.[22]

The Freedmen's Bureau operation always ran on a shoestring, and a transient one at that. It was often short of physicians, at least of physicians willing to be hired to serve the freedpeople. For example, one district superintendent wrote the head of the Freedmen's Bureau in Virginia in December 1865, "Quite a number of Freed People in the Town of Manchester and County of Henrico are suffering for medical attendance." These areas were on the periphery of Richmond. He continued, "I therefore respectfully request that a medical officer be directed to report to me for duty, in the aforementioned parts of my district."[23] The response? The bureau had none to send. It was also short of hospital buildings. The best were prior military hospitals, such as Howard's Grove in Richmond and the Balfour Hospital in Portsmouth. But otherwise, the *temporary* bureau had no interest in building hospitals, much less providing long-term physician contracts. The bureau rented whatever buildings it could find and usually filled them with leftover army cots, bedding, and other furniture. A bed might be simply a "bed tick"—a sack like a long pillowcase—stuffed with straw.

In the dry prose of Freedmen's Bureau reports and letters, one discovers an extent of illness and debility that no one had predicted among the former slaves. After all, propaganda depicted southerners' enslaved men and women as happy, healthy, and well-fed, just like, say, their pigs and horses. And now these emancipated men and women were in a part of the country that was the least likely to feel charitable toward their care. The missionary societies could erect churches and schools, but building a health care system from scratch was beyond the capacity of any nineteenth-century government, much less one determined to tidy up all problems in a year or two and then get out of town. The two years after the war saw the freedpeople of the South exposed to yellow fever, cholera, and smallpox. Their unsanitary shantytowns suffered from contaminated water supplies with the usual sequelae of diarrheal illnesses, especially typhoid fever. In his report for the year ending in June 1868, a bureau inspector told De Lamater that there was much illness in Richmond, including diarrhea. Although Howard's Grove Hospital was meant to be shutting down, in fact that was impossible: "Howard's Grove is full."[24] But the severity of community diseases among the freedpeople did not change the government's course, although it may have slowed it where hospitals were concerned.

Smallpox was a source of great worry to local bureau doctors in Virginia, North Carolina, and South Carolina, although evidence about it in official reports is somewhat scanty. The Freedmen's Bureau chief medical officer, L. A. Edwards, did mention it and lauded the response of bureau doctors. Of this trio of yellow fever, cholera, and smallpox, he wrote in October 1866 that there had been little mortality; "prompt and vigorous measures, both remedial and preventive, have invariably been adopted with energy and zeal by the officers of the bureau, with cheering and successful results."[25] When news of smallpox reached his office, he had written to the Virginia state medical director, Dr. De Lamater, urging rapid care, prevention, and cooperation with local authorities. Such was the case with Portsmouth, in the fall of 1866, when De Lamater was asked to both act and write special reports about the outbreak "from time to time." Edwards was concerned and had called his doctors to step up their efforts.[26]

Edwards boasted of the success of such measures in November 1867. Few cases of cholera or yellow fever had struck the freedpeople; in fact, they seemed immune to the latter, "almost entirely exempt." Smallpox had appeared in some districts, "but, by active sanitary measures and prompt vaccination, these violent and virulent diseases have been entirely subdued or modified." He reported that a "system of vaccination has been extensively practiced in most of the districts."[27] As a result, in the tally of cases and deaths among Virginia freedpeople from September 1, 1866, to June 30, 1867, there had been 72 cases of cholera and 44 deaths, with no reported cases of yellow fever. In that same interval they counted 603 cases of smallpox with 94 deaths, and an additional 124 cases with 10 deaths over the course of the summer months of 1867. Freedmen's Bureau doctors reported that they vaccinated 1,338 freedpeople in the first interval and 362 in the second.[28] Among the freedpeople in the southern states as a whole, the bureau reported 6,552 cases of smallpox for 1866.[29]

Historian Jim Downs has written the most thorough account of this smallpox epidemic among the freedpeople in his book *Sick from Freedom*. His chapter about smallpox is titled "Reconstructing an Epidemic" because this outbreak was so weakly reported at the time and had subsequently been little recognized by historians. He put the story together from fragments of events in North Carolina, South Carolina, and Mississippi (among others) and had little information about the Virginia experience. (At the time of his research, the Virginia Freedmen's Bureau field records were not available to historians, as they were being organized and microfilmed.) One of his findings was that doctors in these states were short on smallpox vaccine and resorted to the older technique of arm-to-arm inoculation with active smallpox virus.[30] This was an effective method but with higher risk to the patient. There was also the risk that the inoculated patient would spread smallpox to others.

The story was different in Virginia. Somehow the Virginia bureau found at least 1,700 doses of vaccine, and probably more, as it is likely that local whites also received the procedure as the epidemic prevailed. Smallpox was uncommon in the South until the Civil War; in fact, southerners accused the Yankees of deliberately exchanging Confederate soldiers sick with smallpox in order to introduce the deadly malady to the South. Whatever the truth of that belief, smallpox had become common in the Confederacy by 1863, especially in Virginia. Such charges of deliberate smallpox dissemination were part of the ongoing propaganda battle between the warring sides that would erupt into a full barrage in the fall and winter of 1864–65. Regardless of intention, smallpox did make horrid inroads into the South during and after the war.[31] Vaccine had been scarce in the Confederate States during the war, but afterward doctors in the Freedmen's Bureau could requisition supplies stored in US Army depots. Vaccine could be transmitted by mail using the practice of drying scabs and then reconstituting them at the point of use. Or the lymph harvested from active pustules could be pressed between pieces of glass and sealed, or dripped into glass ampules, moistened with glycerin, and sealed. In both cases the vaccine material came from *vaccine* sores; no actual smallpox lymph was deliberately used by doctors in the war or after. It was common in the Civil War to vaccinate arm-to-arm, and this was likely done in postwar Virginia as well. The preferable source of vaccine was from young children, who presumably did not yet have other infectious diseases. Experiments had been made in growing vaccine virus on cows during the war, but this largely failed. Successful "farming" of vaccinia would not become common until the 1870s when a new vaccine virus, the "Beaugency Lymph," arrived from France. So, during the war and after, the preferred choice was lymph fresh from a baby, but the high volume of need meant that it went dirty arm to dirty arm, at times, among both troops and freedpeople.[32]

Robert Reyburn, the last chief medical officer of the Freedmen's Bureau and US Army surgeon during the war, summarized the available statistics on diseases among the freedpeople that had been gathered by the bureau. His work showed a steady decline of smallpox from its apogee in 1866 to its near disappearance by 1869. He had particular familiarity with what happened in Washington, DC, among the large population of freed slaves there. "It need scarcely be said that vaccination and revaccination of all the freedpeople exposed to infection was strictly enforced, and ... with the same result which has always attended its proper enforcement, namely, the extirpation of the disease."[33] Indeed the Virginia medical director's report for 1868 listed only ten cases of smallpox, no deaths, and 112 vaccinations, all during the period from July 1, 1867, to June 30, 1868.[34] No doubt Harris did his share of vaccinating as a Freedmen's Bureau doctor.

J. D. HARRIS, DOCTOR IN CHARGE, FREDERICKSBURG FREEDMEN'S HOSPITAL

In the fall of 1865, Dr. Harris moved from Howard's Grove Hospital in Richmond to the Freedmen's Bureau hospital in Fredericksburg. Harris was listed as "on duty" at the hospital as a physician from October 1, 1865, to the end of October 1867, although it is unclear whether he had actually taken up residency in early October. He was the only physician and had as assistant a clerk who presumably kept track of bureaucratic paperwork. There were fifty beds in the hospital, usually divided about evenly between men and women, with eight or ten children. The patients were all African American. The hospital building itself rented for $20 a month. There is no description of size, but Harris did requisition wood for six fireplaces, the mode of heating the hospital wards.[35] That suggests at least two floors, perhaps segregated into male and female wards. The fireplaces each burned two cords of wood a month, at least in winter; a cord of wood cost $5.25, so that these twelve cords cost $63 a month in the cold months, more than the month's rent. Fredericksburg had been a major Confederate hospital center at one point, with many of its warehouses and mills converted to this function. The city's landscape had also suffered severe damage from Union bombardment in 1862 and 1863. So, it is likely that Harris was working in one of these former commercial buildings, captured from the enemy with equipment intact, such as cots and other hospital equipment like bedding, dishes, and cooking pots. Or it may have been empty, with furnishings moved out by the Confederacy or ransacked by

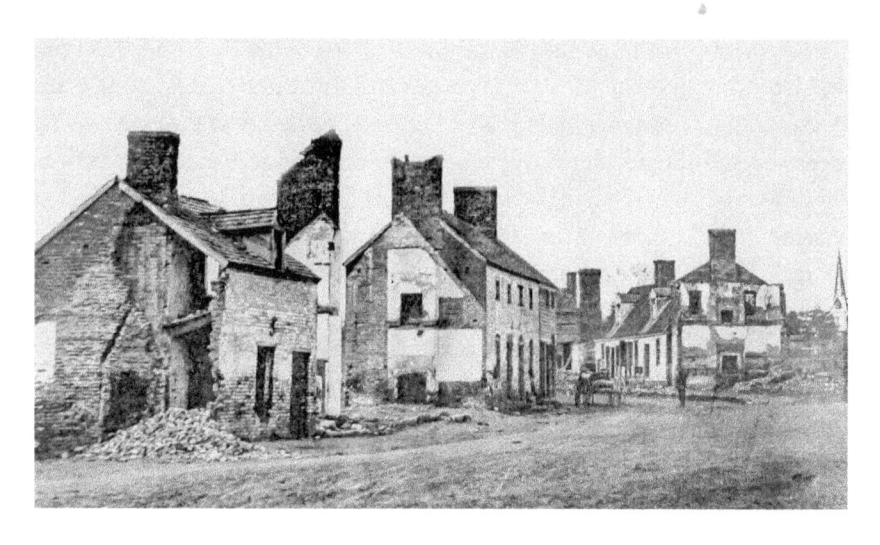

Fredericksburg, Virginia, ca. 1863. An abandoned warehouse such as seen in this photograph housed the Freedmen's Bureau hospital after the war. William H. Allen, *The American Civil War Book and Grant Album* (Boston: William H. Allen, 1894).

the public. There is no overall inventory. In four rooms attached to the main building were a laundry, a dispensary, a kitchen, and an office.[36]

The unrecorded personnel (beyond the doctor and the clerk) and the undocumented hospital furniture and bedding leave us guessing. There is a clue in the fact that Harris ordered 600 pounds of straw for his fifty patients in September 1867, a supply that was expected to last a month.[37] Such straw would have been used to stuff bed ticks and pillowcases, a common practice during the war. When the mattress became soiled, the straw was dumped out, the tick washed, and fresh straw inserted. The unlisted personnel were likely made up of freedmen and freedwomen, either convalescent patients or servants hired from the community. Some may have been family members of patients, who volunteered. Were they paid, perhaps in kind from hospital food? Or from a different community source, such as the AMA or Black churches? Evidence of such payments does not appear in the records so far examined. Another possibility, and a likely one, is that the document set is far from complete and the information we seek here was not saved.

There is no specific mention of smallpox in these monthly reports and requisition orders. Vaccine was not requisitioned, for example. The hospital continued to have only fifty patient beds filled by fifty patients. Remember, however, that there was a room labeled "dispensary" at the hospital. This was a term often used in the era for an outpatient "clinic" for the impoverished.

Harris could have seen any number of community freedpeople via this structure; nowhere does he report patient visits or medicines given, at all, for hospital or dispensary. Somewhere there may be a hospital record book in the National Archives, but when I last sought a particular Civil War hospital, one could only request all the hospital books for a given state and look through them. And it is always possible that the books were lost. If found, they would probably look like Alexander Augusta's records from Savannah, with patients listed in ledger form, with age, date of admission and discharge, and a one- or two-word diagnosis.[38]

The smallpox epidemic became severe in Virginia in 1866. We know from the annual report (see earlier in this chapter) that Virginia had 603 cases spread over the months of September 1866 to June 1867. But we do not know how they were distributed geographically or how they were housed. During the war, army surgeons had learned to isolate smallpox patients in separate hospital buildings or "under canvas" (tents) on the grounds of large hospitals. Howard's Grove, located in the green fields outside of Richmond, had at one time been a Confederate smallpox hospital. And Satterlee Hospital in Philadelphia, with at times 5,000 patients, reserved one corner of the grounds for smallpox tents. In spite of ongoing debates about the contagiousness of cholera, typhoid fever, and yellow fever, there was no dispute that smallpox was contagious person-to-person. So, to the extent possible, smallpox patients and their immediate contacts were isolated in what was called quarantine, even though that phrase had originated in the practice of isolating ships out of port when there were cases of plague, cholera, or yellow fever on board.[39]

It seems likely that some large portion of the Virginia smallpox patients and their contacts were segregated in Fredericksburg during the fall of 1866—and Harris was in charge of them. In late fall Harris suddenly requisitioned supplies for 1,000 persons, on top of his usual orders for maintaining the fifty-bed hospital. He may have thought the need self-evident, but it was mysterious to the Freedmen's Bureau chief medical officer, L. A. Edwards, who in turn wrote J. J. De Lamater, asking for an explanation. Apparently De Lamater sent one back. Edwards acknowledged it, saying, "Your communication ... in explanation of the Requisitions of Dr. J. D. Harris at Fredericksburg, Va. is received and gives a satisfactory statement in reference to your action in the case." Even so, Edwards wanted to seize the teachable moment. "It may be remarked however that the call for supplies for 1000 persons in addition to the 50 beds was very obscurely made. The fact should have been distinctly set forth in the Requisition that a portion of the supplies were for the Sick in Quarantine," chided Edwards. Unsaid but obvious from the word "Quarantine" was the presence of smallpox patients in need of rations. "It is the aim and design of this office to give full discretion to the Surgeons in Chief of Dis[tricts] in their administrative duties," Edwards continued. It was the "apparent excess of supplies allowed in the Requisition" that "demand[ed] an inquiry." He also pointed out, as a general rule, that a surgeon should not order supplies that were not needed at present. It is telling that Edwards's key ambition was to emphasize economy. He did approve the extra supplies but otherwise showed no concern about the persistent smallpox epidemic.[40]

The urgency and willingness to break protocol suggest that Harris was flouting the rules because he, at least, felt the smallpox crisis demanded immediate response. He saw those patients as suffering people, not just figures in a ledger. He should have been applauded by his bosses, not criticized for paperwork abnormalities. Another indication that Harris saw his patients' needs more clearly than the white physicians and officers comes in a small gesture made in August 1867 at the Fredericksburg hospital. He requested "that 100 feet of planks be furnished" for the hospital. Why? "To make seats for the patients." The officer commanding in Fredericksburg endorsed the request and sent it to the quartermaster. Whether those unfortunate men and women soon had somewhere to sit other than the ground is unknown. But Harris was the sort of doctor who noticed the need and did what he could to meet it.[41]

Harris ended his time in Fredericksburg on October 31, 1867. By November 18 he was at the Freedmen's Hospital in Hampton, Virginia, out on the peninsula near Fort Monroe. He likely began that service on November 1, as the bureau liked to keep such contracts by the month. His contract continued to the end of December 1869. The large Freedmen's Hospital in Hampton was one of the last to close. It maintained a census of over 100 patients throughout 1867 and 1868.[42] Even at the end of his service, Harris was still striving to help the Black people who were poorly served by the federal government. This again was revealed in a letter that survived in his endorsement file. Lieutenant M. S. Reed, an associate surgeon in the "African Corps," endorsed and passed on a letter from "J. D. Harris, A.[cting] A.[ssistant] Surg. in charge of Freedmen's Hospital Elizabeth City Co. Va. as to whether he is to admit in Hospital those indigent persons who were not residents of this county in 1861, but who are simply suffering from want of food." Harris was obviously taking the humanitarian approach—feed the hungry. But the Freedmen's Bureau was trying to shut down and to induce civil employers to take over the care of the needy. Many slaves had fled to this part of Virginia, the neighborhood of Fort Monroe, during the war. While social services had long been assigned to one's "home county," the place that by law was supposed to take care of its own, this made little sense when "home" was a former plantation. Still, the bureau persisted and denied the Harris plan of at least feeding these desperate people.[43]

On July 11, 1868, Dr. De Lamater was told to close all remaining Freedmen's Bureau hospitals in Virginia and turn patients in need of continued care over to community care. There were obvious problems with this plan. No hospital was integrated by race, and the impoverished state of Virginia was in no financial condition to take on new construction. And as Reconstruction gradually faded and former Confederates resumed control of government—in Virginia as in other southern states—there was little political will to care for the freedpeople. Patients were first consolidated into two hospitals: one in Richmond and one in Hampton.[44]

These choices (rather than blanket closure) suggested that at least a minimal well of compassion persisted among the Virginia medical bureaucracy. The area around Fort Monroe had the largest Freedmen's Hospital, and it remained open. The medical bureaucracy decided to gather all remaining Freedmen's Bureau patients to hospitals in the Richmond area. This included the cluster of patients diagnosed with insanity. They had originally been sent to the old mental hospital at Williamsburg, then to Howard's Grove (perhaps when Harris was briefly in charge), and then finally the remnant to the federal mental hospital in Washington, DC. Even the bureau's chief medical officer realized that "of course none of the insane inmates can be discharged until a proper place is provided for them.... The aged, permanently disabled etc. must necessarily be included in the same category." This bit of common kindness was countered by the opening lines of the letter, addressed to Dr. De Lamater in late September 1869. In the best military bureaucratese, it said, "Your attention is respectfully called to the fact that Winter is fast approaching and that it would be a most inappropriate season for discharging patients from your hospital." So, he should discharge them now, dropping the population down to no more than 150 patients.[45] It is ironic that the last remnant of patients from the Freedmen's Bureau hospitals in Virginia was sent to the Freedmen's Hospital in Washington, DC. It is possible that patients who had known J. D. Harris in Virginia might again have met him in Washington, where he was an attending physician at this hospital. But we are getting ahead of our story.

THE 1869 ELECTION

As was true for other southern states, Reconstruction brought great political upheaval in Virginia. The Confederate government of the state was condemned as rebellious, and various aspiring replacement politicians, corrupt or well-meaning, poured into the state to fill the political vacuum. One such was Horace Wells of Michigan. A former US Army colonel who happened to be stationed in Richmond after the war, he became General John Schofield's appointee for military governor in the state while the reversion to civilian control was negotiated. In order to return to the Union, the state had to accept the abolition of slavery, accept the franchise for Black men, and vote in the new constitution that established allegiance to the federal government. Any adult males in Virginia who wished to vote had to swear fealty to the Union and disavow all support for the defeated Confederacy. This included newly liberated male slaves, most of them illiterate. Outsiders came to Richmond, either as leaders in the occupying army or as "carpetbaggers" on the make, seeking to find fortune in Richmond's ruins. The many teachers and preachers of the American Missionary Association were there, working to educate the freedpeople. The first gubernatorial election under the new regime occurred on July 6, 1869, on a ballot that included accepting or denying the new constitution.[46]

The prewar Democratic Party was the party of rebellion and the mainstay of the Confederacy; as its members were excluded from politics at this point, the politicians available to form the new government were former Whigs and new Republicans. While the Republican Party prevailed in numbers, it was not uniform in its politics. Some favored Radical Reconstruction, with full liberation of the Black population, public works such as schools and hospitals to help them transition to full citizenship, and protection under the law with unbiased judges. These rights were in accord with the goals of the Freedmen's Bureau, especially the provision of courts to hear cases in which whites abused Black people in property or labor dealings. Others, who called themselves Conservative Republicans or later True Republicans, argued for restoring order and white rule, as well as a return to the stability of Black people in a status as close to slavery as possible. Such legislation would bring prosperity and the end of wartime hardships, they believed.[47]

The Radical Republicans favored Horace Wells, the military governor, for the civilian governor role, even though he was already embroiled in charges of financial corruption involving the construction of railroads and other matters.[48] This reputation, and his carpetbagger origins, made him unpopular with the Conservative Republicans, who nominated someone more sympathetic to their point of view. Their man, Gilbert C. Walker, while also a northerner, was touted as more honest and beneficent than Wells.

Thus, it came to pass that in the spring of 1869 the Republicans gathered at a Black church in Petersburg to discuss whom they would nominate for governor, lieutenant governor, and other high offices in the state. It was the "most disorderly and scandalous assemblage ever held in Virginia!" the (opposition) newspaper headlines cried. Delegates yelled to get the floor, pushed others away from the podium, and jeered when the other side began speaking. They fought over whether delegate representation by county should be proportionate to Black population. They argued about who were proper delegates. They disputed who should chair the meeting and how long each person got to talk. Deputy US marshals and the local police struggled to prevent outright riot. And everyone shouted, "Out of order!"[49]

The Conservatives tried to nominate their own man, but that failed. Wells was the nominee, by acclamation. Those in the Wells faction wanted Henry C. Taylor of Montgomery, Virginia, as their choice for lieutenant governor—but he had to be first nominated to, and then elected by, the convention.[50] It seems the Wells faction never even got a chance to put up his name. The first nominee was Dr. W. W. C. Douglas, of Richmond County, a former Confederate surgeon. And then Black activist Lewis Lindsay grabbed the floor and nominated "Dr. J. D. Harris (mulatto) of Hampton."[51] The question was called; Harris received 85 votes to Douglas's 31. He was thereby chosen by a combination of Black delegates—and politically conservative white ones. Why did the most racist, pro-Confederacy delegates vote for a man of African descent? Because the plan was to weaken Wells with this choice and thus instead elect their preferred candidate, Walker, for governor.

Lindsay was a former slave who probably knew nothing of this devious plot, as he was a firebrand Radical Republican who was always pushing the Republican government to move faster and more completely on issues of equal rights for the freedmen. He was also known for having a hot temper, and at times alcohol contributed to his love of rowdy political demonstrations. One suspects he was urged on to make the nomination by politicians who hid their real motivation (that is, creating a losing Wells ticket) and instead emphasized that it was a great opportunity to raise a Black man to political power. The state also had a US Senate seat to fill, an appointment then in the hands of the state legislature. Why, if Wells was sent to the Senate by the legislature, then Harris would become governor![52]

Indeed, the Harris nomination was widely applauded by the African American delegates. Dr. Bayne said, "The time has come for black men. We are going to have black men on every ticket, and we tell you that if you don't put them on[,] we will split your tickets as sure as there is a God in glory." And Harris was an exemplary man, an educated man. He had served his government as a surgeon in the army. Then, "a negro delegate" said, "The time has come to treat black men without regard to skin or color. [*Applause loud and long*]." Harris was not recorded in the newspaper report as speaking, but one can imagine how thrilled he felt as this acclamation overran the crowd. After more speeches, Harris was duly nominated.[53]

A reporter for the *Richmond Whig* (no friend of the freedpeople) summed up the proceedings. "The Radical state Convention, after a turbulent, disorderly and unharmonious session of two days has at length adjourned," he sighed. "Both factions which took part in its disgraceful proceedings are perfectly aware of the utter weakness of the ticket nominated."[54] This correspondent reported multiple rumors of graft, evident in both sides buying delegate votes. He himself saw a poorly dressed Black man with a twenty-dollar bill, a large denomination for one in evident poverty. The Wells contingent must have bought that Black vote, he concluded, while at the same time planning a whole slate of white men to accompany the governor into office. But a member of the opposition told the reporter that "the Wells party were to receive a vital stab where they least expected it." Members of the anti-Wells partisans had finagled the Harris nomination for lieutenant governor, and the Black delegates raised "a jubilee over the prospect of at last doing the black men justice by putting one upon the ticket."[55] It was too late to convince them of a "better" white candidate.

The manipulation of the Black delegates is clear in retrospect but was less apparent at the time. Harris was said to have accepted the nomination "with a solemnity of tone and earnestness of expression that warmed the colored brethren toward him." The anti-Wells delegates pictured the services of Harris as a surgeon in the hospitals during the rebellion, nursing poor wounded Union soldiers, while his opponent, as a rebel surgeon, "had his collars decorated with stars that vied with Venus, Queen of the Night."[56] Not surprisingly, the "effect was electric," and delegates "stampeded to Harris." There were rumors that the Wells supporters, despairing of this choice, began to conspire to kill or at least kidnap Harris. This roused the Black voters even more in his favor. "After this nomination of Harris, the [white] Wells faction became completely demoralized." If we remember that the reporter was not a man to favor Black elevation, it is still clear what a clever ruse the Wells opposition

FOR CONSTITUTION.

For Governor.
H. H. WELLS, of Alexandria.

For Lt. Governor,
Dr. J. D. HARRIS, of Hampton

For Attorney General,
THOMAS R. BOWDEN, of Richmond.

For Congressman at Large
A. M. CRANE, of Winchester,

For Congress 7th District,
CHARLES WHITTLESEY.

For State Senator 3rd District,
J. J. ROBINSON.

For House of Delegates,
Orange County,
Wm. B. SANFORD.

Republican candidate card for the 1869 election in Virginia.
Courtesy of Library of Virginia.

had pulled off. As he reported, "I heard no one say that the ticket is a strong one, but heard a number of Republicans declare that it was the weakest that could have been nominated."[57]

The most stridently conservative newspaper, the Richmond *Daily Enquirer and Examiner* (hereafter *E&E*), covered the election closely and revealed much about Harris the candidate and Wells, his unwilling partner. "We hear that the WELLS people are a good deal annoyed," the paper reported on March 15, 1869.[58] Over time the paper printed several, at times contradictory, biographical blurbs of Dr. Harris. He was "a ginger-bread colored negro, was born in North Carolina, carried North when a child, raised and educated in Cleveland, Ohio, studied medicine and graduated at a Cleveland institute. During the war he was a doctor in the Freedmen's Bureau."[59] With no note of inconsistency, it reprinted a *Norfolk Examiner* piece four days later, which claimed that Dr. Harris "hails from Hampton, [Virginia,] where he's been living for some years. He is a native of Jamaica, and is a firm believer in the doctrine of miscegenation, having at some period of his life taken to himself a white wife with whom he is now living."[60] The next day, the *E&E* revealed that Mrs. Harris was a "Yankee school-marm" from New Jersey.[61] Yet another biographical account claimed, "Dr. Harris [was] formerly a resident of Mr. Lewis Marshall's plantation, in Fauquier county."[62] It seems the *E&E* editors did not read their own newspaper.

By the end of April, the newspaper's tone began to shift. "It will, perhaps, be necessary to state that Mr. Harris is a colored gentleman, whose scholarship, ability and personal character are unobjectionable."[63] The paper pointed to the irony of the Wells Republicans disliking the nomination, when supposedly they were the ones who were all about Black elevation. In the complexity of this political climate, the paper's strategy was to disparage Wells by praising Harris. This threw the anti-Black faction of the Wells supporters into an inconsistency. These Republicans were "violently opposed to the ticket, because about one part in four of Mr. Harris is negro. The action of these so-called Republicans shows them to be a class of politicians who desire to be hoisted into place and power by the vote of the colored man" while denying him all privileges except voting. It remained to be seen, noted the newspaper, whether the 101,000 colored voters would see through this treatment.[64]

A "Colored Convention" of Virginians met at the end of May 1869. Harris, already the lieutenant governor nominee, was called to the podium to address the convention. One newspaper account said of him, "He is [a] bright mulatto of respectable appearance, and his intelligence cannot be denied." "Bright" is used here to mean "light-skinned." That reporter went on to say, "He is not much of an orator, but possesses a remarkable aptness for illustration by anecdote, and is an interesting talker." I suppose that the reporter meant that he did not shout loudly enough or clearly enough, as the content of the speech was not impugned. On the other hand, his politics followed the Radical Republican line, which the reporter did not favor: "His speech was thoroughly radical, and he counselled his hearers to act upon the principle that they should trust their own race, however ignorant, over the perhaps duplicitous whites." He quoted Harris as proclaiming, "Trust no white man unless he showed by his deeds that he was in earnest! ... [They] must contend for every right that would make the colored man equal, as he deserved to be." Harris affirmed the conference's choice in nominating a Black man; it was a much better strategy than the semi-Confederate doctor presented as an alternative.[65]

Another report on the convention appeared in the May 29, 1869, *E&E*, giving a different emphasis regarding Harris's speech:

> He consumed about three quarters of an hour in a talk in a conversational tone of voice, in the course of which he related many anecdotes, some of them very good and very much to the point. He said little about the canvass, but remarked that he had heard it said that many white Republicans intended to *scratch* their tickets and not vote for him for Lieutenant Governor. He said the negroes had 101,000 votes in the State, and that the white [Radical] Republican vote was about 10,000. If Wells should be elected and he defeated, the colored people would know that the white Republicans didn't intend to allow a colored man to have an office if they could prevent it, and it would be the duty of the colored men to watch and hold them to a strict accountability for their votes in the election.[66]

From this point on, articles in the *E&E* were fairly positive about Harris, all the more to emphasize the fact that Wells had not accepted his own running mate. If Wells was telling voters to scratch through Harris's name and write in another, then he was a scoundrel. The paper's goal was to anger the Black voters against Wells because of his treatment of "poor Harris."[67]

Wells had no choice but to accept his running mate, but he did not have to like him or even be outwardly friendly to him. Harris did not campaign with Wells, nor did he ever visit the governor's mansion. Where and how Harris campaigned is unknown. In the meantime, the conservative opposition from the Republican convention coalesced into a party called the "True Republicans" and nominated a slate against the Radical Republicans. These were the two opposing parties in the 1869 election. While Wells and Harris rather assumed they owned the Black vote, the opposition made a great pitch for it as well, emphasizing how crooked Wells was in his railroad and other business dealings.

The True Republicans and their newspapers jumped on the story that Wells would not entertain Harris at the governor's mansion. Remember that Wells was the acting military governor of the state until the election's conclusion. There was a meeting of Radical Republicans on June 2, 1869, and the question was posed: "Why didn't he [Wells] invite to his house and entertain, while he was in the city, Dr. Harris the nominee for Lieutenant Governor, on the same ticket as himself, instead of allowing him to find quarters at a negro boarding house on Broad St.?" The response? "The interrogatory was a bombshell." A riot followed, requiring the sheriff and appearances before the magistrate for brawling.[68]

The *E&E* had great fun with this story three weeks later. "We have at last an answer to our question why Gov. Wells does not invite his associate (Dr. Harris) [parentheses in original] on the Radical ticket to his house. Wells in a moment of unusual candor has met the enquiry—for which we heartily thank him. We like to understand things, and then we can get along," the paper said agreeably. Wells "admits that he has not invited Harris to his house—although Harris was in Richmond the other day at the State Negro Convention." His answer was to harken back to his predecessor Governor Wise, famous among other acts for hanging John Brown. Wells asked, "Did H. A. Wise, when Governor of Virginia, [allow] *every vagabond Dutchman and Irishman* with whom he acted during the Know-Nothing canvass to stick *their legs* under his mahogany? *Social intercourse* is a matter of taste, and I don't choose to invite Harris to my house."[69]

The newspaper responded with faux indignity: "Don't choose to invite Harris to your house? The Dutch then, and the Irish are 'vagabonds,' and Harris who is on your ticket for Lieutenant Governor, is no better?" The writer was outraged. "Did you know sir, that Harris, colored though he be like Frederick Douglass, drives about, and practices his honorable profession, in a newly painted top-buggy, with new harness, and a sleek, well-fed horse? Are *you* good enough to get 100,000 negro votes, and too good to ask the colored Lieutenant Governor to your table?" Wells had preached equality to Blacks, the writer reminded him. "If Dr. Harris is good enough to be the second officer in this Commonwealth, are you who are looking to *his* race for your promotion to the first office, too good to break a loaf of bread with him?"[70] On the other hand, the writer pointed out amiably, if Wells wanted to argue that all Blacks were vagabonds and unworthy in the state house, then the newspaper was fine with that conclusion. The editors thought so too.

The *E&E* editorial continued to lambaste Wells. "What title have *you* to the Executive Mansion of this proud State? Elevated over the heads of the descendants of the Jeffersons, the Henries, the Randolphs, the Lees. What title have you? Who gave you your commission to run for this office? Who but Dr. Harris and his race?" So, what right did Wells have to judge the Blacks unworthy? With Cassius he wondered, "On what meat hast this Caesar fed that he is grown so fat?"[71] In the referenced scene from Shakespeare's *Julius Caesar*, Cassius is asking why Caesar had been elevated when much better men, from better families, had been left behind.

The July 6, 1869, election was hotly contested; 82 percent of eligible voters cast a ballot. The True Republican Party won the day, with Wells losing by more than 18,000 votes. Harris came in 20,668 votes behind the True Republican candidate, although he did garner 99,400 votes, about 45 percent of those cast.[72] His final known foray into politics came in the fall of 1869, when he was nominated for the position of US senator by a friend in the Reconstruction state legislature. Harris received only 3 votes, while the other two candidates received 20 and 10.[73] With both events, J. D. Harris became the first African American male to run for elected office in the American South.

Although we have no direct report of Harris's emotional state during these tumults, some of his indignation at the shoddy treatment during the campaign comes through newspaper accounts. "Dr. Harris, Well's [sic] associate, demands that hotels in Virginia shall be open to Negroes. Will Mr. Wells define *his* position on this question?" asked the *E&E*.[74] We know Harris had to stay in a segregated boardinghouse in Richmond as no white hotel would take a Black man—no matter how well dressed or politically elevated. He met similar insult after purchasing two second-class tickets on the *Mystic* steamer for himself and his sister Kate on June 17, 1869. But such compartments were reserved for whites, he was told. They would have to stand outside. Harris was not the first, nor of course would he be the last, to demand equal treatment for African Americans on public transportation.[75] Unlike Alexander Augusta, who fought such conventions on streetcars in Washington, DC, and Baltimore, Harris did not have military police on hand to force the breaking of "time-honored" segregation rules. Nor was he connected to Henry Wilson, a Massachusetts senator who brought Augusta's matter to the floor of the Senate.[76] And this was not wartime, when a military uniform commanded respect. Instead of calling for military or political intervention, apparently Dr. Harris did say he would take the matter (and a prior such event, on the steamer *Eliza Hancock*) to court. I wonder whether having his sister as a witness to the degradation made it all the worse. No doubt he wanted his family to be proud of his achievements.[77]

He was dressed as a gentleman, if we can go by the photograph taken in February 1868: suit, tie, neatly trimmed beard. His occupation required a professional degree and carried respect. He was even a candidate for high state office. But none of these markers of class could make him a gentleman—at least according to a Norfolk paper, which revisited the outrage a few days later. In an article labeled "Social Equality," the paper began, "The other day the aspiring 'gentleman of color,' who looks forward to the day when he shall preside over the Senate of Virginia, and succeed Wells in the mansion once filled by the noblest, and purest, and best of our Statesmen . . ." At this point the newspaper man stopped for breath, overwhelmed by the impossibility that a colored man could be a gentleman, much less governor of the state. The story then continued with the events on the *Mystic*, saying that the captain "put an end for the present to his social ambition." Such vanity, such entitlement, was on display in every quarter where Black men had the reins of government, the article continued. In Haiti, for example, the paper claimed that the government was offended when President Ulysses S. Grant appointed a Black man as the US emissary there. Only a *white* man would be high enough for the Haitian government's standards. "Thus Harris, in Virginia, and [President Sylvan] Salnave in Haiti, demand equality with the white race." This could only be stopped, the paper concluded, if every Black demand for equality was met by the cool rejection shown by the bold white captain on the *Mystic*.[78]

The nomination for lieutenant governor was undoubtedly an honor; that moment when he accepted the accolade at the convention in Petersburg must have been highly gratifying. As far as can be told, he held his head up high despite his running mate's scorn. If his job was to appeal to the Black voters, then so be it. If, by his calculation, there were 10,000 white Republicans and 101,000 Black ones, it looks likely that he lost all the whites but only 11,000 Blacks. Yes, it was a loss, but still almost 100,000 people in the state of Virginia acclaimed him as their candidate.

In bouncing back from the despair of John Brown and the failure of his Haiti hopes, Harris came to Virginia fresh out of medical school with a fertile field of service before him. He would elevate his brothers, all right—not out of slavery through armed revolt or by bringing them to Haiti to form a new empire but by healing their bodies from disease and letting their souls grasp the full meaning of the new freedom. We cannot know of the day-to-day slights that would have continually reminded him of his low status in at least some white eyes. Still, the government treated him with a key form of respect, namely a monthly paycheck for the professional work he was doing. Some white men appeared to validate his status as a somber, learned gentleman suitable for state government. And a white woman from New Jersey had the determination and grit to take him as her husband despite the massive cultural imperative against their union. Her love must have been strong indeed. It would be sorely tested in the decade to come, but for the moment we will leave them in that "third house on the right-hand side from the Hampton Bridge," as Dr. Harris returned to his Freedmen's Bureau hospital, where one suspects he was always welcomed by the patients.

10

Finding a Professional Home

After the election loss in July 1869, Harris continued to practice at the Hampton Freedmen's Hospital until his contract expired a few months later. He might have made some money tending to the Black families in the area who could afford to pay, but there were probably not enough of them to support his family. It is likely that Mrs. Elizabeth (Worthington) Harris did not work after her marriage; proper gentlewomen did not, as a rule. What happened next is open to speculation. William D. Harris, J. D.'s brother, was living in Charleston, South Carolina, at this time, which may have been an incentive for J. D. and Elizabeth to move to that state where fewer people would be so aware of the humiliating outcome of the election. At any rate, his political fame must have done him some good, as Radical Republican legislators in South Carolina recommended him for a job as assistant superintendent at the state lunatic asylum in Columbia.[1]

Little formal education in psychiatry was available in mid-nineteenth-century America. Physicians governed the institutions and learned on the job. It is possible that in his few weeks at Howard's Grove Hospital outside of Richmond, Harris had experience with the mentally ill freedpeople assigned to that facility. The most progressive form of psychiatric care at the time involved creating an orderly environment with good nutrition, comfort, and exercise. The older methods of punishment or restraint were no longer considered standard. But the South Carolina asylum was in such miserable repair that none of these positive techniques were possible. The hospital was poorly heated in winter, the stalls that held the patients were squalid and filthy, and there was never enough food. These problems had existed before the Civil War; funding decreased during wartime and dwindled even further with the collapse of the postwar economy.

Politicians treated staffing the asylum as one of the plums of office, and turnover often occurred with change of administrations. This was certainly the case when the Radical Republicans took over South Carolina during Reconstruction. In 1868 they voted to give control over the asylum to the governor, allowing him to appoint all the positions, including the regents who had once been in charge. At first, John W. Parker, superintendent since 1837, remained in office. But in February 1870, the regents named Dr. J. D. Harris of Virginia to be the assistant superintendent, secretary, and treasurer, and another Black man to the role of steward.

The terms of his appointment as assistant superintendent were quite generous, as reported in the minutes of the Board of Regents, minutes that Dr. Harris himself kept as the recording secretary. On February 24, 1870, the board first removed prior attendant and secretary, Dr. Cornwell. Then the trustees "moved that the Governor be requested to appoint Dr. J. D. Harris to the offices of Asst. Physician, 'Head Attendant' and Sec[retar]y treasurer which offices are duly merged into *one* at a salary of fifteen hundred dollars a year, house rent and rations." They also approved a servant for him at $300 a year. In April they discussed the contract for building a house for the assistant surgeon, to be 1,140 square feet.[2] (Housing was likely scarce, as Columbia was, famously, burned after Sherman's march through the city in 1865.) Mrs. Elizabeth Harris wrote a friend at the American Missionary Association about the asylum job and its implications. She reported, "The Doctor is Asst Physician-Head Attendant Treasurer & Secretary in our State Lunatic Asylum—at a salary of $2000 & quite encouraging prospects for the future. I know that you will heartily sympathise with any advancement he may make."[3] Although she might have been putting a gloss on the situation to impress her friend, still it sounds like the couple was quite pleased with the appointment. Her expansion of the salary may likewise reflect mere amplification or be the sum of the actual salary, servant salary, house rent, and other allowances from the job.

The asylum's management swirled amid the broader political maelstrom of South Carolina's Reconstruction. As the postwar economy crashed, public institutions like the asylum deteriorated accordingly. Payment was supposed to come from families who could afford it or from the patient's county if that person was indigent. But with little money coming from those sources, the Reconstruction government of 1870 shifted costs from counties to the state. Now that counties had no fiscal responsibility, their leaders felt free to send to the asylum many mentally disabled former slaves who once would have been kept on the plantation. The Freedmen's Bureau hospital system had been the first to take these folk in, but now that it was shutting down, those unfortunate individuals were transferred to the state asylum.

This population transition in turn helped justify the political steps of putting Black people on the governing board and hiring an African American physician. As historian Peter McCandless summarized,

> The changes at the asylum enraged and alarmed many white South Carolinians. When the new regents were appointed, the *Columbia Daily Phoenix* accused the legislature of sacrificing the insane to the political spoils system and putting their care into the hands of "colored men, and others equally unfitted for their parts." At bottom, the Conservatives' objections to the new regime were based on racial as much as on medical concerns. Many whites feared that the new board, with its black majority, would use its power to mix the races and put the white patients under the control and care of blacks. These apprehensions seemed realized when the new regents appointed blacks to the positions of assistant physician and steward.[4]

Six months later Dr. Joshua Ensor took Parker's place as superintendent.[5] Ensor found the asylum in deplorable condition. "On taking charge of this Institution, August 5, I found it far behind the times, in almost everything that is now considered necessary in a well-appointed Asylum, and many improvements must be made upon it before it can take rank with other Institutions in this country for the insane." He even noted that a visitor found the asylum to be the worst in the country, save one.[6] Ensor appealed again and again for adequate funds to feed, clothe, and house his patients, to little avail.

For the Harris family, life in Columbia held many of the same tensions as in Virginia, and perhaps more so. Famously, General W. T. Sherman either did or did not deliberately set fire to Columbia in the last fall of the war; in any event the town burned, and bitterness against the Yankees and all their works flamed. Daily the landscape declared not only defeat but destruction.

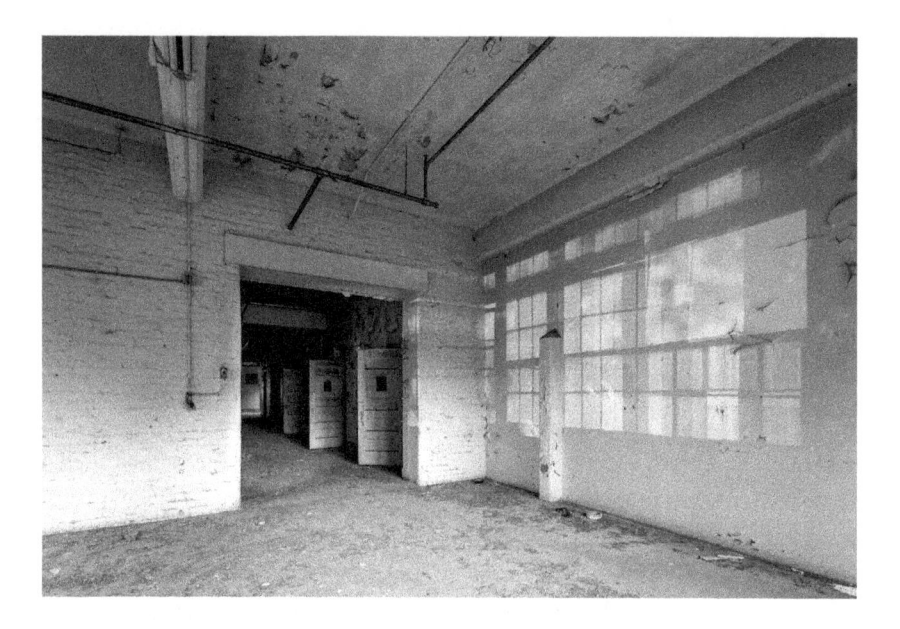

Modern photograph of the interior of Babcock Building, South Carolina Lunatic Asylum, Columbia (now South Carolina State Hospital). The series of doors show the small size of the cells in which patients were housed. Courtesy of Amy Heiden.

There were multiple ongoing philanthropic endeavors to elevate and educate the former slaves, just the kind of work Elizabeth did for the AMA. But the AMA itself was not there. Her husband worked long hours, leaving her alone with perhaps only a servant. In a letter to an AMA friend, she urged a visit. "Columbia is a beautiful town—notwithstanding its devastations by war— and should you ever visit it remember us. It is delightful here in spring & it is a summer resort for wealthy families of Charleston & neighboring towns. I believe you have no teachers in Columbia but you may have occasion to pass through it in visiting other localities where you have schools."[7]

There was a further isolating event to consider, even if it was a blessed one. Sometime in midsummer 1870, Elizabeth realized she was pregnant, and in early fall she would have started "showing." No proper woman would leave the house, or even receive visitors, while she was in such a delicate condition. In Hampton Elizabeth had a circle of friends made over the past few years, at least some of whom probably accepted her biracial marriage. But it is certain that she was scorned by the community of white southern Christian women in Columbia, however impoverished by the war's devastation. She was a Yankee of course, and even worse a Yankee woman married to a Black man. Such women were seen as "of the lowest class," according to one history of the period. Their marriages were excoriated in the newspapers and sometimes met with violence.[8]

Miscegenation was a deep societal fear in the aftermath of abolition. Political opponents had used the supposed Republican promotion of interracial marriage as a campaign accusation against Lincoln in 1864. Historian Joel Williamson has argued that at its core, this fear was always about Black men marrying, raping, or bedding white women. White men had been raping Black women as part of the accepted power hierarchy of slavery since the colonies were born. This behavior might be derided by patrician women such as Mary Chesnutt (whose father-in-law had multiple biracial offspring serving him on the family's plantation), but such racial mixing was commonplace and often accepted. J. D.'s father, Jacob, in fact, was the product of just such a slave owner/slave woman pairing.

A year before Elizabeth first recognized the pregnancy, the supreme court of neighboring Georgia explicitly prohibited the marriage between white and Black persons and declared such marriages null and void.[9] As the months went by, her visible belly may have exacerbated the horror of those viscerally opposed to miscegenation. One might ignore events that happened behind closed doors, but her physical shape testified that she was indeed married to J. D. in word and in action. Daughter Worthie was born on March 11, 1871. The details of delivery and support during the childbirth are unrecorded. Probably, J. D. delivered his own daughter.

Offering Dr. and Mrs. Harris some companionship was his brother William and his family. By November 1868 William was in Charleston, where he was a minister and teaching a freedmen's school. Daughter Lottie was with him.[10] Bishop Daniel Payne, head of the African Methodist Episcopal Church, moved William again in the new year. In February 1869 William wrote the AMA, "Having been assigned to duty in Columbia by our Bishop & Conference I find a large field of missionary work. My daughter who has been teaching successfully in Charleston since May (as I desire to have her with me), is now out of employment." He tried again to get the AMA to hire her and to renew his own commission. He said of the Howard School in Columbia that it was supported by several different associations, and his letter describes a substantial northern presence in the schools of the town.[11] (Multiple schools that opened for newly freed slaves were named after O. O. Howard, commissioner of the Freedmen's Bureau). He perhaps hoped to shame the AMA into also supporting this school, which might have led to his daughter's employment there.[12]

The 1870 census has the William Harris family together in Columbia.[13] The family stayed in South Carolina until 1874, when William took ill with a disease labeled "typhoid dysentery" and soon died, at the age of forty-seven. Typhoid fever was spread via water supplies contaminated with infected feces. Public health workers in the North were already absorbing knowledge from Britain that both explained the disease and its prevention through water purity. But the American South was always behind in such urban improvement designs, as was evident when American troops fell ill of typhoid in droves on their way to fight in Cuba in 1898. Sanitary public water supply systems only began to be instituted in the South in the 1910s and 1920s. Typhoid contamination of wells remained common in the rural South well into the 1960s.[14] William's death was but one indicator that his siblings were unfortunately liable to waterborne disease, as will be discussed later. When William died, he left wife Kitty with four children to support, all of whom lived in Columbia. At least here was a household where Elizabeth would have been "received." Whether Kitty's attitude toward the marriage was frosty or warm, it seems likely that they had some social interaction. William died intestate, so Kitty applied for the right to administer his estate.[15] As we shall see later in the chapter, J. D. and William had invested in Washington, DC, real estate together in the early 1870s, a venture that caused rancor between the two families in later years.

In April 1870, just a few weeks after assuming his South Carolina asylum duties, J. D. Harris took a leave of absence from the hospital, for unknown reasons. The Board of Regents continued his salary with no reduction.[16] Harris was back in June, when he signed the monthly meeting notes, and was present for the rest of the year. The summer was calm, and he cared for all the patients routinely, both Black and white. Nobody seemed alarmed by the arrangement until Dr. Joshua Ensor's arrival as the new superintendent in August. Ensor was outraged that a Black man should treat white persons, especially white women. He reported to the board that the patients found Harris distasteful. Harris resisted but finally resigned, rather than being officially fired, effective February 1, 1871 (with full pay until then).[17]

In the words of Henry Thompson, a historian sympathetic to the Confederate perspective, "The first attempt to apply the doctrine of equal social rights to the public institutions of the State was made, in [Governor Robert K.] Scott's administration, with the State Lunatic Asylum. The board of regents, composed of whites and negroes, sought to have an assistant physician of the institution, who was a negro, treat the white as well as the negro patients."

Scott was, not surprisingly, a Republican. The same regents appointed Dr. Ensor. "Fortunately, they were defeated in their nefarious undertaking by Dr. J. F. Ensor," continued Thompson. Ensor was admittedly a Republican, "but a good man whose service in the Federal army had been creditable, and whose administration of the affairs of the State Asylum had won for him the respect and good will of everyone in the state."[18]

Infuriated by being forced out, Harris took to the public press to express his indignation: "Dr. Ensor has written a statement, now in the hands of the President of the Board of Regents, which affirms that I was relieved of my duties as Assistant Physician *solely* and *purely* because of the prejudices which exist against my color and race." His letter, appearing on the front page of the *Columbia Daily Phoenix*, continued, "On these terms I can afford to suffer both insult and injury. But whether anyone can afford to insult and injure another on account of color, is a question which time will determine. Respectfully yours, J. D. Harris, M.D."[19]

It was racism, pure and simple, but medicine is a very personal business. Some patients in my own Duke primary care practice could not imagine receiving a pelvic exam from a male physician, and some women from very conservative religious faiths would not disrobe at all in front of a male. The patient exposes his or her body to a stranger in the setting of a special professional relationship that makes such behavior possible and appropriate. This is often uncomfortable for the modest person in general; it can be even more difficult if the doctor is of a different gender, race, or nationality. Female nurses in the Civil War struggled with the appropriateness of soldier-patient nakedness and conquered it with metaphors invoking family ties, such as mother and son.[20] But a Black man treating a white woman was, for some, the same as rape. Harris would claim the privilege of his profession provided a shield against impropriety, but social repugnance at Black hands on a white female body was too much for many if not most nineteenth-century Americans. The common tropes of Black men as being oversexed and lusting after white women were just too strong.[21]

ON TO THE DISTRICT OF COLUMBIA

The J. D. Harris family left Columbia after the asylum job ended. And with it, of course, went the right to live in the nice new house. They moved to Washington, DC, near the buildings of Howard University in the northeast section of the District. There they bought a house on the corner of Seventh and Boundary Streets. This area had already become a magnet for middle-class

Blacks, and particularly for African American physicians. By 1870 there was a Black medical association, founded by Alexander Augusta, head of Howard's medical school. It was the center of political maneuvering to acquire recognition by the American Medical Association, or to force the local white society to admit the Black doctors into its circle. Here Harris could revive his passion for political action after the defeats in the South. His old friend Charles Purvis was part of it as well.[22] In DC Harris found political excitement, a return to legitimacy as a salaried doctor in the hospital, and respectable connections for his wife. Nowhere else in America was there such an aggregation of educated, professional Black men who would have shared many of J. D.'s ideas and perspectives.

The large concentration of African Americans was one reason this cluster of middle-class educated families could thrive. In 1860 there were 14,316 "colored" persons counted in the DC census; almost 78 percent of them were already free. Once President Lincoln ordered that all slaves in the District of Columbia be freed on April 16, 1862, the District became a major target for slaves fleeing Virginia and Maryland. By 1870 there were 43,404 people of color living in DC, many of them destitute.[23] The District was also the place where the federal government invested in national institutions, such as the Smithsonian Institution and St. Elizabeths Hospital, which served not only paying psychiatric patients but also mentally ill soldiers from all states and the citizens of the District who needed mental health care. As historian Martin Summers has noted, St. Elizabeths was at once a local and a national institution. In 1862 the government established the first Freedmen's Bureau hospital to care for the many fugitive and freed slaves who had fallen ill in the miserable freedmen's camps in the DC area.[24] Probably most important for the area's medical men was the diversion of funds (legally or not) from the Freedmen's Bureau to help pay for the creation of Howard University, including Howard Medical School and Freedmen's [later Howard] Hospital. These institutions were all seen as national, and not just for local inhabitants. It is no accident that the Harris family bought a house near the school's boundary, an address that has now been absorbed into today's Howard University footprint. Howard University became the center of Black medical care and education in the District.

The middle-class population of educated African Americans created a nexus of friendship and support for the Harris family. Brother William had been an AME preacher in Georgetown not long before, and some of his congregants no doubt called upon Mrs. Dr. Harris. At the university and the medical school, J. D. found old friend John Mercer Langston, now dean of Howard University Law School. Langston, like Harris, was light-skinned and had been a leader in the "Colored Convention" and abolitionist movement in Ohio. Located in Cleveland, Langston and his brother Charles had been key agents in the Wellington rescue and in drumming up local support for John Brown's raid. If not beforehand, Dr. Harris certainly made the acquaintance of Alexander Augusta, dean of Howard Medical School and founder of the local African American Medical Society. The established Black community in northeast Washington, DC, having the largest group of "people like him" in the country, became a safe harbor for the J. D. Harris family. And Mrs. Dr. Harris made friends with Mrs. J. M. Langston, likewise finding acceptance and culture in her circles.

Family memory says that Dr. Harris was a professor at Howard Medical School in these years and that he specialized in teaching obstetrics.[25] He certainly was a practicing physician, as he purchased a professional listing in the city directory for the District of Columbia. In the 1875 volume, he is under the physician listing with an address of "7th nr Howard Univ."[26] This is the same as his home address, so perhaps he set up a consulting room on the first floor. Harris is not listed on the faculty of Howard Medical School in school catalogs from 1871–72 and 1873–74 (if there was a catalog for 1872–73, it is missing now). The definitive history of the school, which details the lecture schedule during the early 1870s, does not include him. Charles Purvis, another African American physician whom we met in an earlier chapter, was the professor of obstetrics in these years.[27]

What did J. D. Harris do to make a living in Washington, DC? First, he had a private practice in his house. Second, he was hired to be a "ward physician" at the Freedmen's Hospital associated with Howard Medical School (about which more below). So, he could admit his private patients to the Freedmen's Hospital if need be. This was one of the structural barriers that limited African American physicians elsewhere. Anyone with a medical license could set up practice, but having "admitting privileges" to a hospital was key to full patient care. Third, he managed his wife's business affairs and investments. Elizabeth Worthington Harris was the only surviving sibling of her generation, and her father gifted her with a modest amount of wealth after her marriage. While her father was alive, J. D. took over the management of some of Mr. Worthington's investments as well. Elizabeth would later discover that her husband had put some of those properties solely in *his* name without telling her. He also made other investments in the stock market and life insurance.[28]

Two key sources give us insight into J. D. the businessman. One is the legal footprint left by several court cases concerning his financial dealings. The other comes from Elizabeth's letters to the superintendent of the asylum to which he was admitted in 1876. These letters reflected her mind and her concerns; she was paying his hospital bills and so had to justify her own handling of finances, including not always being on time with her checks. Her correspondence was sometimes inaccurate, as when she said that J. D. served and traveled with the army as a commissioned surgeon; instead, he was a contract surgeon to the army hospitals and never left the Virginia Peninsula. Likewise, at one point Elizabeth claimed his disease was brought on by failures in business, although later she said the disease *caused* the failure in business. So, keep the saltshaker handy.

Acceptance of Elizabeth's reports about their wealth is complicated by her grievance that he stole her property by putting his name on her deeds and poorly managed her business in the two years prior to his collapse. The document for the competency hearing said that "he owns jointly with your petitioner [that is, his wife] from $5000 to $6000 of real estate in this District [of Columbia] the rent of which amount to between $700 and $800, and aside from said rents he possesses about $300, of personal property consisting of household furniture."[29] The Panic of 1873 had most likely affected the value of their real estate, since failing businesses and impoverished tenants could not pay the rent owed or contract to rent at all. Mrs. Harris at some point took over the management of her father's property (perhaps while he was still alive and living with them), converting his stocks into property. They lived off rents, but only if property was rented and in good repair. Dr. Harris may have aspired to give up medical practice to become a "man of business" or in his failing judgment thought he could do so. The need for him to get to a bank or speak to a man was important to him when confined in the asylum. But then he also wanted to see the surgeon general or see members of Congress about, presumably, a new position. He had created a self-identity that merged entrepreneur with government physician, and in the asylum, he sought to rejoin these manly occupations.

"Business dealings" may well have contributed to the pressure on Dr. Harris in the years leading to his commitment. In 1874 he appeared in the District of Columbia equity court seeking payment from a man's estate for promissory notes that Harris held. The man, Thomas Walter, had purchased property using money borrowed from a second man, who in turn sold the debt to Harris. In the interim Walter had died, payments with interest had stopped, and Harris sought an order for the estate to pay the remainder.[30] This suggests that Harris may have been in the practice of investing in real estate not just by direct purchase but also by loaning money to others for purchases secured by real estate. Such practices, especially after the downturn of 1873, may have left him holding more than one piece of useless paper. The history of his business interests intertwines with the story of J. D.'s mental illness; here we shall talk about business and visit the asylum in the last chapter.

Both Elizabeth's letters and a subsequent lawsuit reveal how a once ambitious property transaction went south in a major way. Not only was the financial investment far larger than expected, but it caused a rift in the Harris marriage. In an 1877 letter to the asylum doctor, Elizabeth Harris described her differences with her husband over control of the property she brought to the marriage. "I told you yesterday that Dr. Harris refused to deed *my property to me*. Years ago, my father put his stock *in my name*, telling me to pay him the interest during his life, and at his death—give $1000 as he directed and have the rest for my own use. I once asked father (at Dr. Harris's suggestion) if I could convert it into real estate, and he said yes if I could be *certain* of the interest." At that point she handed over the stock to J. D. with the plan that he would sell it and invest in property for her. "Then the Dr. was very solicitous to take father[']s property and some of mine for a police station, the deed of which should be *in my name*. With *that* promise, I let Dr. have it *to use for me*." As we will see later, they did indeed buy that land and build or expand a police station on it. But Elizabeth's father was not done; he did not trust his son-in-law's judgment. "Meanwhile my father changed his mind & said he would prefer I should retain the stock as they always had been *paying stocks*. But as the stocks [by] then had been converted into real estate I could not disturb my father by telling him of it."[31] This put her in the uncomfortable situation of deceiving her father in order to support her husband's ventures.

The police station project became more expensive than planned. "In connection with the police station it became necessary to purchase more land and Dr. wanted more money. I promised it to him on the same condition, namely that it should be *in my name* (as my mother had always made her children *promise* that their property should always remain in their *own names*)." So now her deceased mother's ideas, feminist indeed, enter the picture. "There were buildings to be erected on this land & I had not enough money—but Dr. said that he would lend me money at ten percent." Now he was loaning money to his wife, and at a significant rate of interest! She continued, "The rent of my stores and rent from the police station should go towards paying my indebtedness to him—and he would have the back lot and alley *in his name and mine, until my rents* had completed the payments and then it should be deeded to me." That was the plan as she understood it, but he kept changing the arrangements. "He put the alley in *his* name & when the buildings were complete, he said I should *never have it all in my name[;] that my property should be his also*."[32]

These discussions raise the question: Did "coverture" persist in the laws of the District of Columbia in the 1870s? When Elizabeth Worthington married J. D. Harris, did all her property transfer to him by a law that assumed the husband controlled all of the wife's property at marriage? This was an old concept in Anglo-Saxon law and prevailed in most states at the turn of the nineteenth century. But women were increasingly pushing for reform by midcentury and had succeeded in the District of Columbia in 1869. The act announced, "The right of any married woman to any property, personal or real, belonging to her at time of marriage . . . shall not be subject to the disposal of her husband." Henceforth a wife would retain all control of her property.[33] There is no indication that Elizabeth knew about this law, although through her friendship with law professor John Mercer Langston she might have heard of it. Still, J. D.'s actions—mismanagement, theft, deception, grandiosity—all cut deeply into her affection and trust for him.

Four days later she continued, "Do not let Dr. Harris go to the city *on any pretext whatever.* There is no business that I want him to straighten. He has straightened my father and me out of nearly $10,000 all because I trusted him. Do not let him either send or receive letters until I have seen them. I will answer his letter tomorrow. If he will be willing to return to me my property he can write me to that effect. If he will not I had better not see him again."[34] A month later she quoted the opinion of Langston that Harris had "possessed himself of *one half of my own and my father's property* without my knowledge or consent."[35]

In September 1877, when Mrs. Harris had her husband declared insane and incompetent, she was able to reassert her control over the property as she was now appointed his guardian. While the challenges of maintaining solvency while paying his fees at St. Elizabeths would continue throughout his commitment, so did her anger at this betrayal. Two months before his death in 1884, Mrs. Harris asked Superintendent William Godding if it was sometimes true that the insane recover lucidity for spells as they approach the end. "If ever such is the case with Dr. Harris, will you telephone me . . . so I can go at once to see my poor husband. Perhaps he will be able to tell me what first led him to deceive me with regard to my own property. It is a comfort to me to believe that he was in a state bordering on insanity for years before he was taken. But if I am unable to reach him in time—tell him that I freely forgive him for appropriating my property."[36]

Events in the spring of 1876 may have had a more immediate impact on his mood. In her lament about the police station purchase above, Elizabeth Harris described some of the complexity of that transaction. There was more to the story, however. Not only did they purchase land but they paid to have the police station building erected (or perhaps expanded) according to an architect's plans that aligned with specific expectations supplied by the District of Columbia. This included difficulties in excavating a foundation, as it turned out to be situated over a sewer line. The basement readily flooded; initial basement walls buckled and curved; the architectural plans were not followed (and somehow lost); and much extra work was needed to bring the project to completion.[37]

The contractors claimed that Dr. Harris visited the site frequently, approved of the extra work, and said that he would cover the additional costs. One of the contractors also testified that "when Dr. Harris spoke to me about this work he told me that he was acting as agent for Mrs. Harris his wife and the co-defendant in this suit, he told me that it was his wife's money he was using, and he wanted to be as cautious as possible with it." The contractor had told Harris of the changes needed, and "all these things were done by the special orders of Dr. Harris, I told him that all this work would have to be paid for as extra and he replied that he expected nothing else." In his 1876 deposition, Dr. Harris denied that he had said any of these things.[38]

The suit was over the extra money that the contractors claimed was due them for the repairs on the construction. Dr. and Mrs. Harris had paid the amount initially agreed upon ($2,925) but still owed, according to the contractors, an additional $1,926. The court decided that the extra work was due to the fact that the contractors had proceeded in a negligent manner in the first place and ruled that the Harris couple did not owe them the overrun amount. It is interesting that in these descriptions of Dr. Harris and his behavior, there was no report of excess anger or rage of any sort. No discussion of race enters the charges and countercharges, either. Each side in this account had reason to lie for the sake of the case, but the contractor's account of Harris as a man of business, managing his wife's property and making decisions that approved the extra expense, rings true. Such a story lends credence to the claims of Mrs. Harris that his poor judgment cost them thousands of dollars in the years leading to his confinement.[39]

A further illustration of J. D.'s financial acumen (or lack thereof) appeared in court when yet another agreement was disputed. The transaction went back to 1872, when brothers William and J. D. were partners in a real estate agreement with one William H. Hunter. By 1877, when the dispute was heard in equity court, Kitty Stanley Harris was acting on behalf of her husband's estate and Elizabeth was there to represent not only her interest but the interests of her husband's estate, since by then he had been declared insane. In 1872 the Harris brothers had sold Hunter a tract of land in the "Barry Farm" area of the District of Columbia, a postwar Black settlement in Anacostia then under construction. The terms were as follows for this $1,000 lot: $5 down, day of sale; $45 thirty days later; $150 at ninety days, and then four $200 promissory notes payable yearly until settled. There was no mention of interest. These sums amount to the $1,000 purchase price. Before he died, William had J. D. act as his agent; the widow Kitty Harris had him continue this practice. It is interesting that Hunter was essentially taking out a no-interest mortgage. How common or special this was among that community is unknown. But perhaps banks were less willing to loan money to Black citizens.

The Harris brothers could not know that the Panic of 1873 would crash the money markets and cause widespread unemployment. Mr. Hunter appears to have been a victim of such financial distress, as by mid-1876 he had paid off only $416.50 of the $1,000 loan. Under the terms listed in the original promissory note, he should have paid off the loan entirely by that year. The math then gets a bit confusing, but the bottom line was that the J. D. Harris family owed the William D. Harris family $180. Elizabeth had been reluctant to go to court against Kitty ("my dear Sister") because lawyers would just add to the cost. In October 1879 she had offered to start paying off the debt at the rate of $15 a month beginning in January 1880. But she had not followed through even with that small sum. Kitty finally went to court in March 1880, four years after she had received the most recent payment on the loan. The court sided with Kitty Harris and agreed she had waited long enough. Elizabeth was ordered to pay the $180 in full, with interest, and to mortgage property if sufficient cash was not on hand.[40]

Dr. J. D. Harris and his wife, Elizabeth, may well have had other property dealings in his portfolio that did not erupt in court. But it is apparent through her letters that she lacked sufficient funds after he went into the asylum. She asked that his worn-out underwear be returned home so she could use the cloth to make underwear for their son, Thoro (born March 31, 1874). But before Harris was admitted to St. Elizabeths he worked at Howard Hospital. This takes us back in time a few years to cover this side of his life.

HOWARD HOSPITAL

The District of Columbia Freedmen's Hospital (or Freedman's Hospital, in some versions) had a complicated history. It descended from the first hospitals founded in 1862 in Washington, DC, to help care for the flood of slaves fleeing Virginia and Maryland to DC, where slavery was no longer legal. The medical care sites for the freedpeople during the war were never sufficient, and the crowded, dirty conditions of freedmen's camps led to high rates of disease. In 1865 the newly established Freedmen's Bureau took over a military hospital in LeDroit Park. O. O. Howard, the head of the Freedmen's Bureau, then built both the original Howard University structures in 1867 as well as a new hospital nearby with bureau funds. All that accomplished, O. O. Howard donated the buildings to Howard University "on the condition that they be used for the education of the freedmen." The hospital remained tied to the Freedmen's Bureau, and as other bureau hospitals closed across the South, the unfortunate patients who could not be discharged were transferred to this last refuge. Since Harris worked in several bureau hospitals in Virginia, it is possible he saw familiar faces on the DC hospital's wards.[41]

Some said that O. O. Howard went beyond his authority, in this governmental support of Howard University and its hospital. As the historians of the school put it, "A few years later, General Howard would be severely criticized for this extreme generosity to a private institution with which he was so intimately connected."[42] After an investigation, the government took the hospital back, but on the condition that it paid Howard University $5,000 of annual rent for its use. This provided a major continuing funding source for the university. The hospital cared not only for Black people but also for indigent whites of the area. It was a community hospital for DC, "a poor man's retreat," and the city paid toward its support.[43] Students from Howard Medical School attended clinical rotations in the hospital, and Howard sent postgraduate resident physicians to work there. Howard professors admitted their own patients to the facility. But wards of the hospital also had independent doctors, separate from the Howard faculty. There was intermingling—Howard faculty could lecture at the hospital and do teaching rounds; ward physicians in turn might well teach Howard students as they studied at the bedside. But the first commitment of the faculty was to the students, while the primary commitment of the ward physicians was to the patients. The hospital included male and female patients on separate wards, and it is quite possible that Harris delivered babies among his other duties.[44] He probably made around $100 a month, the same sort of salary that contract surgeons made in the army and when working for the Freedmen's Bureau.

So, when was Harris on the staff of the Freedmen's Hospital in DC? He would have moved to DC sometime in 1871, after the South Carolina asylum position ended early in the year and Mrs. Dr. Harris had time to recover from daughter Worthie's birth in March. One 1900 source with access to hospital records placed Harris in the Freedmen's Hospital from April 1 to August 1,

1873.[45] This is evidence that, yes, Harris was a physician at the hospital in those months but does not demonstrate that this was his only stretch of employment there in the first half of the 1870s. The records of the hospital for its early years are sketchy. Another piece of information suggests that Harris remained on staff at least ten more months. Times were tough after the business crash of 1873 ushered in years of depression and the hospital was short of funds. Surgeon-in-chief of the Freedmen's Hospital, Dr. G. D. Palmer, must have been aghast to learn in the spring of 1875 that his budget had been reduced by $5,000 by the secretary of the Interior for the coming fiscal year. He wrote back saying that "a saving may be made in the heating arrangements also in the subsistence and Medical Departments and in the Chaplaincy without detriment to the interests or welfare of the inmates." One wonders if those inmates would have been so optimistic. He then continued, "We can dispense with the services of ward physician Dr. J. D. Harris."[46] A year before his breakdown, Harris was again out of work.

Palmer was new in his job as surgeon-in-chief to the Freedmen's Hospital. He replaced Dr. Robert Reyburn, who had been both the first dean of Howard Medical School in 1870 and surgeon in charge of the Washington, DC, Freedmen's Hospital from 1868 to 1875. He was also professor at Georgetown Medical School and medical director of the Freedmen's Bureau in its last two years.[47] The compilation of diseases of freedpeople during Reconstruction, mentioned earlier in the discussion of smallpox in 1866, was his work. Reyburn comes into our story here because of a comment in a letter from Mrs. Dr. Harris written after Harris was confined at St. Elizabeths. "Dr. Reyburn testified that Dr. H. was losing his mind for a year before he was sunstruck, that he observed the effect of his spasms."[48]

If Reyburn's observation was correct, then we have one explanation for why Harris was not more quickly incorporated into the Howard Medical School enterprise, especially since he was a well-known figure among African American physicians. Purvis met him as a fellow student at Western Reserve Medical School in 1863–64. Augusta is likely also to have known him and sympathized with his difficult path to acceptance as an African American doctor. Certainly O. O. Howard knew of him from the Freedmen's Bureau, where he was kept on in Virginia when the hospitals shrank and merged. In that position he had a favorable reputation. But was his performance in DC already subpar? Reyburn's comment, via Mrs. Dr. Harris, is our only evidence, and it is hearsay. Once J. D. was hospitalized and his disease became more evident, then Elizabeth remembered that he had suffered spasms eleven months before the sunstroke completely disabled him. In those days she also saw him stand in the street and gesticulate wildly at nothing at all or be easily disturbed and sometimes frightening over minor issues.[49] It is rather likely that colleagues also saw some odd symptoms, and his business acumen faltered in these months preceding the major disease event.

These few years of practice in DC were the final ones of J. D. Harris's medical career. Like his brothers William and Robert, his work was cut short by severe illness. Tragically, in his case, it was his brain that suffered attack. His children would have little memory of him and his persistent search for a homeland of freedom and recognition for himself and fellow African Americans. In the next chapter we'll turn to his life in the asylum, a time we are able to glimpse intimately from his wife's letters to the asylum doctors (and a few missives from the failing man himself, offering opinions about his care). There is no moral to be drawn from this denouement of a remarkable life. The hero did not triumph as in his romantic poem, but the opponent was none so flagrant as the evil Mr. Cory. Perhaps it was a tiny creature, no bigger than a pin, who brought down this remarkable man.

11

A Roaring Fire, a Fading Light

Something dramatic happened to Dr. J. D. Harris during the mid-1870s. We know of this period mainly through letters his wife wrote to the asylum doctors where he was ultimately hospitalized, as well as through the legal documents committing him there. Many questions remain about the causation of his illness. Ever since I first saw his death certificate, which listed "chronic mania" and "epileptic apoplexy" as the causes of death, which was "instantaneous," I have wondered what exactly went wrong with his splendid intellect and fiery ambition.[1] Gradually during the mid-1870s, J. D. Harris began to change. By 1877 his wife was in despair. "When I saw you last your brain seemed all ablaze," wrote Elizabeth in 1877. "I never saw you so nervous and so restless, so irritable—and so dissatisfied. It is your *disease* that makes you so."[2] Harris was admitted to St. Elizabeths Hospital for the insane in 1876, after a weeklong episode of seizures and threats of physical violence. His wife blamed the stress of business failures, including the loss of nearly $10,000 early in the 1870s. Home was probably noisier and more crowded as well; their son, Thoro, had been born in 1874. J. D.'s moods became volatile, he was quick to anger, and more than once he attacked Elizabeth physically. He may even have made sexual advances on their female servant. His character had changed radically.

Think about the multiple stressors on this man. Most immediate was the embarrassment of being driven out of South Carolina by the resurgence of the Redeemer politicians. Before that he had lost the lieutenant governor's race in Virginia and was to some extent humiliated by those who used him to force failure on the Republican ticket. Remember his aspirations in the Haiti years and that letter of 1865 asking for service in Savannah—he had strong inclinations toward service to his race, but also a sense of superiority over that race since he was "colored," not Black. Neither emigration nor Reconstruction had worked out as he had hoped. Despite that valuable medical degree and his consequent ability to serve the freedpeople in DC, his sense of heroic identity must have been fading. He had seen the horrors of mangled bodies up close in his wartime hospital roles, as well as starving freedpeople and untreated smallpox patients forgotten by a government that was turning away from Reconstruction. Could all these stressors have combined to cause his breakdown? One African American historian at the 2014 meeting of the Society for Civil War Historians (where I presented a paper on Harris) postulated that the accumulated racism endured by any intelligent Black man who lived in the mid-nineteenth-century United States was enough to cause insanity.[3] Another sympathetic reader of the Harris story suggested his doctors just did not understand the difference between epilepsy and insanity, and Harris had only the first and not the second. In considering the Harris biography, the asylum years are among the most fascinating—as well as the saddest.

THE COLLAPSE

How did his epilepsy/insanity first emerge? According to Harris himself, it began with an episode of heatstroke. Instead, it seems likely that the first symptoms were behavioral, and it probably began in a way less obviously disease-related. Mrs. Harris described a change in her husband's behavior toward her. "The Doctor while in health was uniformly a kind considerate husband and I was quite proud of his intellect. . . . But he was in a poor way before he was sunstruck. Indeed he had spasms eleven months before, and from that time he has been *easily disturbed* and sometimes dangerous. He had been known to stand still and gesticulate wildly in the street. My excellent girl who has lived with me five years says were he to come home she would leave *for her own safety*."[4] She also wrote, probably in late 1876 or 1877, "I feel that I must tell you that some time before Dr.'s sunstroke he was becoming excited—twice attempted to take my life—once by choking and once by stabbing by a lance[t?]. I was saved only by the determined *persistent efforts* of my excellent girl (Bettie Lee)."[5] From these letters, giving only Mrs. Harris's side of events to be sure, we can gather that his behavior had changed radically; he had not always been quick to anger, paranoid, or violent. As the sunstroke event occurred in July 1876, this account would place the initial symptoms a year or two before then.

In the petition to have him declared insane, Elizabeth Harris, through her lawyer, described the sunstroke and its aftermath.

> That on or about the second of July 1876 he received a sunstroke from exposure which seemed sensibly to impair his mind; and that for one year previous to this date he had suffered from spasms, convulsions and fits which were brought about by some losses in business. In the fourth day after the sunstroke, he became so violent that it took three men to hold him. This paroxysm continued for one week when his physicians Doctor Palmer, surgeon in charge of Freedmen's Hospital and Dr. Robert Reyburn said that they could do nothing more for him, and advised that he be sent to the Government Asylum for the Insane. On [the basis of] their certificate of examination he was sent to the said Asylum where he has since remained.[6]

Two affidavits from the physicians who treated him at St. Elizabeths, Drs. C. H. Nichols and A. H. Witmer, confirmed that J. D. Harris was not "capable of managing his business, or even of taking care of himself."[7] There are no hospital case notes or prescription orders to add depth to the diagnoses and treatments offered by his physicians.

Elizabeth Harris met her husband sometime in the mid-1860s, and they married in 1868. While it is possible that he was already suffering from violent rages at that time, it seems likely that he changed from being a "kind considerate" person into a violent one sometime after their marriage. In another letter to the asylum doctor in May 1877, she wrote of her growing fears of him: "At home he throws all restraint off, and he is another man. I would not now *trust* myself alone with him. I who know him well, know his extreme, excitable temper. He never *told* me of the insanity in his family. I never knew *what caused* his fits, his spasms, and his unwarrantable excitement at times. Now I know that he was *insane*."[8] This description is interesting. It reflects an experience of intermittent frightening behavior but also interludes of normality. This intermittency, and with it the hope during the quiet periods that all was well, must have kept her on edge and her emotions raw.

LIFE IN THE ASYLUM

When the doctors at Howard Hospital, his colleagues and friends, could do nothing more for him, Joseph Dennis Harris was taken to the Government Hospital for the Insane, known from the late 1850s as St. Elizabeths.[9] The hospital was founded in 1855 to care for mentally ill citizens of the District of Columbia, soldiers stationed in the District who might become deranged, and private patients from elsewhere who could afford to pay for their care. During the war, regular medical patients were housed there, including Black soldiers from the Union army beginning in 1863. The hospital had extensive grounds, covering more than 400 acres on the Anacostia River in the southeast quadrant of the District by the 1870s. Working-class patients were expected to tend the fields and farm animals, work in the kitchens, sew and repair the linens, and maintain the cleanliness of the wards. Such work not only reduced the hospital's costs but was thought to be therapeutic in itself, as it exhausted nervous irritability and taught regular habits of order and discipline. Patients were segregated by race, class, and gender through assignment to designated wards and hospital buildings.[10]

The first superintendent of St. Elizabeths was Dr. Charles Nichols. He earned his medical degree at the University of Pennsylvania and trained under Amariah Brigham at Utica State Hospital. Brigham shared with the other founding members of the Association of Medical Superintendents of American Institutions for the Insane a commitment to a certain style of psychiatric care called "moral therapy." One of its leading proponents in the United States was Thomas Kirkbride, a friend of Nichols and superintendent of the Pennsylvania Hospital for the Insane.[11] In fact, Kirkbride's ideas were instrumental in planning the design and construction of St. Elizabeths. Proponents of moral therapy believed that mental illness resulted from malignant environmental causes, such as marital difficulties, strong emotions, overwork, setbacks in life, and intemperance. The urban landscape with its hurried pace, noise, pollution, and all-around nervous pressures was particularly to blame for exhausting the susceptible temperament. The cure was a peaceful, orderly environment with plenty of fresh air, beauty, regularity of schedule, and minimal stress. Regular work was also part of the routine, adjusted to the gender and social class of the patient. Nichols strove to create just such a model institution at the hospital in Washington.[12]

As Thomas Otto, author of a recent history of the hospital, has pointed out, Charles Nichols was progressive in his approach to the care of African Americans but still held the usual attitude of his age toward the dangers of racial mixing. In his annual report for 1856, Nichols was proud of the new West Lodge, designated for Black male patients, bragging that it showed government beneficence to the locality's Black population. Still, he insisted that the races must be housed separately: "Opinion and practice vary somewhat in regard to the propriety of associating white and colored insane persons in the same wards of the same institution; but I believe the majority of practical men decidedly condemn the association, and resort to it, if at all, only as a choice of great evils."[13] Historian Martin Summers, in his recent book on race and mental illness in the nation's capital, places much greater stress on the racist side of the psychiatrists at St. Elizabeths. He accuses them of believing that Blacks were primitive, savage, and lacking in sexual control and thus required different therapies from those the more culturally advanced white patients underwent. William Whitney Godding, the second psychiatrist to head St. Elizabeths during Harris's stay there, even blamed emancipation for the abrupt rise in Black mental illness. Released from the stern guidance and disciplinary regimen of their owners, slaves, especially male slaves, he believed, were incapable of managing freedom and constructing effective self-management.[14]

Nichols was superintendent until 1877; he was then succeeded by Godding, who came from the state hospital in Taunton, Massachusetts, and had worked as an assistant physician at St. Elizabeths before the 1877 appointment. Godding summarized his recommended treatment in the mid-1880s as favoring a mix of moral therapy and somatic interventions. He cautioned that the treatment of mental illness required that therapy be customized to the patient without allegiance to the rules of any system. But there were general guidelines that he could lay out. Above all else, patients needed plenty of sleep, plenty of exercise in the open air, occupation, and diversions and entertainments. If necessary, the patients should be restrained for their own safety and that of others. The goal in giving medicines was to restore physical vigor, calm the overly agitated patient, and to produce sleep when not obtainable by other means. He preferred alkaline bromides, chloral hydrate, and other hypnotics over the use of opium as a sedative. Godding recommended baths both for general hygiene and as a distinct therapy. He also used electric treatment via a galvanic battery in a few cases.[15] Harris, it turned out, would be one of those "shocked" patients.

Godding appointed the hospital's first pathologist in 1884, Isaac W. Blackburn. As Harris died at the end of 1884, it is possible that Blackburn performed his autopsy—or, also likely, not, since perhaps the paying patients were not as readily autopsied as the charity cases paid for by the District or the army. In 1903 Blackburn reported that he had completed 1,642 autopsies on the 2,807 deaths that had occurred during the past eighteen years (that is, 1884–1902). Among those he had found twenty-nine intracranial tumors. Each patient was identified with initials and case history; none of the biographical details (including age) or initials matched Harris's.[16] Blackburn's St. Elizabeths autopsy records are now housed at the National Museum of Health and Medicine; librarians there tell me that there is no recorded case from 1884 or the spring of 1885 that matches the details of Harris's case. While the cause of his epilepsy might have been evident from a dissection of his brain, Mrs. Dr. Harris made sure that her husband was not "interfered with" and was safely lodged in a proper cemetery.

Harris was admitted to St. Elizabeths in the late summer of 1876, a year when crowding at the institution had become a real problem. There were three categories of male patients at the hospital in that year: soldiers—Black and white—who had been sent by their communities for government-funded care; local poor people, also Black and white, who qualified for indigent care; and paying patients. Harris was a paying patient, an all-important attribute that raised him to the top of the patient hierarchy. This meant that he had a private or semiprivate room, access to the nicely furnished and much less crowded wards, and attendants who were less likely to treat him with brutality.

The subject of paying for her husband's care was prominent in Elizabeth Harris's letters to the asylum superintendent. In 1880 his quarterly "board" was sixty-five dollars, which she had increasing difficulty meeting over time. Often she fell behind, waiting, for example, for money coming due in rents so that she could, in turn, pay the superintendent. Nichols was known for his leniency in this regard. During the Civil War, when the rates for wealthy southern patients housed at St. Elizabeths could not be paid by their Confederate families, Nichols let the debts accumulate rather than expel the patients who, without benefit of private pay, had no right to the free services of the institution. Godding also tolerated late payments.[17]

So where was this private African American patient housed? St. Elizabeths had a large central building with multiple wards where white patients lived, men and women in different wings. Black male patients had a separate building. Harris mentioned the names of his wards in some of the letters he himself wrote to the superintendents. The wards named after trees (Walnut, Poplar, Sycamore) were in the central building. These were the more elite wards, where patients lived in private rooms with use of an elegant parlor (Poplar Ward had a piano) and a low ratio of attendants to patients.

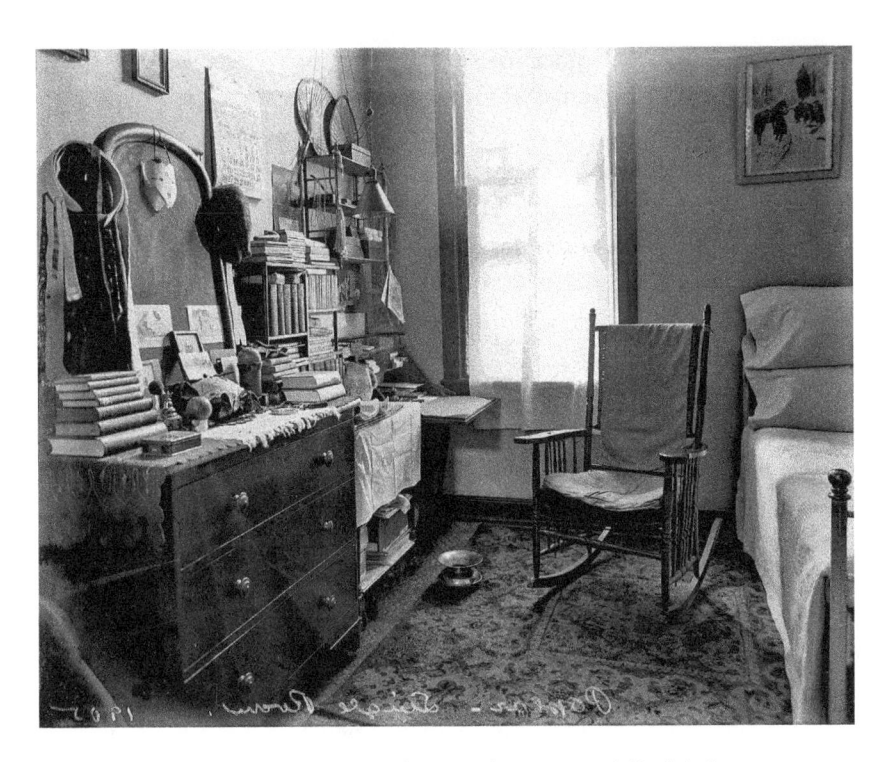

A room in the Poplar Ward, the wing where J. D. Harris lived during part of his stay at St. Elizabeths Hospital in Washington, DC.
Courtesy of National Archives, Washington, DC, NAID 5664628.

For example, in a letter to Dr. Godding, Thanksgiving 1879, Harris said, "I am well now, thanks to electricity and to you under the Almighty. To be sure, I am unable to endure the sun, or heat, in bedrooms of Poplar Ward, but in the Sycamore have shown what was told you long ago, that my convulsions are due *purely* to *heat* and exhaustion."[18] A few weeks later he asked to be moved back to Poplar Ward (it being January, perhaps the sun was less of an issue). The reason was that he was disturbed in his sleep by a roommate. "I have endured so long as I can, the foul language of this eloquent old man from Virginia (Col. Drinkard—I believe he is named).... He constantly awakens me in the night by calling out the names of those places [that Harris knew in Virginia].... He sometimes startles me by yelling as he does; it may be in my ears: 'You bald-headed negro scoundrel etc. etc.'" Harris believed that Drinkard meant no insult but found that the disruption of his sleep required medication with chloral hydrate.[19] He asked to be transferred back to Poplar Ward or elsewhere, or to be discharged to escape the situation. He was still in Sycamore Ward at the end of 1881.[20]

These details tell us something remarkable: Harris was housed as a white man. He was not committed to the building where other Black men were housed and was considered not only white but elite white in the hospital due to his paying status. Colonel Drinkard recognized him as Black and seems to have objected to living next to him, but Harris dismissed that fact without commenting on the racial overtones specifically. It is the *only* mention of his race in these letters. He was a paying patient and therefore, for all intents and purposes, *white*. Mrs. Harris emphasized these pleasant surroundings in an 1877 letter in which she tried to soothe her husband. "You are not in a prison, but in a Hospital that is much like a large family. Every effort is made there to make you contented and happy. You have evening entertainments with no extra expense."[21]

He also had the privilege of walking the grounds, attending church on Sunday in the chapel, and taking the wagon into town on business or to visit his family. One physician asked him to sing in the choir.[22] His wife came to see him and was received in a parlor, where he might also speak to the wives of other men if they were visiting. In one letter to Dr. Nichols, Mrs. Harris complained that her husband was free to talk to these visitors, adding to his potential as a flight risk. "When I went over to see Dr. Harris last Friday, he told me that a few days previous he was sitting near walnut ward window when he saw Mrs. Thomas in the front parlor, and he came around to where she was. Then when I called over with Mrs. Langston, he saw Mrs. Cook in the front parlor and he came around to where she was."[23] Mrs. Harris reported these encounters because she feared her husband would send secret messages out through these possibly sympathetic women, but the information also displays a culture more akin to a boardinghouse than to a tightly regulated or crowded asylum. She may also have feared that he would make romantic gestures toward them. Dr. Harris was accorded dignity by this environment, despite his violent temper and susceptibility to seizures.

This tenuous social status entirely depended upon the family's affluence. When they first moved to the District, Dr. Harris had a salary working at the Freedmen's Hospital as well as money from private patients. His wife and her father, Albert Worthington (who lived with them), brought the household substantial income. Albert Worthington advised his daughter on property investments. John Mercer Langston was a constant friend and source of financial advice. It was the expected thing that affluent Blacks in DC invest in the Freedman's Savings and Trust Co., founded in 1868. Frederick Douglass was its figurehead leader, although he knew little about the bank's management. The Panic of 1873, as the global depression of that year is known, began with the failure of Jay Gould's bank in New York, followed by runs on banks across the country. Freedman's Savings and Trust entered bankruptcy, paying most depositors mere pennies on their accounts. Douglass offered a $10,000 loan to shore up the establishment, but it was not enough. Elizabeth Harris and J. D. Harris had at least some of their money there.[24]

That Harris was treated as a gentleman in the hospital hierarchy was also evident in concerns about his clothing. Paying patients bought their own clothes, and the clothes Dr. Harris wore were hardly those of a working man. For example, in March 1879 Mrs. Harris told Dr. Goddard that her husband wanted "a *pair of shoes*, a *necktie*, a *hat*, and perhaps some shirts." She asked the superintendent to see that the clothes were bought but that the bill not exceed ten dollars. "I am much straitened but the Dr. must be comfortable."[25] So concerned was she with clothing costs that she declared, "With regard to his underwear that is past mending[,] I can make it over for my children. I find myself obliged to economise this year as I have never done before and if he has any articles of clothing unsuitable or unfit for him to wear please have the things done up in a bundle and directed to me."[26] Still, she speaks of supplying him with suits, ties, a hat, and formal shirts—clothing such as he is wearing in the one photograph we have of him. He was not dressed to work on the farm, on new hospital construction, or in the greenhouse. Even in the asylum, his clothes marked him as a gentleman.

By 1880, Mrs. Harris was having increasing difficulty in meeting the costs of her husband's confinement. Enclosing her quarterly payment, she wrote to Godding, "My own and my father's income have assisted in supporting my husband who has been in the Asylum nearly four years (3 yrs & 9 mo.) and in supporting his family at home. I am in danger of losing some of my property. I am in arrears on taxes nearly $600 and a lawsuit is already in court to compel me to meet a claim against the Dr. of from between two and three hundred dollars." She wondered if it would be possible for him to qualify as a US Army veteran rather than as a paying patient. "Dr. Harris went through the *entire war* as surgeon in the army—which position he filled with great acceptance. I am moved to ask can he be retained as your patient with the *same care and bill of fare* as he receives now—*at government expense?*"[27] As we do not have the answer from Godding, we can only guess what his reply was to this suggestion. But there is no doubt that, in general, the patients paid for by the government received a poorer quality of care than the paying patients. The story Elizabeth told as to his army service was false. There is no way to know whether she was deliberately lying or whether he misled her as to his army service.

In 1876 Charles Nichols's stewardship of St. Elizabeths was the subject of a congressional inquiry upon accusations of, among other things, cruelty.

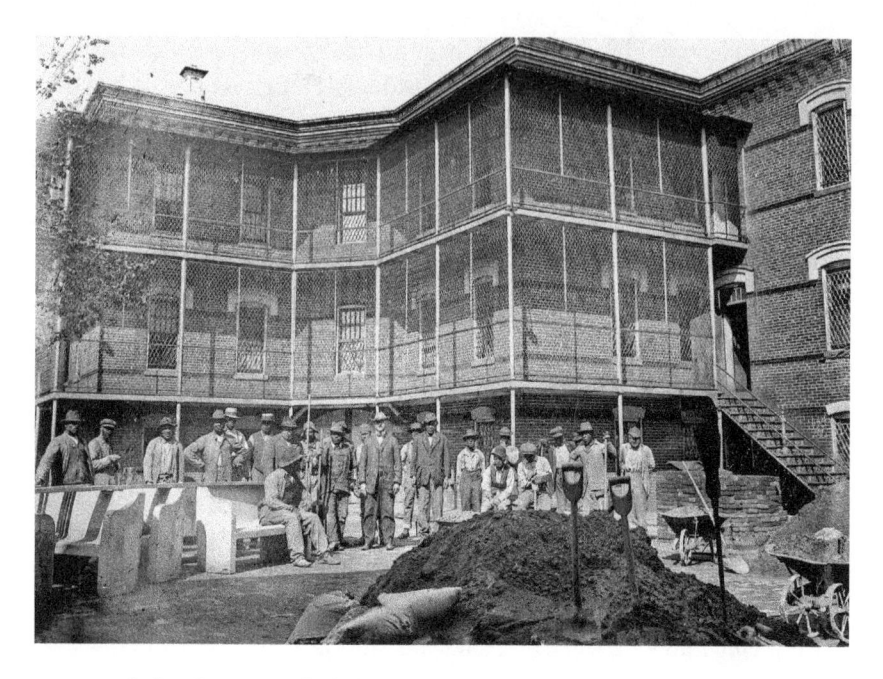

Black patients at St. Elizabeths Hospital, preparing to work on the grounds.
Courtesy of National Archives, Washington, DC, NAID 5664743.

Stories of attendants beating patients were investigated. In one case it was said that a white Irish attendant struck a Black patient with a club that was kept on the ward for just that purpose. The resulting investigation showed that the poorly paid attendants had a high ratio of patients to care for and had few means other than violence to maintain order. The wards stank with the smells of patient feces and urine, and the attendant turnover rate was high. Later photographs of the poorer wards show great crowding and a lack of amenities as compared with the better class of patient wings. Harris might even have been forced into manual labor if moved to such wards.[28] He may have been listed as a blacksmith at age seventeen in the 1850 census, but he had left manual labor behind for decades. His wife was desperate that he should remain categorized as a gentleman, but she was equally desperate to find help in paying the quarterly rate.

A further problem for Elizabeth Harris was that in order to claim her husband as a veteran, he must have been enrolled in the Union army. As far as my research has revealed, he never did so. He was a contract surgeon, to be sure, but neither enlisted nor commissioned in the army. So even if the wards offered to veteran Black patients were acceptable, he was not a veteran and was not eligible to be there. Later she explored the possibility that contract surgeons might be entitled to a pension, which would help to pay for his care. In January 1883 she wrote Godding, "I am glad to tell you that contract surgeons if disabled in the service *do* draw pensions when this condition renders them unable to support themselves and their families." This idea will be familiar to those connected to modern US medical care for veterans. Was his disability service-connected? And did that disability prevent him from pursuing his usual occupation? Mrs. Harris put on her bonnet and went straight to the top. "I have seen the Surgeon General who seemed very favorably inclined and who sent me to the chief clerk of pensions to get the needed blanks. Now I have lived through these years of Dr. Harris['s] affliction and I have practiced economy in every possible way. I have spent five years winter and summer in Washington without it ever occurring to me that he is entitled to a pension."[29] Why didn't she think of that before?

There were several components of such eligibility. She had to prove he was a contract surgeon and document when and where he served and who supervised him. Second, she had to demonstrate that he was injured *during* the war. For any Union soldier, if he broke his leg in battle and was left crippled, he was eligible for a pension. If his leg was, on the other hand, run over by a streetcar in 1878, he was not eligible (at least until the law changed in 1890).[30] So she had the hard task of proving that J. D.'s current condition—epilepsy and insanity—was caused by wartime events. Accordingly, she asked Godding, "Since he is able to converse will you ascertain *when* he entered the service and *in what company* and *regiment* and *by whom commanded* and *when* he *left* the service *what* hospitals he closed and what is *his height?*"[31] In another letter she begged that Godding would prod him for details: "Will you ask him what he witnessed and how he was affected by it? And will you ascertain from him in *what Div.* he served and who *were* the physicians or *Surgeons over* him? I surely have been careless that I have not thought of this before."[32] This detail was necessary for the all-important form, which would in turn allow pension money to flow from the government to St. Elizabeths.

Elizabeth Harris summarized her assumptions about how the war could have affected her husband's nerves early in 1883. "I do not know that I ever told you that Dr. Harris went through the war and was *on the field with the Army* when Richmond was taken. I have been asked were not the seeds of insanity sown *when he was on the field* and he saw the distress and suffering of our Army? He never shrank from duty and he was a faithful and efficient contract surgeon. Were not his nerves afflicted by what he saw and what he was obliged to go through with? Perhaps it was so, and if so, is he not entitled to a pension?"[33] She bolstered this statement of fact with her own personal observations. "I remember Dr. sometimes would commence narrating some of the scenes that he witnessed as surgeon both in the Hospital and on the field and then he would shudder and close his eyes and say he could not tell them and [I] never pressed it. He was always very reticent about telling me anything that would affect me and now as I think of it I believe that the seeds of disease were sown while he was connected with the army."[34] Disingenuously she closed, "Now *if he is not entitled* to a pension God knows I do not want it, but if he is, why should he not have it?"[35]

It is unlikely that Dr. Harris was ever actually "in the field." His first known appointment was to the hospital in Portsmouth and, in the summer of 1865, to Howard's Grove Hospital in Richmond. He would have seen plenty of wounded, sick, disfigured, and dying men—trauma enough, to be sure, but not battlefield experiences. Every surgeon who served during the war would have had this same exposure to the bodily horrors created by shot and shell. Service in the hospital might well have set him up for some sort of post-traumatic stress disorder. But there is no evidence that he was exhibiting the behaviors or symptoms of that problem in the ten years between leaving army service and the onset of his disease. Whether Mrs. Harris really believed that his disease had its origins in the war or was instead deceiving the doctor and herself that he had a just case for renumeration is hard to tell. She may have talked herself into believing it. In any case, her application failed, as her difficulties paying the fees persisted until the end.

But J. D. Harris never did descend to the indignities of the charity patients. He was never in the poor wards, white or Black. His attendants were not faced with the crowding that made these wards so unmanageable, and his category—paying patient—protected him from their violence. Surely his white wife, who visited him, would have raised a ruckus if there was any indication that he was being brutally treated. And if the paying patients were not treated with kindness, they would have taken their fees elsewhere, so it behooved the administration to be sure that these patients, at any rate, received care and consideration.

NINETEENTH-CENTURY MEDICAL KNOWLEDGE ABOUT EPILEPSY AND INSANITY

In South Carolina, Harris had treated patients in an asylum; as a doctor in Virginia, he had treated general medical patients in the military and Freedmen's Bureau hospitals. He might have seen some mental patients in the freedmen's hospitals and at Howard. What knowledge of epilepsy and insanity would he have acquired? What can we conclude about the general level of knowledge about his diseases among well-educated American doctors of the time? How did his two diagnoses—epilepsy and insanity—relate to each other? And how did Harris understand his disease and its treatment?

It is always difficult for a historian to gauge what level of knowledge about a medical issue any given physician has at any given time. Still, in this case we have a well-read physician, Harris, cared for by two leaders in the field of mental illness, Nichols and Godding. The influence of the concept of "moral therapy" was pervasive among the top tier of asylum superintendents in the 1870s, and there is direct evidence that Nichols and Godding were familiar with it. But what of their attitudes toward epilepsy and mania? As a proxy for contemporary knowledge, let me introduce here two experts: Edward Sieveking and William A. Hammond. Sieveking's book, *On Epilepsy and Epileptiform Seizures* (1858), based on his work at St. Mary's Hospital in London, was a major neurology textbook in the nineteenth century. Hammond published his *Treatise on Diseases of the Nervous System* in 1871, the first neurology textbook written by an American. Both works were influential and likely well known to the doctors at St. Elizabeths.

The association of insanity and epilepsy was uncommon in the mid-nineteenth century. The superintendent at the South Carolina asylum reported that only 22 out of 322 patients had the two diseases in 1870.[36] As secretary to the Board of Regents, Harris signed that report. In Sieveking's book on epilepsy, he mentioned that cases of epilepsy often ended up in asylums but implied that this was because the disease tended toward imbecility. "We would observe that a lunatic asylum is generally made the ultimate resort to epileptic patients in whom the usual remedies have been exhausted, and in whom incipient mental fatuity has already indicated organic intracranial lesion." This was unfortunate for the newly admitted patient since seeing others with the disease would be depressing and "exercise a baneful influence."[37] Sieveking's experience with epileptics was heavily tilted toward children, however, and he did not describe any patients with personalities as angry and occasionally violent as Harris was.

Sieveking's explanation of the causation of epilepsy was in accord with the Harris case. He said, "I believe that, in the great majority of instances of epilepsy, the first attack is due to an irritation produced by derangement in the amount or quality of blood circulating in the brain. In a person predisposed we frequently find over-fatigue, a long walk, carrying heavy loads, prolonged mental exertion, the manifest cause not only of the first, but of many succeeding seizures." Sieveking referred to "cerebral congestion" and promoted the therapy of counter-irritation as a way to draw off excessive blood from the head. He also divided causation between predisposing causes, such as heredity, and exciting causes, such as a blow to the head or an infectious event like meningitis. He did not mention sunstroke, but then he practiced in London, not Washington, DC. He did use an interesting analogy. "If we apply a lighted taper to a muslin curtain, the boarding of a wooden hut, or solid masonry of a church, the effect will vary with the greater or less inflammability of the different substances. The curtain will speedily take fire and flare away; the planks may be scorched but will probably not inflame; while the stones will show no traces of the influence of a destructive agent which the first shower will not wash away."[38] The exciting cause was the taper; the "fuel" in the analogy represented the underlying constitution of the individual.

Then he expanded this situation to the human acquisition of nervous disorders. Some people were very susceptible to disease from a slight stimulus, while others were immune from any but the severest blow. Still, once begun, the disease was the same. He thought it was important to remove the stimulus, if possible, but was less impressed with the need to divide epilepsy into nosological categories based on causation. Sieveking also described the failure to find any specific cerebral lesions on autopsy; while he listed a long catalog of abnormal findings, they were without a pattern or consistency. After all, he pointed out, people rarely died of epilepsy, making immediate clinicopathological correlation difficult.[39]

In his discussions of therapy, Sieveking began with praise of the hygienic approach. He noted that in general medicine it was well known that treatment of diseases may be difficult, so prevention through hygiene was paramount. He talked about the "moral treatment" of epilepsy, picking up on the phrase from the "moral treatment" of the insane, as summarized above. Sieveking particularly emphasized the importance of hope. "Confidence begets confidence, and if the physician feels it in himself, he will probably beget it in his patient. . . . This moral element should never be lost sight of in the treatment of disease, but least of all in a disease of the nervous system like epilepsy." His meaning in using the word "moral" becomes clearer in his next statement. "Everything that can be done, consistently with justice and propriety, to raise the *morale*, to strengthen the will, to rouse the moral energies of the patient, comes within the sphere of the physician. His duty is to treat the patient in all his relations; to have a regard to his moral, his intellectual, his physical nature."[40]

Sieveking also promoted the use of tonics, as "among these we find especially the mineral tonics to deserve and hold a high rank." Tonics were substances thought to strengthen the body. He particularly favored preparations of iron and zinc but also liked strychnia. While he mentioned bromide of potassium, a known sedative, he did not give it a strong endorsement. Overall, Sieveking argued that drugs had been both overused and applied indiscriminately. "In fact, there is not a substance in the materia medica, there is scarcely a substance in the world, capable of passing through the gullet of man, that has not at one time or other enjoyed a reputation as being an anti-epileptic." Under hygienic treatment, Sieveking advised attention to pure air, water, food, sexual function, and social situation. Most important was rest. "Rest of body and mind, as we all know, is one of the most certain restoratives to a healthy state; but nowhere is its beneficial influence more palpable than where disease of an exhausting character has fastened upon the nervous system." The key therapeutic step here was to avoid mental stimuli, especially stressors such as the pressure of work and the "harassing cares of a large family," as well as late-night social gatherings when "the patient ought to have given himself up to Morpheus."[41]

Where did Harris's doctors get their information about the cause and treatment of epilepsy? They may have read Sieveking or heard his ideas summarized in journals or papers. Certainly, the removal of Harris from the stresses of work, business, and family met Sieveking's dictum. His doctors also drew on William Hammond's 1871 neurology text, which included a chapter on epilepsy and another on insanity. Given Hammond's fame as surgeon general of the Union army and leadership in the founding of the American Neurological Society (1876) and its initial journal, it is quite likely that this work would have been consulted by any well-read asylum physicians and considered a prime source for them on the treatment of epilepsy.[42]

Hammond began by characterizing epilepsy as a disease marked by paroxysms "of more or less frequency and severity, during which consciousness is lost, and which may or may not be marked by slight spasm, or partial or general convulsions, or mental aberration, or by all of these circumstances collectively." While Hammond then claimed that the "essential element of the epileptic paroxysm is loss of consciousness," he also recognized gradation in the symptoms, which could range from "*petit mal*," or slight attack, to the "grand mal," or severe seizure: "The first is unattended by marked spasm or agitation; the latter is characterized by more or less tonic and clonic convulsions." His gradation schema began with "momentary unconsciousness without marked spasm" and proceeded to greater severity of spasms and longer extent of loss of consciousness.[43] He allowed that this range of symptoms might all occur in the same individual at various times.

Spasms are mentioned frequently in the J. D. Harris asylum letters. Hammond offered a clear explanation of how the term was used. "The spasms may be very slight. Sometimes there is momentary strabismus [crossed eyes], at others retraction of the angles of the mouth." The patient might stick out his tongue, tense the neck muscles, or suddenly bend forward in his chair. Other behaviors appeared volitional. "A patient ... tugs violently at his hand; another walks about the room, but without taking any determinate course; a young lady leaves her chair and stands upon another ... [while] another talks all kinds of gibberish." What these spells had in common was that they were not under the conscious control of the patient, the events were brief, and the patient usually had no recollection of what had happened. Such events could frighten the onlookers. It was as if, for a moment, the person was possessed. No wonder older theories posited just such a cause for epileptic behavior.[44]

Hammond was clear about the relationship between epilepsy and mental illness. He admitted that for some epileptics, their "minds are as healthy as their lungs," but "in the majority of cases, it will be found that the mind sooner or later becomes involved, and it sometimes happens that a single attack causes marked intellectual deterioration." The mental derangement frequently accompanying epilepsy was mania, "a combination which, as every insane asylum shows, is not uncommon. The mania of epilepsy was usually of a very exalted character, and during its existence the subject may commit homicide or other crimes."[45] By mania he was referring to a condition of overexcitement or arousal, violence, and agitation. The word "mania" here was not used in the modern sense of bipolar disorder.

Hammond's epilepsy chapter, published thirteen years after Sieveking's book, frequently drew on Sieveking's ideas and departed from it mainly in its therapeutic recommendations. Hammond's review of the causes of epilepsy resembled Sieveking's, with the addition of 2 cases of sunstroke etiology in his survey of 206 cases from his own practice. Like Sieveking, he found most epilepsy to commence in childhood and the teenage years. Occurrence in the forties and beyond was relatively rare (Harris was forty-three when his sunstroke event occurred). But while Sieveking emphasized a hygienic regimen for epilepsy, with support from medications, Hammond gave central place to medical intervention. "First among remedies are the bromides of potassium, sodium, or lithium," he argued. He preferred the lithium compound but found it costly and felt that potassium or sodium bromide worked nearly as well. Like Sieveking, he also supplemented this course with zinc oxide or strychnia, the latter "for the purposes of a tonic, and for counteracting, to some extent, the debilitation produced by the bromide."[46] Potassium bromide and lithium bromide were used in the treatment of both mania and epilepsy, just as lithium carbonate is used today. Medicine now understands that the substances act by stabilizing neuronal membranes, resulting in reduced nerve transmission; the older remedies could be effective but also had significant side effects.

The most novel suggestion in Hammond's text, compared to Sieveking's, was the recommendation of electric therapy. "When the opportunity affords, I always make use of the constant galvanic current, applying it to the brain and sympathetic nerve." He advised three sessions a week, of about ten minutes each. "For one-third of this time I pass the current antero-posteriorly, one pole being placed on the back of the neck, and the other on the forehead; for another third, one pole is placed on each mastoid process, and for the other, one on the sympathetic nerve in the neck, and the other on the spinal column at about the first dorsal vertebra." He found that of 130 cases given the treatment, 59 were "entirely successful."[47] His definition of fully cured was the lack of a seizure over a six-month span. Depending on how painful the electric treatment was, one wonders whether the patients reported their symptoms accurately.

HARRIS AS A DOCTOR/PATIENT

It is very likely that Harris was familiar with Hammond's ideas on therapy for epilepsy. He would have shared with the asylum doctors a common set of assumptions about mental disease and the varieties of options for treatment. He had himself been an asylum physician for a year in South Carolina. We learn, from the court documents, how Dr. Harris came to be a mental patient—he had a prolonged seizure episode (days of intermittent convulsions) accompanied by behavior so violent that it took several men to hold him. Yet once he came out of this initial period of frenzy, he was often rational, was able to interact with family members and physicians, and took an active role in the understanding and management of his case. We know this because at times he wrote letters to the asylum superintendents. Perhaps there were many more, now lost, but the ones we have are remarkable.

In the spring of 1877, nine months or so after he was admitted to the asylum, some sort of episode happened in the presence of Dr. Nichols. Harris felt that he needed to explain his side of things and to diminish the significance of the events as circumstantial. "When you unexpectedly called yesterday[,] I had just been exhausted by too much exercise in walking over the grounds & up the stairs," Harris apologized to the doctor. "Petit mal is, of course, my present disease. I meant to say the cause of my coming here was something more called 'sunstroke,'" he concluded.[48] Harris was using a classification system for seizures first devised in France by J. D. Esquirol in 1815, although he merely gave labels to the well-known phenomena with which the disease could present.[49] While the variations among grand mal, petit mal, and absence seizures were defined differently by different writers, on the most simple level it was clear that grand mal was characterized by loss of consciousness, flailing limbs, loss of bowel and bladder control, and self-damage, such as tongue biting. Petit mal was milder, being revealed by local muscle twitches, such as facial tics or the jerking of a hand. Absence sometimes appeared like a loss of attention or lack of engagement with surroundings.

Harris displayed two goals here. First, he argued that his seizures were temporally connected to sunstroke. So, if he was protected from the heat, then the seizures would not be a problem. He also wanted to say that his seizures were trivial events, easily managed. Both arguments were probably incorrect, as was clear in observations from his wife's letters. His initial hospitalization in the setting of prolonged paroxysms obviously went beyond petit mal. She may have had reason to exaggerate the severity of his illness, but as she was writing to the asylum superintendent this seems unlikely. He would have ample opportunity to directly learn of Harris's symptoms, from either his own observation or that of the caregivers at the asylum. The most detailed letters come from the summer of 1877, when the court proceeding to have him declared insane and incompetent was about to go to trial. Mrs. Harris needed the asylum physicians to declare him incompetent so that she could assume control both of his body (he must remain in the asylum) and of his finances.

She summarized recent events to Dr. Nichols in June. "You will remember that there was an excessively warm Sunday a few weeks ago. Dr. was sitting in the Chapel with his thick coat on and he felt the heat very sensibly, and after he returned to his room he became unconscious." So, again, the association with heat. "Then on June 6th," she continued, "a brother in law of the editor of the Republican [newspaper], he said, gave him a cigar, and he smoked half of it. Shortly after he had a spasm of some length, and became unconscious and his saliva ran down his beard and ruined his linen." This was echoed the following day by another "spasm," not as severe and without loss of consciousness. She suspected that Dr. Harris did not tell her of all these episodes because he wanted to come home and so tried to convince her that he was recovered.[50] The following summer she likewise reported to Dr. Witmer, one of the ward physicians, "I found Dr. Harris not quite as cheerful as he was at my last visit. He had had another fit—which he called a seizure—and he found in the morning that he had bit his tongue. He told me that he was better, but his appearance indicated that he had suffered considerably."[51] From such references it seems likely that Harris did have grand mal seizures at times, although the focal seizure activity (the "spasms") were more common.

Harris was a physician, and he tried to take an active role in the management of his case. In 1878 he expanded his theories about his condition. "Experience is necessary to comprehend the diseases of the sympathetic system for by experience we know clearly where the body suffers. My disease was cerebral congestion, resulting from nervous debility caused by heat & excitement."[52] In using the word "sympathetic," Harris was referencing the concept that disease in another organ can lead to the brain responding in "sympathy" with a seizure. Mechanical irritation in the big toe, for example, might generate a general sympathy and lead, somehow, to irritation of the brain.[53] Such theories underlay the notion that removing (possibly) diseased ovaries would cure epilepsy or mental illness in women.[54] Harris also talked directly about the "sympathetic nerve" in his neck as being key to his case.[55] Finally, both Sieveking and Hammond make use of the concept of "cerebral congestion" in explaining seizures and other disorders.

Harris became convinced that using topical electric current would improve his condition. This was not entirely a quackish notion; Hammond considered the application of electric current as especially valuable in neurological diseases featuring spasm and muscle paralysis, such as multiple sclerosis, and the muscle weakness that could follow strokes. Harris had talked to a purveyor of an electric belt and was anxious to try it, although his wife remained skeptical. "The expenses of the Galvanic belt you mentioned is I am told $25. A belt of another patent is $6.00," she told Dr. Godding in February 1878. "I have heard by those who should know something about Dr. Bosworth of 918 E St N. W. that he is a '*quack* and a *humbug*.'" Bosworth was anxious to sell her a belt available from New York that he thought would be "a sure cure for all of Dr. H's complaints—and most all insane people ailments—by giving better circulation."[56] She was quite worried about cost.

A year later, Mrs. Harris continued to be skeptical but apparently gave in and paid for a belt. She told Dr. Godding, "If you see any probably permanent good resulting from the use of Henry Maloy's galvanic belt for Dr. Harris and you choose to get it for him, I can pay for it next April (when I pay his board bill). Dr. H. M. Maloy's address is No. 205 East 14th St, NY and the price of the belt less the discount is $4.20."[57] This or some other belt was in Dr. Harris's possession two months later, and he evidently enjoyed experimenting with it. First, he tested its effect upon a familiar problem of his, the digestion of cheese. "To prove the effect of cheese which hitherto has made me sick at night, I ventured on Friday evening last to eat a considerable piece," he told Godding. "Before mid-night I awoke with a burning sensation in my stomach to which I applied a battery of the Belt I am wearing[,] which immediately relieved the disorder and I was asleep again within five minutes."[58]

Harris drew broad conclusions from his experience with the belt. "More important is the fact that my convulsions were proven to be caused by the sympathetic nerve. It is true my delirium was caused by sun. Heat—year before last, and again last year, from needless exposure. I shall therefore be careful hereafter. So should everyone who has had cerebral congestion." But Harris believed that the impact of the galvanic belt on his epileptic condition had broad implications for understanding its etiology. "I now accept, as being deserved, what you were kind enough to say last Sunday. For the fact is demonstrated that the current of magneto voltaic electricity evolved by the belt I am wearing is a cure for what has hitherto been called *Epilepsy* but which I have now proven to be a function disorder of the *Sympathetic Nerve.*" So convinced was Dr. Harris of the power of the belts that he proposed that he should reveal this vital information to the surgeon general as well as to physicians and surgeons at hospitals in the city. "But as regards this Hospital [I] would accept no compensation other than that intimated." He had worked out a special deal with Dr. Maloy in New York to supply belts to St. Elizabeths for half the usual charge. He left the matter "now entirely at your disposal."[59]

Two weeks later Harris asked his wife to buy yet a stronger belt. She told Godding, "A letter from Dr. Harris of April 27th is rec. in which he says, *in order to hasten his recovery*, he desires his belt of 4 batteries exchanged for one of 12 batteries costing $3.30 additional. I suppose by this that his belt has not benefitted him as he expected and as the *agent promised*. Of course I know that the expensive belt will not benefit him any more than the one he has, and it may be then he will hear of and desire one of 100 batteries and where will it end?"[60] In early May she put the matter in Godding's hands: "If he still desires the belt, and the thirty days in which one may change belts has not expired—*and you think it advisable* for the sake of keeping him happy, to get the belt, and you can advance the money to get it, I will settle for it next July. But I had so much rather get him the hat, shoes, etc. which he *really needs*."[61]

Once the new belt was purchased, she inquired of Godding, "On the whole, is he better or worse? I have sometimes noticed that if I make a *short* call on him he appears very well, while if I remain *long*, his mind is very weak." Apparently, Dr. Harris still had faith in the electric device and showed some outward signs of improvement. "Some of his letters are very pleasing," she reported. "I am glad that he has his new belt, and one of a higher power than he expected for the money."[62]

Such optimism was short-lived. A few months later she wrote, "I suppose Dr. Harris is failing and his mania is more frequent than formerly." From this point he apparently made no further demands on electric devices but had fixed on a transfer from one ward to another as the best means of improvement. "I presume he does not realize his condition but imagines that a change of residence could relieve him. If you can make any little change in his room, which he so much desires, I dare say that it will work wonders in his imagination."[63]

There was no description of the medical therapies that Harris may have received while he was in the asylum, except that he did comment on using chloral hydrate to sleep while being bothered by a noisy roommate.[64] As seen in the discussion of Goddard's therapeutic philosophy, using chloral hydrate to promote sleep was an innovation over using opiates, one that he considered progressive.[65] But what of potassium bromide, the anti-epileptic promoted by Hammond and in common use as an anti-seizure medicine? The only evidence we have comes from Dr. Harris's opposition to its use, an opinion he summarized in a document called "Sympathetic Diseases, 1878" found in his patient files so presumably sent either to his wife or to Godding.

Harris began by introducing the common framework of diseases being conditions of either overexcitement or debility. Thus, medications acted either to calm overexcitement or to stimulate the weakened body. This was common medical thought in his period. He was sure that "my disease was cerebral congestion, resulting from nervous debility caused by heat & excitement." He echoed here the accepted wisdom of his time, including Sieveking and Hammond. So, he was first overstimulated by heat and excitement, which created a condition of debility, and now he needed restoration to baseline through the use of stimulants.[66] He did not recommend potassium bromide, for "all who use the Bromides only, in nervous diseases are inexperienced. They serve to modify life's forces stored in vegetable and animals from which sources medicines should chiefly be drawn. The body may also need mineral tonics, for they are necessary to vital force." Harris went on to give the recipe for a proper nerve tonic, suitable for his case and others.

> The tonic I prefer is as follows (for general debility of the nervous system):
>
> Rx
> Strychinia sulph gr j
> Ferri pyrophosphatis
> Quinia Sulph aa zj
> Acid. Phos. Dil
> Zingerberis syrup aa Zij
> M fr mist
> S: teaspoonful in a little water three times a day.[67]

As was evident in the discussions in Hammond and Sieveking, such ideas were mainstream among physicians treating epilepsy. Quinine (quinia sulph) and iron (ferri pyrophosphatis) were stimulants used commonly for non-neurological debility diseases. Hammond and Sieveking mentioned strychnine, while ginger (zingerberis) added (literally) zing.

One sort of stimulant in common use in Civil War hospitals was absent from his formula: medicinal alcohols such as brandy, whiskey, or other spirits. While Harris may have prescribed alcoholic therapeutics during the war, by the early 1870s he was attending temperance meetings in DC. His wife never mentioned drinking as one of his weaknesses and expressed her own temperance views in letters from the early 1880s. One of their empty rental properties was in an area increasingly occupied by bars and retail liquor establishments. "Now you want your money and you ought to have it," she told Godding. "I have been offered $80 a month by liquor dealers for it if I would consent to have the store part used as a restaurant but my *whole nature revolts* at the idea." She related that when her sister died, she left a crippled child. The child's father ran through the money in dissipation and drink. "No I have not come down so low as to rent for liquor."[68]

Whatever his own position on the use of medicinal alcohol to treat epilepsy, Dr. Harris was sure he knew the proper course for epileptic management. He was so confident of this that he offered to provide care for fellow inmates at the asylum.

> I venture a suggestion for which your patient and favorable consideration is requested.

> *i* Give me all epileptiform cases male and female on one floor both sides:
> *ii* Give Dr. Cleaver the second floor for such cases as he may elect male and female
> *iii* Then you select the one or two physicians who shall have charge of the remainder
> *iv* No argument is necessary for this proposition, but you will find me entirely liberal respecting lung disease if it be preferred I should have my share of those to attend. Etcetera etcetera.[69]

So, Harris saw himself as a medical expert, not only for his own case but in treatment of epileptic patients in general. His plan harkens back to one tried by Ira Russell in St. Louis, where he assigned one ward to a physician sympathetic to Black patients and one to another who scorned them. Regardless of the severity of patient illnesses, the racist physician's outcomes were worse. Perhaps they discussed this experimental approach when Russell met Harris in 1865. But, more to the point, one can see in this document the typical delusion and grandiosity of the manic patient, only in this case he saw himself as a doctor, not Napoleon. His wife noted this sort of posturing as well. She wrote to Superintendent Nichols about an unfortunate visit: "He mortified me exceedingly by his egotism and vanity."[70]

It is clear both from his wife's letters and from this sort of document that Harris retained significant cognitive abilities even as his brain failed him, and he used his residual brain power to cope with his tragic situation. We have seen how central concepts of self-identity were to him. In his Haiti period he was to be a leader of Black men; during the US Civil War he served the Union cause and his own people as a surgeon; in 1869 he ran for political office. He struggled to escape from his childhood status in North Carolina when free Blacks were less than full citizens and when men of his skin color were vulnerable to kidnapping into slavery. Now he was imprisoned in the asylum. His attempts to escape, either through legal means or by enrolling his siblings in plans to get him away from there, indicate that on some level he felt trapped, not treated. These letters about treatment indicate that another coping mechanism was to transform his identity from patient to doctor, not only by offering advice on his own diagnosis and directions for his care but also by assuming the role of doctor to his fellow inmates. In other letters he similarly asserts the importance of his financial dealings and the need to get out and see his lawyer or banker. He is a doctor, a man of business, even an advisor to the surgeon general. This was not just the delirium of a proto-Napoleon; he really had been, and to some extent still was, all those things.

In 1877 Dr. Harris made multiple attempts to leave the asylum and enlisted his family members to help him. At times he was so determined to leave that Mrs. Harris instructed his doctor not to let the patient be alone with visitors, as he might convince them to take a letter to his brother or to a lawyer. "He told me last Friday that he was determined to get out and if I would not help him he would get some one who would; he *could* do it, and *would* do it."[71] One could imagine a conspiracy here, that for some reason Elizabeth kept him confined for nefarious reasons of her own. Certainly, he wrote letters to his North Carolina family that begged them to come and get him out. From his wife's correspondence we learn that two brothers and his mother, Charlotte, visited him at the asylum.[72] She also discovered that J. D. had written to his brother Robbie (then in Fayetteville, North Carolina) to come rescue him. Elizabeth realized that at times he could appear quite lucid and reasonable. But she was afraid to have him at home, since this quiet, reasonable man could so quickly transform into an angry, violent one. He also tried to go to court and force a writ of habeas corpus to lead to his release. This was reflected in Elizabeth Harris's letters warning the doctors not to let him correspond with his lawyer or his family.[73]

Dr. Harris repeatedly told his wife that "he *must* go south."[74] His brother Robert; Robert's wife, Mary Harris; and his mother, Charlotte, all lived in Fayetteville, and that was his favored destination. Elizabeth Harris found the North Carolina branch of the family to be a particularly bad influence. "Dr.'s mother has a peculiar nervous temperament," and her son Robert "has done Dr. a great deal of harm—by writing him since he has been in the asylum."[75] Other family members also suffered from insanity, raising the likelihood of a hereditary cause. Elizabeth Harris asked Dr. Nichols in March 1877 to block his relatives' letters. "I think that letters or calls from his relatives would only make him *dissatisfied* and *miserable*. They have no sympathy with me, and they have no better judgement than to worry him."[76]

J. D. Harris had relied on his extensive family network for aid and support all of his life. When he made an expedition away from them—to Iowa, to Haiti, to New York—within a year or two he was back in a community that included some family members. The strength of that family network sustained him. He had made the decision to marry Elizabeth Worthington on his own, and we have only one measure of his family's response—the fact that brother William married them. It is sad to see his futility in seeking escape from the asylum, escape that would allow him to go home to (at least) his brother and mother. William, who had been his companion in the hostile world of South Carolina, was dead by the mid-1870s. J. D.'s wife admitted that he desperately wanted to come home to her, but she feared his physical attacks. Far from a conspiracy to constrain him against his will, I see the tragedy of a great man brought down by disease that no family intervention could remedy.

FINAL YEARS

As late as 1881, when he had been in the asylum more than five years, Dr. Harris was still arguing for his release. He wrote Dr. Godding, "I have the honor respectfully to inform you that I cannot remain longer in this Hospital of my own accord. My reasons will be given you if desired. Please send this note to Mrs. Dr. Harris and cause me to be relieved as a patient. Very truly yours. J. D. Harris, M.D."[77] A week later his wife asked Godding, "I am anxious to know *just his condition* and if he has any sane moments as he used to. I would like to see him at such a time if only for ten minutes."[78] At this point, when his wife considered him insane most of the time, he could still summon the dignity and coherence to politely request release, although presumably his assumption that this was possible was itself a sign of delusion. Nine months later she wrote, "Occasionally letters from him are sensible or partly so. I think it must be very sad to him to realize his condition, as I suppose he sometimes does."[79] Indeed.

Although Dr. Harris repeatedly sought discharge, there is no evidence to support the idea that he was wrongfully committed. Multiple physicians at the Freedmen's Hospital and the doctors at St. Elizabeths were witness to his illness and agreed to his need for involuntary commitment. Were they all racists somehow controlling or demeaning a Black man and his aggressions? At the time of the commitment hearing, Frederick Douglass was the US marshal for the District of Columbia. It was the duty of the marshal to convene a jury to consider whether J. D. Harris was a "lunatic." Frederick Douglass judged the evidence, and Frederick Douglass signed his commitment order in September 1877.[80] Harris was surrounded by a social network of Black professionals who could have freed him if he had been inappropriately incarcerated, but none of them stepped forward.

John Mercer Langston, his friend from Ohio and now Howard Law School dean, told Mrs. Harris that J. D.'s mind was "shattered," and this was reinforced by the patient's surety that Langston and Mrs. Harris were in a conspiracy to prevent his access to his money.[81] Elizabeth Harris cited Langston as an authority when countering Dr. Harris's claims. Elizabeth told one of the doctors that Professor Langston says "he should not be allowed home again."[82] Three months later Langston averred (as reported by Elizabeth), "His mind now is a total wreck."[83] No one benefited by his being in the asylum, if indeed it was some sort of plot. And his subsequent medical history after commitment supports the severity of his disease.

Lacking medical records from the subsequent years up to his death, we can see only his gradual decline through Elizabeth's eyes. "The six years that his disease has progressed has made such a difference in him that it makes me miserable to see him in such a condition. . . . I would prefer to remember him as he was."[84] By 1883 she spoke of his illness with resignation. "To me there is something very sad in the thought that Dr. Harris is always disturbed in mind with scarce a probability that he will ever be in a condition to have one more conversation with me."[85] She was sad not just for herself but for her children, who would never know their father. "I have heard nothing from the Dr. for some time. Does he ever mention his family?" she wrote in 1883.[86]

To return to the question with which the chapter began: How should we understand the interrelationship between his two diagnoses, epilepsy and mania? In the words of a 1998 textbook, "Little in the field of epilepsy over the past several decades has engendered so much controversy as the concept of an 'epileptic personality.'" This concept was believed in during prior decades, was somewhat deflected by a study that found no evidence of it in the early 1960s, and is now ardently opposed by those defending patient rights. "Only through a concerted and generally successful effort to alter this image [of the dangerous epileptic] have most patients been accorded full social rights. The effort to remove the clouds of social ostracism from these patients has been ongoing and deserved. However, some contend that one of the primary results of this effort has been the outright denial of the concept of an 'epileptic personality.'"[87]

Some of the symptoms that Harris demonstrated, such as the "petit mal" seizures that were observed on occasion, are more commonly seen in seizures of the temporal lobe. Much of the debate about the "epileptic personality" has focused on patients with seizures in that part of the brain. Sigmund Freud himself commented, in an essay on Dostoevsky, that "we know that epilepsy produces these remarkable changes in the personality."[88]

Harvard physician Norman Geschwind (and his student David Bear) are credited with resurrecting the concept of the epileptic personality in the 1970s and 1980s. Their list of "TLE [temporal lobe epilepsy] behaviors" included hyper-religiosity, hyper/hypo-sexualism, aggression, deep thoughts about the cosmos, and so on. The model never worked very well, and the system has often been derided since. Still, "Geschwind's writings and lectures stimulated a generation of physicians, psychologists, and scientists to reassess behavior in epilepsy. It remains a field mired in controversy," said neurologists Julie Devinsky and Steven Schacter at a Geschwind symposium in 2009. "It is no longer controversial that behavioral changes are common among patients with epilepsy. The prevalence of depression in epilepsy is common, yet many neurologists fail to ask 'how are your spirits?'" The moral of the story? "Geschwind opened the door, but many in neurology have failed to walk through."[89] Geschwind argued that the rejection of the epileptic personality was part of psychodynamic psychiatry's rejection of all organic causes of mental illness. The intense turn toward brain anatomy and function that accompanied the "Decade of the Brain" (1990–99) and continues to the present may, someday, offer new answers to these questions.

THE END

Whatever disorder troubled the mind and soul of Dr. Joseph Dennis Harris came to a close on Christmas Day in 1884. He died that day at St. Elizabeths Hospital for the insane. In the last few years of his life, he became uncommunicative, at least with his wife. Her scant letters from that period are all about paying bills, with few references to her husband other than that she hoped for him to have a short period of lucidity, one that apparently never came. She had him buried in Graceland Cemetery, Washington, DC, on December 27. He was fifty-one years old.[90]

Conclusion

This study asked from the beginning how such a man as J. D. Harris, a mid-nineteenth-century African American, was able to acquire a medical degree and accomplish so much in medicine as well as in other fields. From his story we can glean a few answers.

Family support was key to much of what he and his siblings were able to achieve. His mother was literate, in both French and English. She instilled a strong moral and religious sense in her children. They also learned that it was important to cultivate respectability and to serve the needs of their less fortunate neighbors. "Elevating their race" through education, Christian teaching, medical care, and provision of occupation were all steps central to the properly lived life. For the Harris children, service was a calling, and its accomplishment justified their life choices. From both parents, J. D. learned the value of hard work and contribution to society. Temperance was also a family value, one the Harris sons both practiced and preached in adulthood.

Family support furthered J. D.'s career through financial contributions. If the boys had stayed in Fayetteville with their father and his network of free Black craftspeople, they would likely have gone to work as apprentices at twelve or so, and their labor would have contributed to household prosperity. This is the path the earliest Harris children followed, and they took those skills with them to Ohio. William was able to buy a farm and likely put some of his siblings to work there. But at age thirty J. D. went to medical college, which meant living at home with his mother and being a *drain* on family finances, not a contributor to them. Cicero and Robert went to high school in Cleveland, likewise postponing their productive years. How did mother Charlotte scrimp and save so these children could get an education? Her affluent son-in-law Cicero Richardson probably helped, although how the money flowed is unclear. What is crystalline is the dedication to higher education at the cost of traditional teenage salary contribution. This may be the most important family value that enabled J. D. to become a doctor.

The intelligence of this brood of children shines throughout their life stories. William began as a laborer, ran his own farm, and then moved, self-taught, into ministry and education. Sister Sarah was a printer—she had a job requiring literacy and careful attention to detail—while also raising nine children of her own. The younger boys Robert and Cicero graduated high school in Cleveland and went on to found colleges in North Carolina. For Robert it was a normal school—a school that trained teachers—which developed over the years into Fayetteville State University. For Cicero it was Livingstone College, a school that graduated preachers. The tradition of creating teachers and preachers who would in turn promote literacy among the Black citizenry of North Carolina illustrates the drive to "fill the pipeline" with literate Blacks who could go on to careers unimaginable to their enslaved ancestors. "Elevation of their race," indeed, carried out one student at time with an ever-broadening scope.

J. D. Harris had not only intelligence but also passion and courage, traits that drove him to Iowa, to Cleveland, and to the Caribbean, all in search of a place where he could make his name and his fortune. His fictional avatar Minor Larry, from his poem *Love and Law, South and West*, revealed his response to the overt racism and violence that Black people experienced in America. But the poem also showed Larry overwhelming his foe and claiming his rightful place and his bride. The Black man was not helpless! He could take action and succeed. The Wellington rescue and John Brown's raid electrified Harris. It was time to begin anew, in a tropical homeland where Black colonists would flourish and the American immigrants would take their place as the natural leaders of the island and even the Caribbean as a whole.

But then, suddenly, his direction changed. Disease had ruined the colony he had led, but again, all was not lost. He would go home, learn to be a doctor, and find a place in the new America of Abraham Lincoln's administration. And indeed, in 1864, Harris achieved his dream. He was a doctor, paid by a benevolent government, and heartened by his abilities to help his own people. In his marriage to Elizabeth Worthington, he acquired a life partner who shared his dedication to service and to religion. She gloried in her own title as "Mrs. Dr." The digression to the Virginia lieutenant governor's race must have been both exhilarating and quite satisfying. Yes, he lost, but he garnered nearly 100,000 votes. The family gloried in their literacy and sense of service to God and their people.

J. D. Harris continued to seek gainful employment. He had been able to make a living as a doctor after medical school only because his employer was the US government, but that opportunity faded as the Freedmen's Bureau wound down. Through political connections he acquired the post as state asylum doctor in Reconstruction South Carolina. But, as elsewhere in the South, the resurgent Confederates were regaining power, and that Black doctor had to go. J. D. retreated to the only place left for him to treat Black patients and live in a professional community—Howard University, Howard Medical School, and that northeast corner of Washington, DC. There he both maintained a private practice among the growing Black middle class and had appointments at Howard Hospital and the last remaining Freedmen's Bureau hospital. He also engaged in "business"—buying properties, renting them, and at times renovating them for resale. Business was booming, until it was not. The Panic of 1873 and particularly the failure of the Freedmen's Savings Bank severely battered his financial well-being, just as disease attacked his brain.

The timing of these events corresponded to enormous transitions in American society. J. D. Harris found unlikely doors of opportunity and walked through them. To be certain, the first impulse was a shove: the great expulsion of free Black people from a southern society determined to defend their "peculiar institution" at all costs. The Harris family moved to Ohio, where social factors both liberal and conservative pushed Black people to mobilize in the Colored Conventions and the Wellington rescue. The location of Ohio as a central hub of the Underground Railroad radicalized some free Blacks, both in the direction of open revolt (John Brown) and external colonization (transporting free Blacks to new homes in Haiti or Canada). J. D. Harris was there to experience it all, with a side trip to Iowa that disillusioned him about the hopes of free Black people for settlement of the American frontiers.

Nothing so accelerated J. D. Harris's transition to the practice of medicine as the American Civil War. Lincoln's 1863 decision to enroll Black men, including former slaves, into the colored regiments created immediate needs for medical care. Harris was able to rush through medical training and find paying positions as a direct consequence of this societal revolution. The institutions established to care for such soldiers offered government pay for doctors, including Black doctors, who had few other sources of income. The Freedmen's Bureau continued this federally sponsored health care for African Americans and thus gave rise to yet another locus for Harris to practice, with both acceptance by patients and a steady paycheck.

The South Carolina Lunatic Asylum was a new practice opportunity for Harris, albeit a tenuous one. His position depended in turn on the persistence of the postwar Reconstruction government voted in before white South Carolinians had regained the right to vote. Once they recaptured the franchise, the Black Republicans were voted out, and Harris lost his job. The Harris family then transferred to Washington, DC, the last remaining locus of African American medical institutions: Howard Hospital and Howard Medical School. Even there, government support for the Black medical community of physicians and patients was waning in the mid-1870s, when J. D. Harris fell ill. Howard University would struggle amid accusations of financial malfeasance and waning federal support in the 1880s and 1890s, although it did manage to survive into the twentieth century.

How to tie the trajectory of J. D. Harris's life into this discussion of social capital and family values? Certainly, he benefited mightily from the free Black networks and family framework outlined above. But even he could not escape from the infected environment brought about by poor people crammed together in communities that lacked adequate sewage control. This was certainly an accurate description of many of the camps where freedmen and freedwomen lived during and after the war, where they received the ministrations of the Harris brothers. Haiti, if anything, was perhaps even worse, as Flight I, the Harris colony, bordered a river that still suffers major pollution problems today. The family value that pushed the Harris boys to serve underprivileged African Americans likewise pushed them into dangerous disease environments. This is clear for William, who died of dysentery, and also for Robert, who likely died of amoebic dysentery, liver failure, and ascites. But does this hold true for J. D.? Could poor environmental hygiene cause seizures?

A SPECULATION AND POSSIBLE EXPLANATION

What was this illness that caused seizures and atypical behavior that was at times violent and at other times seemed to recede, revealing his usual personality? Most infectious causes (syphilis, meningitis, tuberculosis, and so on) would have progressed much more rapidly than this disease, which lingered over nine to ten years, with only gradual worsening. Answering this question becomes a matter of "retrospective diagnosis." I realize that some historians deeply dislike the exercise of using present medical knowledge and categories to try to understand the past. But every time I have presented the story of Dr. Harris, someone in the audience wanted to know: What did he have? So I shall boldly speculate here.

Let us begin with the early symptoms. His wife reported that he had been acting oddly for six to nine months before his major breakdown in July 1876 and was even violent toward her twice. The cleaning girl was afraid to be in his presence, for reasons unspecified. His occupational skills seemed to be slipping—he was making bad financial moves and lost his medical practice appointment at Howard Hospital. It was at least partly in response to austerity measures, to be sure, but his performance at the hospital may also have been to blame. How much of his odd behavior was noticed at the time and how much "remembered" afterward is hard to judge, clouding our diagnostic lens.

His major breakdown began with seizures that went on for days (a condition known as status epilepticus). After the doctors at Howard could not help him, he was moved to the St. Elizabeths mental hospital, where the seizures slowly subsided and consciousness returned. No infectious symptoms, such as fever, were recorded. Later his wife, Elizabeth, said he could be alert and oriented sometimes and then would fall into spells of agitation and confusion. Some of these spells began with "spasms," facial twitches or jerky movements of an arm or leg. During these spasms the patient seemed oblivious to his surroundings. Elizabeth also thought it important to note that two of his sisters were admitted to mental asylums in middle age and diagnosed with "insanity." Brother Jarvis had "idiocy" from childhood.

Common diseases of the time that caused "insanity" included neurosyphilis, pellagra, and brain tumors. Chronic alcoholism can also cause seizures and decline in mental function over years of indulgence. The family were committed temperance folk, however, and if J. D. drank surreptitiously, it is likely that Elizabeth would have known and objected before severe effects could follow. Remember, she refused to rent her property to a business that served alcohol. Pellagra, caused by malnutrition, was common at the South Carolina mental hospital where he had worked and continued to be so well into the twentieth century. But the attendants ate better, and were never affected. The long slow decline is not typical of neurosyphilis or brain tumor.

And as to Elizabeth's suspicion of familial epilepsy, such diseases mostly manifest in children, not in adults in their forties or fifties.

The infection I consider most likely (and I thank my colleague Dr. Jeffrey Baker for this suggestion) is neurocysticercosis. This disease, along with head trauma and perinatal brain damage, is currently the most frequent cause of epilepsy in the developing world, including Haiti. The biological agent of the disease is the pork tapeworm. Such parasitic disease is "related to poverty, illiteracy, and deficient sanitary infrastructures," said one recent review. In fact, global epidemiologists see it as "a 'biologic marker' of the social and economic development of a community."[1] This parasite's life cycle explains the association between such unfortunate conditions and disease occurrence. To put it in simplest terms: (1) human ingests tapeworm eggs in undercooked pork; (2) tapeworm develops in gut and sheds eggs in stool; (3) other eggs spread into the bloodstream and travel to multiple sites in the body, including the brain; (4) in the brain, an egg may lodge and try to grow into a new worm.[2] Pigs are the natural hosts of these parasites; they may eat the human or porcine feces standing uncovered in a farmyard and grow new tapeworms in their gut. These eggs may then burrow into porcine muscle. And in turn these forms of the parasite may infect the human when the meat is handled or ingested, or if cooking is inadequate. Over time, multiple brain infections can lead to dementia and death. A significantly infected brain, as seen in CT scans, can look like someone has taken a hole punch to it.

The epidemiology of neurocysticercosis stems from this life cycle. In Muslim countries, however poor, pigs are rarely eaten due to dietary laws, and pork tapeworm is accordingly rare. But otherwise the disease is located in places where human feces are disposed of on open ground and pigs roam freely. This certainly could have described the neighborhood in Fayetteville where the Harris children grew up. J. D. Harris may have amplified his "tapeworm load" while in Haiti (where cysticercosis is still a major problem) or in the unsanitary freedmen's encampments after the war. The syndromes and symptoms vary as the implanted cysts take up occupancy in different locations, including the brain. There they can sit inert or grow and become inflamed, thus becoming a focus for seizure activity. These seizures may be partial—the "spasms" or petit mal movements seen in J. D.—or tonic-clonic general seizures in which the patient thrashes and falls unconscious. Most cases of cysticercosis appear among patients in their thirties or forties. None of this information linking pork tapeworm to epilepsy was known in the nineteenth century; the connection was first made in the 1930s. So the St. Elizabeths doctors would have fallen back on the stressors of his life, including business failures, and accordingly recommended rest and tranquility. The course of cysticercosis is quite variable. Some patients have no seizures at all, and the worm is found only at autopsy or by means of modern cranial imaging for another reason. Paroxysms of prolonged seizures can happen when an embedded egg breaks through the "shell" around itself, spilling new irritants that elicit a dramatic response.

This diagnosis matches the timing and symptoms of not only J. D. Harris but also his sisters Mary and Kate. The variable presentation—changes in personality, waxing/waning course ending in dementia and death, and relatively slow progress of the disease—is consistent. When middle-aged and older adults are diagnosed with new onset epilepsy, the modern medical response is a brain imaging study, as the assumption is strong that there is a focus in the brain that is generating abnormal electrical signals. In modern-day America that focus is most likely a tumor, although with increasing global connectivity neurocysticercosis is becoming more common in developed countries. If Harris had a metastatic or primary cancer in his brain, it is unlikely he would have lived nine years. But that course is quite possible with cysticercosis. The presence of some sort of space-occupying lesion in the brain is consistent with his course. The family expression of seizures is also consistent here. His brothers Robert and William died of bowel diseases that are also dependent on fecal-oral spread. There is not enough information about Jarvis to say one way or the other. But altogether it makes sense that this "family" disease was caused not by heredity, as Elizabeth believed, but by a common environmental cause. I welcome criticism of this argument and speculation on alternate diagnoses.

EPILOGUE

Elizabeth Harris buried J. D. Harris in the Graceland Cemetery in Washington, DC, in January 1887, next to her father, Reverend Albert Worthington. In her will of 1898, Elizabeth stipulated that her husband and father should be moved to Woodlawn (Graceland was closing) and that she should be buried beside them. Their children, Worthie and Thoro, both attended the Battle Creek College in Michigan, a Seventh-day Adventist school. Worthie Harris married William B. Holden in 1896; both are listed as white in the 1900 census. Thoro's first wife was Agnes Hart Harris. They were grandparents to Greg Harris, who remembers meeting Thoro in 1955, shortly before Thoro's death.[3]

Worthie published a small book of religious poems in 1920. Thoro made quite a name as a composer and publisher of religious hymns. He worked with famed evangelist Aimee Semple McPherson to create and publish her popular hymns. Thoro's wife died of smallpox in March 1922, and he remarried three more times. He moved with his family to Eureka Springs, Arkansas, where he continued publishing hymnals, which he sold door-to-door out of a canvas satchel. All this time, he was recognized as a white man in his adopted town. As others looked more deeply into the family history, Thoro came to be demarcated as "Black." He is now the center of the Eureka Springs Town Museum's celebration of Black History Month.[4]

The first generation of the Jacob and Charlotte Harris family, born 1824 to 1844, had no doubt of their "colored" status. It is likely that they lived near siblings or other family members of their father and mother who were still in slavery. Jacob may have bought his own family members out of slavery where possible. Life became increasingly hazardous for them in Fayetteville in the 1840s. As John Hope Franklin explained, free southern Blacks were an unwanted people, people who were always suspected of fomenting slave rebellion. Their race was never in question and always a source of danger for them. In his lengthy poem, J. D. laid all this out. A slave owner could whip his slaves to death; a free Black person could be falsely arrested as a runaway slave; a man of color could not take advantage of the new lands in Iowa and Minnesota under the homestead laws; and the fairest "octoroon" maiden could find no protection from predation. The final blow was the verdict of the *Dred Scott* case—a Black man had no rights in the United States, as he could never be a citizen.

Even as Worthie and Thoro, J. D.'s children, emerged as white, I hope their mother impressed upon them the struggles and achievements of their father's life within the maelstrom of American racism. His accomplishments were extraordinary. He was indeed part of the cadre of early African American surgeons who lived, as their biographer Jill Newmark proclaimed, "courageous lives."[5] J. D. never gave up, despite his many disappointments; he asserted his intelligence and strong opinions even in the asylum. He never shied from the good fight, no matter how bitter the outcome.

NOTES

ABBREVIATIONS

AMA Archives   American Missionary Association Archives, Amistad Research Center, Tulane University, New Orleans, LA
BRFAL M1913   Records of the Field Offices for the State of Virginia, Bureau of Refugees, Freedmen, and Abandoned Lands, 1865–72, Microfilm Collection M1913, National Archives and Records Administration, Washington, DC (online guide at www.archives.gov/files/research/microfilm/m1913.pdf)
CCP   Colored Conventions Project, http://coloredconventions.org
NARA   National Archives and Records Administration, Washington, DC
Personal Papers   Personal Papers of Medical Officers and Physicians, Records of the Adjutants General's Office, US Army, RG 94, box 249, National Archives and Records Administration, Washington, DC
SANC   State Archives of North Carolina, Raleigh
SCDAH   South Carolina Department of Archives and History, Columbia
SEH   Records of St. Elizabeths Hospital, Washington, DC, RG 418, Case Records of Patients, 1855–1950, box 19, entry 66, J. D. Harris, File #4117, National Archives and Records Administration, Washington, DC
USSC Records   United States Sanitary Commission Records, 1861–79, New York Manuscripts and Archives Division, Public Library, microfilm

INTRODUCTION

1. Humphreys, *Intensely Human*, 88–91.

2. Ira Russell, "Report on Hospitals in Richmond, Norfolk, etc.," [1865], reel 3, frames 154–55, USSC Records.

3. See, for example, Butts, *African American Medicine in Washington, D.C.*; Long, *Politics of African American Medical Care*; and Savitt, *Race and Medicine*. I discussed Dr. Harris briefly in *Intensely Human*, 64–66.

4. Newmark, *Without Concealment*.

5. Reverby and Rosner, "Beyond 'the Great Doctors,'" 3.

6. Reverby and Rosner, "Beyond 'the Great Doctors,'" 3.

7. Humphreys, "The Social History of Medicine—Some Thoughts (and Questions)," quoted in McKay, "Why Do We Do What We Do?," 11–12.

8. Humphreys, "Social History of Medicine," quoted in McKay, "Why Do We Do What We Do?," 12.

9. Newmark, *Without Concealment*.

10. Kibre, "Faculty of Medicine," 1–20.

11. Drachman, *Hospital with a Heart*; Tuchman, *Science Has No Sex*; Morantz-Sanchez, *Sympathy and Science*; Rothstein, *American Physicians in the Nineteenth Century*; Wilkinson, "1850 Harvard Medical School Dispute."

12. S. Harris, *Dr. Mary Walker*.

13. Lett et al., "Trends in Racial/Ethnic Representation."

14. Valerie Montgomery Rice, "Investiture Address," Morehouse College, Atlanta, Georgia, September 11, 2014, www.msm.edu/Administration/office_president/Documents/InvestitureSpeech.pdf.

15. Anonymous, "Summary," 1–2, in Smedley, Stith, and Nelson, *Unequal Treatment*. For the persistence of the problem, see Chanoff and Sullivan, *We'll Fight It Out Here*.

16. Northup, *Twelve Years a Slave*.

17. Olivarius, *Necropolis*. See also Willoughby, *Yellow Fever*; and Hogarth, *Medicalizing Blackness*.

18. Long, *Doctoring Freedom*, 32–33.

19. Blight, *Frederick Douglass*.

20. Boyer and Nissenbaum, *Salem Possessed*; Ginzburg, *Cheese and the Worms*.

21. Robisheaux, *Last Witch*.

22. Nasaw, introduction to "Historians and Biography," 575.

23. Jessica Hauger, "What Is Microhistory?," 8 (unpublished manuscript, July 7, 2021, Microsoft Word file; used with Hauger's permission).

24. Banner, "Biography as History." See also Kessler-Harris, "Why Biography?"

25. Richmond, "Microhistories of Slavery and Racism."

26. Long, *Doctoring Freedom*, 8.

27. Williamson, *New People*, 64.

28. G. Harris, *Harris Family History* (copy in author's possession, gift of Greg Harris).

29. Smail, *On Deep History and the Brain*.

30. See Bonilla-Silva, *Racism without Racists*; and Pettigrew and Martin, "Shaping the Organizational Context."

31. Franklin, *Free Negro*.

CHAPTER 1

1. All references to the US Census rely on its pages as reproduced in Ancestry.com.

2. George Dismukes, Last Will and Testament, July 31, 1827, Chatham County Wills, 1771–1968, C.R. 022.801.12, SANC.

3. Bishir, *Crafting Lives*, 7–8.

4. Gordon-Reed, *Hemingses of Monticello*, 28–32.

5. Bishir, *Crafting Lives*, 11.

6. John D. Whitford, quoted in Bishir, *Crafting Lives*, 47.

7. Bishir, *Crafting Lives*, 49.

8. Bishir, *Crafting Lives*, 54.

9. Beckert, *Empire of Cotton*.

10. Wagstaff, prefatory note to *Harris Letters*, 5.

11. Jacob Harris to Donum Montford, deed of indenture, June 10, 1807, Craven County, Apprentice Bonds and Records, C.R. 022.101.1, SANC.

12. J. Oates, *Story of Fayetteville*, 208–12.

13. North Carolina, Marriage Index, 1741–2004, SANC. Charlotte is often spelled "Charlott" by Jacob, but to avoid confusion and for consistency, I have modernized her name.

14. "Sheriff's Sale for Taxes," *Carolina Observer* (Fayetteville), January 8, 1829.

15. Jacob Harris, sale of property on Hillsborough St., Fayetteville, to Joseph Hostler, November 15, 1834, Records of Deeds, Cumberland County, NC, C.R. 029.40015, vol. 42, p. 475, SANC; Matthew Leary, executor of Jacob Harris estate, sale of property on Hillsborough St. to William Overby, September 14, 1850, C.R. 029.40018, vol. 50, p. 324, SANC.

16. Jacob Harris, Fayetteville, Cumberland, NC, p. 93, Fifth Census of the United States, 1830, M19, roll 120, Records of the Bureau of the Census, RG 29, NARA.

17. Apprentice indenture, September 6, 1831, Jacob Harris, master, and William Burnett, apprentice; deed of indenture, September 8, 1831, Jacob Harris, master, and Owen Clinton Artis, apprentice, Cumberland County, Apprentice Bonds and Records, C.R. 029.101.1, SANC.

18. Identity pass for Cicero Richardson, signed in New Bern, February 17, 1832, in Cumberland County, Apprentice Bonds and Records, C.R. 029.101.1, SANC.

19. Bishir, *Crafting Lives*, 98–100.

20. See Jacob Harris, deed of indenture to Donum Montford, as well as, for example, the deeds for William Burnett and Owen Artis.

21. Perry, "Negro in Fayetteville," 698. Leary was his ancestor. Perry, writing in 1950, was a physician.

22. Charlotte Huntington to Jacob Harris, deed of property transfer, January 5, 1843, Records of Deeds, Cumberland County, NC, C.R. 029.40016, vol. 45, p. 197, SANC.

23. Jacob Harris, sale of ten acres of land that borders Rowan and Chatham Streets, to Benjamin Robinson, January 30, 1846, Records of Deeds, Cumberland County, NC, C.R. 029.40017, vol. 46, p. 308, SANC; Benjamin Robinson, declaration that land sale by Jacob Harris to him is null and void, January 30, 1846, Records of Deeds, Cumberland County, NC, C.R. 029.40017, vol. 47, p. 370, SANC.

24. Franklin, *Free Negro*, 140.

25. Apprentice indenture, December 8, 1837, Jacob Harris, master, and Thomas Brimage, apprentice, to learn plastering, Cumberland County, Apprentice Bonds and Records, C.R. 029.101.1, SANC.

26. Pierre Bourdieu first coined the term "symbolic capital" for that family wealth that is built into relationships "to be kept up and regularly maintained, representing a heritage of commitments and debts of honor." The capital might consist of no more than kind speech, handshakes, compliments, gossip, or scientific information. Bourdieu, *Outline of a Theory of Practice*, 171–79. Later scholars have emphasized the ties between social capital and social networks, such that a given community of connections can be mapped and understood. As such, one's social capital can perhaps be measured by how many lines to others who offer value one person has. As a node in a net, is he or she well supported, or alone? See Lin, Cook, and Burt, *Social Capital*.

27. Jacob Harris, Fayetteville, Cumberland County, NC, p. 307, Sixth Census of the United States, 1840, M704, roll 30, Records of the Bureau of the Census, RG 29, NARA.

28. Franklin, *Free Negro*, 160.

29. John McCaskill, "Notice," *Fayetteville Observer*, July 26, 1845.

30. Daniel, "Two North Carolina Families," 4.

31. Demos, *Little Commonwealth*.

32. W. D. Harris to the Executive Committee, February 13, 1864, AMA Archives.

33. "Dismukes Family History," Ancestry.com.

34. E. Taylor, *Original Black Elite*, 35; "Fayetteville Reminiscences: Mrs. Deming Writes of the Past," *Fayetteville Observer*, August 25, 1897, 2; Régent, *Les Maîtres de la Guadeloupe*.

35. Childs, *French Refugee Life in the United States*, 90. Although Childs's work is predominantly about refugees from the French Revolution, he expanded that category to include those fleeing the Haitian Revolution.

36. W. D. Harris to George Whipple, April 6, 1865, AMA Archives.

37. Brodhead, *Journals of Charles W. Chesnutt*, 40–41.

38. Robert Harris to Samuel Hunt, February 2, 1866, AMA Archives.

39. Ball, *To Live an Antislavery Life*, 5. Ball's footnote to this sentence reviews the historiography of mid-nineteenth-century Black activism in the United States.

40. Franklin, *Free Negro*.

41. Franklin, *Free Negro*, 58–120.

42. Franklin, *Free Negro*, 169.

43. Franklin, *Free Negro*, 180.

44. *Goldsboro Patriot*, reprinted in *North Carolina Standard*, November 20, 1850.

45. Franklin, *Free Negro*, 210. For a similar account of skilled free Black workers being forced out of Charleston, South Carolina, see Starobin, *Madness Rules the Hour*, 97–105.

CHAPTER 2

1. Matthew Leary, executor of Jacob Harris estate, sale of property on Hillsborough St. to William Overby, September 14, 1850, C.R. 029.40018, vol. 50, p. 324, SANC; Records of Deeds, Cumberland County, NC, SANC; Matthew Leary, executor of Jacob Harris estate, sale of property to Melinda Carman on Frink's Alley, September 10, 1850, vol. 50, p. 126, SANC. The advertisement was placed on August 27, 1850, and published on September 10, announcing that the sale would take place by auction on September 14, 1850. Before the auction took place, it appears that at least one of the lots had been sold. "Notice," *Fayetteville Observer*, September 10, 1850.

2. Daniel, "Two North Carolina Families," 3–4. See also Logan, *Liberating Language*, 49; and Walls, *Joseph Charles Price*, 273.

3. Brodhead, *Journals of Charles W. Chesnutt*, 134.

4. Brodhead, *Journals of Charles W. Chesnutt*, 134.

5. Langston, *From the Virginia Plantation*, 13.

6. Langston, *From the Virginia Plantation*.

7. Langston, *From the Virginia Plantation*; Cheek and Cheek, *John Mercer Langston*.

8. Langston, *From the Virginia Plantation*, 27–32, quotation on 31.

9. Jordan, *Slavery and the Meetinghouse*, 20.

10. Weeks, *Southern Quakers and Slavery*, 198–285.

11. N. Taylor, *Frontiers of Freedom*; Jordan, *Slavery and the Meetinghouse*, 18.

12. Quoted in Jordan, *Slavery and the Meetinghouse*, 19.

13. *New York Times*, September 7, 1853, quoted in Foner, *Gateway to Freedom*, 6.

14. Jordan, *Slavery and the Meetinghouse*.

15. Griffler, *Front Line of Freedom*, xi.

16. LaRoche, *Free Black Communities*, 2.

17. LaRoche, *Free Black Communities*, 82.

18. Langston, *From the Virginia Plantation*, 32–36, quotation on 35.

19. Langston, *From the Virginia Plantation*, 90.

20. West, "Harris Brothers," 126–27.

21. Daniel, "Two North Carolina Families," 4.

22. *Report of the Proceedings of the Colored National Convention Held at Cleveland, Ohio, on Wednesday, September 6, 1848* (Rochester, NY: John Dick at Star Office, 1848) 13, CCP.

23. *Report of the Proceedings of the Colored National Convention*, 13.

24. *Minutes and Address of the State Convention of the Colored Citizens of Ohio, Convened at Columbus, January 10th, 11th, 12th, & 13th, 1849* (Oberlin, OH: J. M. Fitch's Power Press, 1849), CCP.

25. *Minutes and Address of the State Convention*, both quotations on 8.

26. Litwack, *North of Slavery*, 20–29.

27. *Minutes of the State Convention of the Colored Citizens of Ohio, Convened at Columbus, January 9th, 10th, 11th, and 12th, 1850* (Columbus, OH: Gale and Cleveland, 1850), CCP.

28. Fiske, Brown, and Seligman, *Solomon Northup*.

29. *Minutes of the State Convention of the Colored Citizens of Ohio, Convened at Columbus, Jan. 15th, 16th, 17th, and 18th, 1851* (Columbus, OH: E. Glover Printer, 1851), 6, CCP.

30. *Proceedings of the Convention, of the Colored Freemen of Ohio, Held in Cincinnati, January 14, 15, 16, 17 and 19, 1852* (Cincinnati: Dumas and Lawyer, 1851), CCP. Quotations on pages 4, 6, and 7, respectively.

31. *Official Proceedings of the Ohio State Convention of Colored Freemen, Held in Columbus, January 19th–21st, 1853* (Cleveland, OH: W. H. Day, 1853), CCP. On this argument, see Horton and Horton, *In Hope of Liberty*, esp. 58–71 and 185–86.

32. *Memorial of John Mercer Langston for Colored People of Ohio to General Assembly of the State of Ohio, June, 1854* (Rochester, NY: Frederick Douglass' Paper, 1854), 298, CCP.

33. *Proceedings of the National Emigration Convention of Colored People Held at Cleveland, Ohio, on Thursday, Friday and Saturday, the 24th, 25th and 26th of August, 1854* (Pittsburgh: A. A. Anderson, 1854), 20, CCP.

34. *Proceedings of the State Convention of Colored Men, Held in the City of Columbus, Ohio, Jan. 16th, 17th, & 18th, 1856* (n.p., n.d.), 6–7, CCP.

CHAPTER 3

1. J. Harris, *Love and Law*.
2. J. Harris, *Love and Law*, 70.
3. Raimon, *"Tragic Mulatta" Revisited*, describes this genre.
4. Daniel, "Two North Carolina Families," 4.
5. *Report of the Proceedings of the Colored National Convention Held at Cleveland, Ohio, on Wednesday, September 6, 1848* (Rochester, NY: John Dick at North Star Office, 1848), 280, CCP; *Address to the Constitutional Convention of Ohio from the State Convention of Colored Men Held in the City of Columbus, January 15th, 16th, 17th and 18th, 1851* (Columbus, OH: E. Glover Printer, 1851), 598, CCP; *Proceedings of the Convention, of the Colored Freemen of Ohio, Held in Cincinnati, January 14, 15, 16, 17 and 19, 1852* (Cincinnati: Dumas and Layer, 1852), 252, CCP.
6. *Official Proceedings of the Ohio State Convention of Colored Freemen, Held in Columbus, January 19th–21st, 1853* (Cleveland, OH: W. H. Day, 1853), 5, CCP.
7. Merry, *History of Delaware County*, 217–30.
8. J. D. Harris, Delhi, Iowa, *The Census Returns of the Different Counties of the State of Iowa for 1856*, Iowa City, 1857, 105–10, on Delhi, Iowa, in general; J. D. Harris listing, pp. 628–29; all on Ancestry.com. Robinson is listed as being resident for twenty years, which may be an error.
9. Title phrase from Dykstra, *Bright Radical Star*.
10. Dykstra, *Bright Radical Star*, 1–15.
11. Dykstra, *Bright Radical Star*, 26.
12. Dykstra, *Bright Radical Star*, 109–18.
13. Alexander Clark, "Petition to Allow Immigration of 'Free Negroes' into Iowa, 1855," State Historical Society of Iowa, accessed December 7, 2023, https://history.iowa.gov/history/education/educator-resources/primary-source-sets/iowa-leader-civil-rights-and-equality/alexander-clark-petition.
14. Dykstra, *Bright Radical Star*.
15. *The Census Returns of the Different Counties of the State of Iowa for 1856*, Iowa City, 1857, 28–29.
16. Merry, *History of Delaware County*, 150–51.

17. Lawrence, "Iowa Physicians," 151.

18. Lawrence, "Iowa Physicians," 166.

19. Lothrop, *Medical and Surgical Directory of the State of Iowa*, 133–34.

20. Lawrence, "Iowa Physicians," 168; "The Next College Session," *Iowa Medical Journal* 2 (1855): 72–73; "Close of Session and Graduating Exercises," *Iowa Medical Journal* 2 (1855): 225–27. The curriculum described in these 1855 sources is very similar to that expected in the mid-1870s and described by Lothrop.

21. Anonymous, preface in Harris, *Love and Law*, 5–6, quote on 5. The Alcott quotation is found in Alcott, *Familiar Letters to Young Men*, 15.

22. Anonymous, preface in Harris, *Love and Law*, 5–6.

23. Campbell, *Fighting Slavery in Chicago*.

24. Cheek and Cheek, *John Mercer Langston*, 171.

25. J. Harris, *Love and Law*, 18.

26. J. Harris, *Love and Law*, 21.

27. J. Harris, *Love and Law*, 22.

28. J. Harris, *Love and Law*, 22–23.

29. Raimon, *"Tragic Mulatta" Revisited*.

30. J. Harris, *Love and Law*, 14.

31. J. Harris, *Love and Law*, 15.

32. J. Harris, *Love and Law*, 15; Cecelski, *Waterman's Song*.

33. J. Harris, *Love and Law*, 16.

34. Perry, "Negro in Fayetteville," 711–12.

35. J. Harris, *Love and Law*, 17–19.

36. J. Harris, *Love and Law*, 23.

37. J. Harris, *Love and Law*, 24.

38. J. Harris, *Love and Law*, 25–26.

39. J. Harris, *Love and Law*, 26.

40. J. Harris, *Love and Law*, 27.

41. J. Harris, *Love and Law*, 30–32.

42. J. Harris, *Love and Law*, 33–34.

43. Joshua McSimpson, "Away to Canada," *Liberator*, December 12, 1852, 200.

44. J. Harris, *Love and Law*, 36–37.

45. J. Harris, *Love and Law*, 35–39.

46. J. Harris, *Love and Law*, 40–41.

47. Ernest, *Liberation Historiography*. Ernest discussed Harris's *Summer on the Borders* book but did not reference the *Love and Law* poem.

48. Ernest, *Liberation Historiography*, 50; Bell, editor's note to J. Harris, *Summer on the Borders*.

49. Berlin, *Slaves without Masters*, 66; Franklin, *Free Negro*, 48.

50. J. Harris, *Love and Law*, 42–44.

51. J. Harris, *Love and Law*, 45–48.

52. J. Harris, *Love and Law*, 49–50.

53. J. Harris, *Love and Law*, 51–53.

54. J. Harris, *Love and Law*, 54–55.

55. Priest, *Slavery, as It Relates to the Negro*; Priest, *Bible Defence of Slavery*. On the large proslavery literature, see Tise, *History of the Defense of Slavery*. My thanks to Larry Tise for directing me to the Priest volumes as the most likely source in the Harris footnote. See also Sloan, *Crimsoned Hills of Onondaga*.

56. Priest, *Bible Defence of Slavery*, 178.

57. Priest, *Slavery, as It Relates to the Negro*, 183.

58. Priest, *Slavery, as It Relates to the Negro*, 185.

59. Priest, *Slavery, as It Relates to the Negro*, 197.

60. Priest, *Slavery, as It Relates to the Negro*, 191.

61. Priest, *Slavery, as It Relates to the Negro*, 191–92; repeated in Priest, *Bible Defence of Slavery*, 230.

62. Priest, *Slavery, as It Relates to the Negro*, 199–200.

63. Haller, *Outcasts from Evolution*; Frederickson, *Black Image in the White Mind*.

64. J. Harris, *Love and Law*, 57.

65. J. Harris, *Love and Law*, 58.

66. J. Harris, *Love and Law*, 58–59.

67. J. Harris, *Love and Law*, 61.

68. J. Harris, *Love and Law*, 62.

69. J. Harris, *Love and Law*, 62.

70. J. Harris, *Love and Law*, 66.

71. J. Harris, *Love and Law*, 67–70.

72. Aptheker, *American Negro Slave Revolts*, 343.

73. "Contentment of the Slaves," *Liberator*, October 10, 1851, 163.

74. S. Oates, *Fires of Jubilee*.

75. C. Morris, "Panic and Reprisal," 29.

76. C. Morris, "Panic and Reprisal," 36. No other "heads on poles" are recorded in Morris, but full information for each eruption of panicky response is not available. It is possible that Harris had also heard about a massive slave uprising that occurred in New Orleans in 1811, when some 100 Black rebels had their heads impaled on poles, a grisly display that decorated the Mississippi levee from the Place d'Armes in the center of New Orleans forty miles up into the plantation district. Rasmussen, *American Uprising*, 147–48. Rasmussen argues that posting opponents' "heads on poles" was a familiar instrument of terror in the Atlantic World of the eighteenth century.

77. C. Morris, "Panic and Reprisal," 42.

78. J. Harris, *Love and Law*, 71. On branding as a form of punishment, see Franklin, *Free Negro*, 124.

79. J. Harris, *Love and Law*, 72.

80. J. Harris, *Love and Law*, 74–75.

81. J. Harris, *Love and Law*, 75–76.

82. Franklin, *Free Negro*, 124.

83. Glass, *Textile Industry*, 14–19.

84. J. Harris, *Love and Law*, 22.

85. Glass, *Textile Industry*, 21.

86. J. Harris, *Love and Law*, 78.

87. J. Harris, *Love and Law*, 79–80.

88. J. Harris, *Love and Law*, 84.
89. J. Harris, *Love and Law*, 84.

CHAPTER 4

1. Abraham Lincoln, quoted in "Conclusion of the Republican State Convention. Speech of Hon. Abraham Lincoln," *Chicago Tribune*, June 19, 1858, 2.
2. Delbanco, *War before the War*, 2.
3. Delbanco, *War before the War*, 5.
4. Northup, *Twelve Years a Slave*.
5. US Supreme Court, Roger Brooke Taney, John H Van Evrie, and Samuel A Cartwright, *The Dred Scott Decision: Opinion of Chief Justice Taney* (New York: Van Evrie, Horton & Co., 1860), Library of Congress, Washington, DC, www.loc.gov/item/17001543/. In this printing of the decision, the quoted text is on p. 3.
6. Fehrenbacher, *Dred Scott Case*, 349.
7. *Dred Scott Decision*, 33.
8. On Van Evrie's racist beliefs, see *Negroes and Negro "Slavery,"* first published as a pamphlet in 1853 and expanded into a book in 1863.
9. Van Evrie, introduction to *Dred Scott Decision*, 1–2.
10. "The Oppression of the Buchanan Administration towards Colored Citizens," reprinted from the *Boston Daily Bee* in *Liberator*, April 16, 1858, 62.
11. "Base and Unnatural Proscription," *Liberator*, April 27, 1860, 66.
12. *Cleveland Leader*, Sept. 21, 1858, as quoted in J. Morris, *Oberlin, Hotbed of Abolitionism*, 214.
13. Langston, "Oberlin Wellington Rescue." On Langston, see Cheek and Cheek, *John Mercer Langston*. On Harris and his participation in antislavery societies, see "Anti-Slavery Societies, Black," *Encyclopedia of Cleveland History Online*, accessed December 7, 2023, http://ech.case.edu/cgi/article.pl?id=ASB1.
14. "Charles Langston's Speech at the Cuyahoga County Courthouse," May 12, 1859, reproduced at Electronic Oberlin Group: Oberlin through History: The Oberlin-Wellington Rescue, https://isis2.cc.oberlin.edu/external/EOG/Oberlin_Wellington_Rescue/c._langston _speech.htm.
15. *Proceedings of a Convention of the Colored Men of Ohio, Held in the City of Cincinnati, on the 23d, 24th, 25th and 26th days of November, 1858* (Cincinnati: Moore, Wilstach, Keys and Co., 1850), CCP.
16. *Proceedings of a Convention of the Colored Men*.
17. *Proceedings of a Convention of the Colored Men*.
18. *Proceedings of a Convention of the Colored Men*.
19. The story of John Brown's raid has been frequently told and retold. One particularly useful and recent source is Earle, *John Brown's Raid on Harpers Ferry*.
20. "Revelations of John, from His Carpet Bag," *Cleveland Plain Dealer*, November 1, 1859, 2.
21. "Revelations of John, from His Carpet Bag."
22. On Copeland, see Lubet, *"Colored Hero" of Harper's Ferry*.
23. Cheek and Cheek, *John Mercer Langston*, 353, describes this misattribution and assigns identity properly to J. D. Harris.

24. "Revelations of John, from His Carpet Bag."

25. "Revelations of John, from His Carpet Bag."

26. John Brown Jr. to Friend Henrie [J. Henrie Kagi], September 8, 1859, *"His Soul Goes Marching On," The Life and Legacy of John Brown* online exhibit, West Virginia Archives and History, Charleston. On Harris and his participation in antislavery societies, see "Anti-Slavery Societies, Black."

27. "Revelations of John, from His Carpet Bag."

28. R. Plumb to John Henrie, August 28, 1859, in "Revelations of John, from His Carpet Bag."

29. John Copeland, facsimile transcript of handwritten interview in jail by US Marshal Matthew Johnson. Copy includes statement explaining that it was to be printed in the *Daily National Democrat* on October 31, 1859. This manuscript draft is in the John Brown Manuscripts, 1839–1943, Rare Book and Manuscript Division, Columbia University, New York, New York. See also Lubet, *"Colored Hero,"* 116–17, 134–43.

30. Copeland, transcript of interview.

31. Gobat, *Empire by Invitation*.

32. Blair, *Speech of Hon. Frank P. Blair, Jr.*

33. Blair, *Destiny of the Races*.

34. Blair, *Destiny of the Races*, 24.

35. Blair, *Destiny of the Races*, 23.

36. Blair, *Destiny of the Races*, 28.

37. Thompson to Blair, June 5, 1858, reprinted in Blair, *Destiny of the Races*, 33–34.

38. Blair, *Destiny of the Races*, 23.

39. J. D. Harris to F. P. Blair, Cleveland, Ohio, December 10, 1858, reprinted in Blair, *Destiny of the Races*, 34–35.

40. J. D. Harris, "The Central American Land Company," *Cleveland Morning Leader*, June 2, 1859, 2; Wikipedia, s.v. "Justin Holland," last modified January 9, 2024, 22:38, https://en.wikipedia.org/wiki/Justin_Holland.

41. J. Harris, "Central American Land Company."

42. J. Harris, "Central American Land Company"; Miller, *Search for a Black Nationality*, 237–38.

43. Joseph Wilson, J. Holland, and F. W. Morris, "Notice—To the Public," *Cleveland Morning Leader*, April 18, 1860.

44. Miller, *Search for a Black Nationality*.

45. Miller, *Search for a Black Nationality*, 235–36. On Redpath, see McKivigan, *Forgotten Firebrand*.

46. *Cleveland Morning Leader*, November 20, 1860.

47. *Cleveland Morning Leader*, November 20, 1860.

48. Dubois, *Haiti*, 135.

CHAPTER 5

1. Phillips, *Lesson of the Hour*, 27.

2. Phillips, *Lesson of the Hour*, 1.

3. Quoted in Starobin, *Madness Rules the Hour*, 4.

4. Phillips, *Lesson of the Hour*, 17.

5. Redpath, *Echoes of Harper's Ferry*. Wendell Phillips's *Lesson of the Hour* is on 43–66. This version includes (65) an additional clause after the word "to-day"—"as Emerson says"—that was not published in the original pamphlet. I cannot find those precise words in Emerson's writings, but similar ideas are included in Ralph Waldo Emerson, "Circles," first published in 1841 and reprinted in Emerson's *Essays*, 188.

6. H. H. S. [J. D. Harris], "The Anglo-African Empire," *Anglo-African Magazine*, March 1860, 88–95. Hereafter cited with author as J. Harris.

7. Hamilton's comment at the end of J. Harris, "Anglo-African Empire," 94.

8. Hamilton, comment at the end of J. Harris, "Anglo-African Empire," 95.

9. Phillips epigraph in J. Harris, "Anglo-African Empire," 88.

10. On the dominant importance of cotton production to the world economy, especially in the nineteenth century, see Beckert, *Empire of Cotton*.

11. J. Harris, "Anglo-African Empire," 88–89.

12. May, *Southern Dream of a Caribbean Empire*.

13. J. Harris, "Anglo-African Empire," 89.

14. J. Harris, "Anglo-African Empire," 89.

15. J. Harris, "Anglo-African Empire," 90.

16. J. Harris, "Anglo-African Empire," 90.

17. [Hunt], *Remarks on Hayti*.

18. Anonymous, "Obituary. Benjamin P. Hunt," *Philadelphia Inquirer*, February 3, 1877, 1.

19. Hunt, *Report of the Committee*. Hunt is listed as the treasurer of the group.

20. Hunt, Benjamin P., Papers, Catalogue of Books . . . , p. 100, mss. No. 4297.63, Rare Book and Manuscript Department, Boston Public Library. Hunt had two copies of the book in his donated collection. My thanks to Kimberly Reynolds, who generously provided documents from this collection when the department was closed for renovation.

21. [Hunt], *Remarks on Hayti*, 25; quoted verbatim in J. Harris, "Anglo-African Empire," 90–91. Hunt does note one exception to this eradication claim, a small French colony (unnamed) that had subsequently again liberated its slaves.

22. [Hunt], *Remarks on Hayti*, 21, quoted verbatim in J. Harris, "Anglo-African Empire," 91, italics added in Harris.

23. [Hunt], *Remarks on Hayti*, 27–28; J. Harris, "Anglo-African Empire," 91.

24. [Hunt], *Remarks on Hayti*, 30; J. Harris, "Anglo-African Empire," 91–92. The Spencer translation of Moreau de Saint-Méry's book (*A Civilization that Perished*) includes this material on 76 and 78. In the French original (*Description topographique*), the quotations are drawn from 76 and 90.

25. J. Harris, "Anglo-African Empire," 92; [Hunt], *Remarks on Hayti*, 33–34.

26. [Hunt], *Remarks on Hayti*, 35–36; J. Harris, "Anglo-African Empire," 92.

27. J. Harris, "Anglo-African Empire," 92; [Hunt], *Remarks on Hayti*, 36.

28. *Proceedings of a Convention of the Colored Men of Ohio, Held in the City of Cincinnati, on the 23d, 24th, 25th and 26th days of November, 1858* (Cincinnati: Moore, Wilstach, Keys and Co., 1850), CCP.

29. J. Harris, "Anglo-African Empire," 93.

30. J. Harris, "Anglo-African Empire," 93. The original Zouaves were North African Berbers, but some units included darker-skinned Africans as well.

31. J. Harris, "Anglo-African Empire," 93.

32. J. Harris, "Anglo-African Empire," 94.

33. *Proceedings of a Convention of the Colored Men*, 12–13. This quotation makes Walker sound like he is familiar with the trade in food commodities. I also found him in a reference about the "colored citizens of Cincinnati" in 1850, a group of which he was chair. So presumably he too was "colored," but whether he meant that, as Harris does, to be the equivalent of "mulatto" I do not know. He supports immigration to Liberia in Christy, *Lecture on African Civilization*. Appendix signed by Elias P. Walker on 51.

34. Hamilton, comment at the end of J. Harris, "Anglo-African Empire," 94.

35. On this complex topic, see Williamson, *New People*, esp. chap. 2.

36. Hamilton, comment at the end of J. Harris, "Anglo-African Empire," 95.

37. Dubois, *Avengers of the New World*, 60–90.

38. Hamilton, comment at the end of J. Harris, "Anglo-African Empire," 95.

39. J. Harris, "Anglo-African Empire," 94.

40. J. Harris, *Summer on the Borders*, 77.

41. Reproduction of Redpath's *A Guide to Hayti* (1860) at The Online Books Page University of Pennsylvania Library, accessed December 8, 2023, https://archive.org/details/guidehaytiooredp/page/n3/mode/2up. On Redpath, see Boyd, "James Redpath."

42. J. Harris, *Summer on the Borders*, 76.

43. The following bibliographical information is taken from Howard Bell's introduction to the 1970 edition of *Black Separatism and the Caribbean*, which reproduced J. Harris's *Summer*. The bibliography list is on p. 12. Rainsford, *Memoir*; Edwards, *History, Civil and Commercial*; Coke, *History*, vol. 3.

44. Bell, introduction to *Black Separatism*.

45. J. Harris, *Summer on the Borders*, 79.

46. Quoted in Coke, *History*, 3:234.

47. J. Harris, *Summer on the Borders*, 82.

48. J. Harris, *Summer on the Borders*, 82.

49. J. Harris, *Summer on the Borders*, 84.

50. J. Harris, *Summer on the Borders*, 85–86.

51. J. Harris, *Summer on the Borders*, 85–86.

52. J. Harris, *Summer on the Borders*, 88–89.

53. J. Harris, *Summer on the Borders*, 89, 92.

54. J. Harris, *Summer on the Borders*, 93–94.

55. J. Harris, *Summer on the Borders*, 95.

56. J. Harris, *Summer on the Borders*, 96, 97.

57. J. Harris, *Summer on the Borders*, 99; Edwards, *Historical Survey*, 74.

58. J. Harris, *Summer on the Borders*, 98; Edwards, *Historical Survey*, 74–75.

59. J. Harris, *Summer on the Borders*, 99; Edwards, *Historical Survey*, 75.

60. J. Harris, *Summer on the Borders*, 99.

61. Edwards, *Historical Survey*, 75–76.

62. J. Harris, *Summer on the Borders*, 100–101.

63. J. Harris, *Summer on the Borders*, 104.

64. J. Harris, *Summer on the Borders*, 104, italics in original.

65. Edwards, *Historical Survey*, 92; J. Harris, *Summer on the Borders*, 104. The poem, titled "Tit for Tat," was included in one of the earliest English books of children's poetry, first compiled by John Aikin in 1796 and reprinted multiple times. See, for example, Aikin et al., *Evenings at Home*. "Tit for Tat" is on 195–96. According to a Wikipedia article on the book, it was one of the most common children's books owned by families in the nineteenth-century Anglophone world—so also, perhaps, in the Harris household. Harris misquotes it by one word—"our" should be "your."

66. J. Harris, *Summer on the Borders*, 115, italics in original.

67. J. Harris, *Summer on the Borders*, 118, italics in original.

68. J. Harris, *Summer on the Borders*, 123, 124.

69. J. Harris, *Summer on the Borders*, 126, 127.

70. J. Harris, *Summer on the Borders*, 127.

71. Howe, "Battle Hymn of the Republic."

72. J. Harris, *Summer on the Borders*, 127.

73. J. Harris, *Summer on the Borders*, 128.

74. J. Harris, *Summer on the Borders*, 131.

75. J. Harris, *Summer on the Borders*, 132.

76. J. Harris, *Summer on the Borders*, 132.

77. J. Harris, *Summer on the Borders*, 136.

78. J. Harris, *Summer on the Borders*, 138.

79. J. Harris, *Summer on the Borders*, 145.

80. Cohen, *Fish That Ate the Whale*, 31–38.

81. J. Harris, *Summer on the Borders*, 144.

82. J. Harris, *Summer on the Borders*, 150.

83. J. Harris, *Summer on the Borders*, 157, italics in original.

84. J. Harris, *Summer on the Borders*, 159–60.

85. Dixon, *African America and Haiti*, x.

CHAPTER 6

1. J. D. Harris, letter, *Cleveland Morning Leader*, May 2, 1860, 1.

2. Dixon, *African America and Haiti*, 192–93.

3. J. Harris, *Summer on the Borders*, 55–56.

4. *Weekly Anglo-African*, March 16, 1861, back cover.

5. George William Curtis, introduction to J. Harris, *Summer on the Borders*, vii–xi, x.

6. J. Harris, *Summer on the Borders*, 15.

7. J. Harris, *Summer on the Borders*, 14, 17.

8. J. Harris, *Summer on the Borders*, 18, 22, 27–28, 14.

9. J. Harris, *Summer on the Borders*, 23–24. James McCune Smith, the first African American MD in the United States, published "Civilization: Its Dependence on Physical Circumstances," in 1859; it is reprinted in Stauffer, *Works of James McCune Smith*, 246–51.

10. J. Harris, *Summer on the Borders*, 16–17, 24.

11. J. Harris, *Summer on the Borders*, 25–26. Here Harris draws on Courtney, *Gold Fields*.

12. J. Harris, *Summer on the Borders*, 29–30, 63.

13. J. Harris, *Summer on the Borders*, 30. Curtis, in the introduction, said apologetically, "I think we may pardon the author that he does not love the government of his native land," xi. Curtis wrote in September 1860 and closed that paragraph with words of praise for the Republican Party that was to bring change to the status of the colored man. Harris likewise noted the onset of new hope in the closing letter/chapter of his book.

14. John Mercer Langston, "An Address to the Legislature of Oho," railed against this law and urged that all references to color be removed from the state constitution. Appended to the *Proceedings of the State Convention of the Colored Men of the State of Ohio, Held in the City of Columbus, January 21st, 22d and 23d, 1857* (Columbus, OH: John Geary and Son, 1857), 18–23, CCP.

15. J. Harris, *Summer on the Borders*, 34–35.

16. J. Harris, *Summer on the Borders*, 36–37.

17. J. Harris, *Summer on the Borders*, 40–41.

18. J. Harris, *Summer on the Borders*, 43–44.

19. J. Harris, *Summer on the Borders*, 44.

20. J. Harris, *Summer on the Borders*, 44–45.

21. J. Harris, *Summer on the Borders*, 46.

22. J. Harris, *Summer on the Borders*, 47.

23. Nathaniel Banks, quoted in *Congressional Globe*, 1855, 103.

24. J. Harris, *Summer on the Borders*, 47.

25. Harris apparently was quoting from "O, Get Along Home, My Yaller Gals," a "Negro song" according to a collection published in 1851. Google Books contains an excerpt from this book, but only pages 841–940. WorldCat notes no other copies. The song appears on 906–7. See www.google.com/books/edition/Old_Uncle_Ned_s_Cabin_Melodies_etc/fDZYAAAAcAAJ?hl=en&gbpv=1&dq=O,+Get+Along+Home,+My+Yaller+Gals&pg=PA906&printsec=frontcover.

26. P. T. Barnum's "What Is It?" is described in Wikipedia, s.v. "Zip the Pinhead," last modified 30 August 2023, 3:57, https://en.wikipedia.org/wiki/Zip_the_Pinhead.

27. J. Harris, *Summer on the Borders*, 47.

28. J. Harris, *Summer on the Borders*, 49.

29. J. Harris, *Summer on the Borders*, 48.

30. J. Harris, *Summer on the Borders*, 50.

31. J. Harris, *Summer on the Borders*, 51–53.

32. J. Harris, *Summer on the Borders*, 55–57.

33. The modern location of Porto Cabello is uncertain. Ports in the Dominican Republic are now labeled "Puerta" (as in "door, entryway"), not "porto." "Porto" means "port" in Portuguese; in Spanish, "porto" means "I carry." There is no port visible on the Dominican Republic map that is about sixteen miles from Puerta Plata and bears anything similar as a name. It is not clear here if Harris envisions a port where at the time (1860) there was none, perhaps a port awaiting dredging by American ingenuity.

34. J. Harris, *Summer on the Borders*, 66–67.

35. J. Harris, *Summer on the Borders*, 55.

36. John Adams to William Stephens Smith, December 26, 1787, Founders Online, National Archives, accessed December 1, 2019, https://founders.archives.gov/documents/Adams/99-02-02-0298.

37. John Adams to Abigail Adams, July 3, 1776, Adams Family Papers, Massachusetts Historical Society, accessed December 1, 2019, www.masshist.org/digitaladams/archive/doc?id=L17760703jasecond.

38. J. Harris, *Summer on the Borders*, 68–71.

39. Dubois, *Haiti*, esp. chap. 3.

40. J. Harris, *Summer on the Borders*, 73–74.

41. J. Harris, *Summer on the Borders*, 73. He is drawing on Courtney, *Gold Fields*, 102.

42. See Dubois, *Haiti*.

43. Pons, *Dominican Republic*, 197–206.

44. J. Harris, *Summer on the Borders*, 157, 158.

45. "W. E. A." of Cleveland to *Weekly Anglo-African*, January 10, 1861.

46. "Emigration Meeting," letter from Toledo, *Weekly Anglo-African*, February 5, 1861.

47. Jackson, "Cultural Stronghold."

48. Fielder, Smith, and Spires, introduction to "Weekly Anglo-African."

49. "Resolution," *Christian Recorder*, May 25, 1861.

50. "The Haytian Movement Out West," *Weekly Anglo-African*, March 23, 1861, 2.

51. "The Haytian Movement," *Weekly Anglo-African*, April 13, 1861, 3. John Brown Jr. is mentioned in the March 23, 1861, issue.

52. James Redpath, letter, *Weekly Anglo-African*, March 23, 1861.

53. Parker T. Smith to the *Christian Recorder*, October 26, 1861.

54. Fielder, Smith, and Spires, introduction to "Weekly Anglo-African," 5.

55. "Haytian Emigration," *Weekly Anglo-African*, October 6, 1861.

56. McKivigan, *Forgotten Firebrand*, 71.

57. See, for example, Moses A. Herse to Mr. Jones, reprinted in the *Pine and Palm*, dated January 24, 1862, but "mislaid" (per the editor) and only printed on September 4, 1862, p. 9.

58. J. D. Harris writing as Peregrine Cope, "Three Weeks at the Capital," *Pine and Palm*, at about January 25, 1862 (estimated from content), published March 6, 1862, 6.

59. See Holly, *Vindication*.

60. J. D. Harris to the Director General of Immigration, Haiti, "List of Immigrants arrived at St. Mark," January 29, 1862, printed in *Pine and Palm*, March 6, 1862, 5.

61. For details of this complex disaster, see especially Dixon, *African America and Haiti*, 177–216; and McKivigan, *Forgotten Firebrand*, 61–83.

62. Dixon, *African America and Haiti*, 208.

63. Harris to the Director General of Immigration, "List of Immigrants Arrived at St. Mark."

64. N. B. Harris to *Pine and Palm*, January 23, 1862, advised the stateside purchase of farming tools. This man named Harris was the agent for a group from Oberlin and advised friends to send mail c/o J. D. Harris, but he and J. D., were not relatives, as far as is known.

65. J. D. Harris, "A View of Things in and around St. Marks," *Pine and Palm*, January 2, 1862, 7. Harris had submitted the manuscript under the pen name Peregrine Cope, but the editor thought it better to use his real name to add verisimilitude to his letter.

66. J. Harris, "View of Things."

67. J. Harris, "View of Things."

68. J. Harris, "View of Things."

69. P. Hall, "Letter from Hayti," St. Marks, December 24, 1861, *Pine and Palm*, February 13, 1862, 5.

70. J. Harris writing as Peregrine Cope, "Three Weeks at the Capital."

71. J. Harris, "Three Weeks at the Capital."

72. J. Harris, "Three Weeks at the Capital."

73. J. Harris, "Three Weeks at the Capital."

74. Henry Melrose, "The Emigrants at St. Mark," report to James Redpath, April 1862, printed in *Pine and Palm*, May 29, 1862, starts on p. 4 and continues on p. 2.

75. "Public Meeting at St. Mark," held April 15, 1862, and published *Pine and Palm*, July 17, 1862, 9.

76. "Public Meeting at St. Mark," 4.

77. "Public Meeting at St. Mark," 4.

78. "Public Meeting at St. Mark," 2.

79. "Public Meeting at St. Mark," 2.

80. "Public Meeting at St. Mark," 2.

81. Henry Melrose, "The Emigrants at St. Mark," report to James Redpath, April 1862, continued in *Pine and Palm*, June 5, 1862, 4.

82. Melrose, "Emigrants at St. Mark," *Pine and Palm*, June 5, 1862, 4.

83. Henry Melrose, "The Emigrants at St. Mark," report to James Redpath, April 1862, continued in *Pine and Palm*, June 12, 1862, 4.

84. Melrose, "Emigrants at St. Mark," *Pine and Palm*, June 12, 1862, 4.

85. McKivigan, *Forgotten Firebrand*, 78.

86. James Redpath, "Resignation of the General Agent, &tc. A Farewell Address," *Pine and Palm*, September 4, 1862, reprinted in Fielder, Smith, and Spires, introduction to "Weekly Anglo-African," 47.

87. Redpath, "Resignation," 49.

88. Redpath, "Resignation," 38, 40, 43.

89. Redpath, "Resignation," 40.

CHAPTER 7

1. Morais, *History of the Negro in Medicine*, 36–37.

2. Newmark, *Without Concealment*, 168–80.

3. Alexander, "John H. Rapier," pt. 1, 38.

4. Alexander, "John H. Rapier," pt. 1.

5. Alexander, "John H. Rapier," pt. 2.

6. J. D. Harris, "Autobiography," in J. D. Harris, Personal Papers.

7. Anonymous, "Sketches of Deceased Members: Dr. Martin Luther Brooks," *Annals of the Early Settlers' Association of Cuyahoga County, Ohio* 4 (1899): 173–75. See also Woodward, "Historical Sketch." Woodward discusses Brooks's contributions on 294–95.

8. J. Morris, *Oberlin, Hotbed of Abolitionism*, 196–97.

9. Anonymous, "Sketches of Deceased Members," 174–75; Anonymous, "Biographical Record of Brooks, Martin L., M.D. (1813–1899)," in the Dittrick Medical History Center, Case Western Reserve University, Cleveland, Ohio.

10. Anonymous, "Biographical Record of Brooks, Martin." According to the Marine Hospital Service records, Brooks was appointed surgeon to the Marine Hospital Service, Cleveland, March 11, 1861, and served until 1865. Woodward, "Historical Sketch," 291–96. Martin Luther Brooks is mentioned on 294–95. The hospital served the army as well as the Marine Hospital Service during the Civil War.

11. The Marine Hospital Service was a government-sponsored health system for seamen, working on both interior lakes and rivers as well as on maritime duty. The seamen and the vessel owners paid into the system on a regular basis. The Marine Hospital Service would later form the basis of the US Public Health Service. See Humphreys, *Yellow Fever and the South*.

12. McMullan, *Plagues and Politics*.

13. "US Marine Hospital," *The Encyclopedia of Cleveland Online*, accessed December 7, 2023, https://case.edu/ech/articles/u/us-marine-hospital.

14. Waite, *Western Reserve University*, 5.

15. Waite, *Western Reserve University*, 34–35. Erie Street is now Ninth Street; the name survives in the Erie Street Cemetery.

16. Tuchman, *Science Has No Sex*, 63.

17. Tuchman, *Science Has No Sex*, 69–70.

18. Waite, *Western Reserve University*, has short biographies of the faculty who taught at Western Reserve Medical School during Harris's attendance there in his chapters on the early years of the school; see 55–170.

19. J. D. Harris, "Autobiography," in J. D. Harris, Personal Papers.

20. Helen Conger, Archivist, Case Western Reserve University Archives, Ohio, confirmed that Joseph D. Harris attended the medical department of Western Reserve College in 1863–64. If he had completed the full course of two years of study, he would have graduated in 1865. He is not listed among the 1865 graduates.

21. Waite, *Western Reserve University*, 5.

22. Waite, *Western Reserve University*, 565.

23. Waite, *Western Reserve University*, 140.

24. Waite, *Western Reserve University*, 143–44, quote on 144.

25. J. D. Harris, "Autobiography."

26. McClintock, "Medical Education in Iowa," 238–52.

27. J. D. Harris, "Autobiography."

28. "History," Carver College of Medicine, University of Iowa Health Care, accessed December 7, 2023, https://medicine.uiowa.edu/about-us/history.

29. McClintock, "Medical Education in Iowa."

30. McClintock, "Medical Education in Iowa," 241.

31. Lawrence, "Iowa Physicians," 168.

32. University of Iowa, Alumni Association, Bureau of Information, "Alumni Register: 1847–1911," *Iowa Alumnus* 8, no. 10 (September 1911). Harris is on p. 169 and Rapier on p. 172. I am grateful to Denise K. Anderson, University Archive, University of Iowa, for this information.

33. McClintock, "Medical Education in Iowa," 243.

34. Humphreys, *Intensely Human*.

35. "Faculty and students at the College of Physicians and Surgeons, State University, Keokuk, Iowa, 1860," University of Iowa College of Medicine Historical Photographs, Iowa Digital Library, accessed December 7, 2023, https://digital.lib.uiowa.edu/islandora/object/ui%3Acofmed_102. There are no Black students, although lighting in the portrait is dim.

36. J. D. Harris, "Autobiography".

37. J. D. Harris, "Autobiography."

38. Warner, *Therapeutic Perspective*, 17–36.

39. J. D. Harris, "Examination," J. D. Harris, Personal Papers.

40. Warner, *Therapeutic Perspective*, 221–24.

41. J. D. Harris, "Autobiography."

42. LOOK IN, "Letter from Virginia, July 2, 1864," *Christian Recorder*, July 9, 1864.

43. W. D. S., "A Letter from Richmond, Nov. 7," *Christian Recorder*, December 23, 1865.

44. See Humphreys, *Marrow of Tragedy*.

45. Humphreys, *Intensely Human*, 74.

46. Humphreys, *Intensely Human*, 74. Ira Russell, "Report on Hospitals in Richmond, Norfolk, etc." [1865], reel 3, frames 154–55, USSC Records.

47. Ira Russell, "Report on Hospitals in Richmond, Norfolk, etc." [1865], reel 3, frame 155, USSC Records. "Painting of Howard's Grove Hospital in Richmond, VA," Chicago Historical Museum, accessed December 7, 2023, https://images.chicagohistory.org/search/?searchQuery=howard%27s+grove. Howard's Grove Hospital was located near the current Martin Luther King, Jr. Middle School in Richmond.

48. Russell, "Report on Hospitals," frames 155–56; and frames 154–55.

49. Russell, "Report on Hospitals," frame 156.

50. Ira Russell, "Hygienic and Medical Notes," reel 5, frame 290, USSC Records.

51. Russell, "Hygienic and Medical Notes," frame 284.

52. Schwalm, *Medicine, Science*, 75.

CHAPTER 8

1. Lawlor, "Fort Monroe's Lasting Place in History."

2. Engs, *Freedom's First Generation*, is a detailed account of the Civil War and Reconstruction in the area where Harris, his brothers, and his wife-to-be carried out their educational, religious, and medical efforts with the freedpeople. See also Hollyday, *On the Heels of Freedom*; Richardson, *Christian Reconstruction*; and De Boer, "Role of Afro-Americans in the Origin and Work of the American Missionary Association." Richardson said on p. 223 of his text that it was W. D. Harris who was married to Elizabeth Worthington. He cites De Boer's dissertation (p. 423). De Boer's mistake is understandable, given the extant AMA correspondence from Elizabeth about Lottie, W. D. Harris's daughter.

3. W. E. B. Dubois, "On the Training of Black Men," *Atlantic Monthly* 90 (September 1902): 294.

4. J. J. De Lamater, "Medical Department," Report on the Freedmen's Bureau in Virginia, pp. 163–64, in "Letter of the Secretary of War, communicating, In Compliance with a resolution of the Senate of Dec. 17, 1866, reports of the assistant commissioners of freedmen,

and a synopsis of laws respecting persons of color in the late Slave States," Senate Executive Doc. No. 6, 39th Congress, 2nd Session, vol. 1276, available online at American Memory, Library of Congress, https://memory.loc.gov/cgi-bin/query/r?ammem/aaodyssey:@field (NUMBER+@band(llmisc+ody0517)).

5. Hollyday, *On the Heels of Freedom*, 1–3.

6. William D. Harris to the Executive Committee of the AMA, February 13, 1864, AMA Archives. William makes his birthdate explicit in this letter. The Harris family tree on Ancestry.com lists his birth year as 1830. The US Census for 1860 has him at thirty-two, which would be accurate if taken before his birthday on June 6.

7. North Carolina Marriage Bond for William D. Harris and Kitty Stanly, October 5, 1850, State of North Carolina, *An Index to Marriage Bonds Filed in the North Carolina State Archives* (Raleigh: North Carolina Division of Archives and History, 1977), Ancestry.com.

8. On Stanly and the New Bern free Black people, see Bishir, *Crafting Lives*.

9. William D. Harris, Draft Registration, Delaware, Ohio, 1863, NARA; Consolidated Lists of Civil War Draft Registration Records (Provost Marshal General's Bureau; Consolidated Enrollment Lists, 1863–1865), RG 110, Records of the Provost Marshal General's Bureau (Civil War), Ancestry.com.

10. William D. Harris to George Whipple, March 1, 1864, AMA Archives.

11. William D. Harris to Prof. Woodbury, April 1, 1864, AMA Archives.

12. Harris to Whipple, May 31, 1864, AMA Archives. Historian Jim Downs has described how devastating smallpox was among the freedpeople, especially those living in the dismal conditions of refugee camps. Downs, *Sick from Freedom*.

13. W. Harris to Whipple, July 1864, AMA Archives.

14. W. Harris to Whipple, April 30, 1864, AMA Archives.

15. W. Harris to Whipple, August 31, 1864, AMA Archives.

16. Matthew 19:14.

17. William D. Harris to W. S. Bell, July 5, 1866, AMA Archives.

18. William D. Harris to M. E. Strieby, July 26, 18[65], AMA Archives.

19. W. Harris to Strieby, July 27, 1865; W. Harris to Strieby, August 1865; W. Harris to Whipple, September 3, 1865, all in AMA Archives.

20. William D. Harris to Samuel Hunt, July 5, 1866, AMA Archives.

21. W. Harris to Whipple, December 1, 1865, February 17, 1866, both in AMA Archives.

22. W. Harris to Bell, July 5, 1866, AMA Archives.

23. W. Harris to Whipple, February 17, 1866, AMA Archives.

24. W. Harris to Whipple, December 11, 1866; unknown newspaper clipping dated December 13, [1866,] in the AMA files, AMA Archives.

25. W. Harris to Whipple, May 29, 1867, AMA Archives.

26. W. Harris to Whipple, September 18, 1867, AMA Archives.

27. W. Harris to Whipple, November 7, 1868, AMA Archives.

28. William D. Harris to E. P. Smith, February 15, 1869, AMA Archives.

29. W. Harris to Smith, March 1869, AMA Archives.

30. William D. Harris, census listing, Year: *1870*; Census Place: *Columbia, Richland, South Carolina*; Roll: *M593_1507*; Page: *168A*; Image: *333412*; Family History Library Film: *553006*; William D. Harris, death record, *South Carolina, Death Records, 1821–1961* [database online];

William D. Harris, Probate Administration Papers, *Richland County, South Carolina Miscellaneous Estate Records, 1799–1955*; Author: *South Carolina. County Court (Richland County)*; Probate Place: *Richland, South Carolina*; Original data: South Carolina, *South Carolina Death Records* (Columbia: South Carolina Department of Archives and History), Ancestry.com.

31. Robert Harris to George Whipple, August 26, 1864, AMA Archives.

32. R. Harris to Whipple, August 26, 1864, AMA Archives. See also West, "Harris Brothers," 127, which first alerted me to the AMA Archives.

33. R. Harris to Whipple, November 29, 1864, AMA Archives.

34. R. Harris to Whipple, December 29, 1864, February 3, 1865, March 1, 1865, AMA Archives.

35. R. Harris to Whipple, April 1, 1865, AMA Archives.

36. R. Harris to Samuel Hunt, January 1, February 1, and March 1, 1866, AMA Archives.

37. R. Harris to Hunt, May 2, 1866, AMA Archives.

38. Daniel, "Two North Carolina Families," 5.

39. The complete list of donors is David Bryant, Nelson Carter, Andrew Chesnutt, George Grainger, Matthew Leary, Thomas Lomax, and Robert Simmons. See "Our History," Fayetteville State University, accessed August 8, 2016, www.uncfsu.edu/about-fsu/our-history.

40. Brodhead, *Journals of Charles W. Chesnutt*, 7.

41. Robert Harris to E. P. Smith, December 1868, AMA Archives.

42. West, "Peabody Education Fund," 8.

43. West, "Peabody Education Fund," 10. See also Knight, *Public School Education*, 238–93, discussing Reconstruction and the Peabody Fund. Knight was hostile toward the Freedmen's Bureau and nostalgic for the Old South.

44. West, "Peabody Education Fund."

45. R. Harris to Smith, April 3, 1869, AMA Archives.

46. R. Harris to Smith, June 15, 1869, AMA Archives.

47. Peter Turner, census listing, Year: *1870*; Census Place: *Cross Creek, Cumberland, North Carolina*; Roll: *M593_1133*; Page: *194B*; Image:*122494*; Family History Library Film: *5526321870 United States Federal Census* [database online], Ancestry.com.

48. See note 53 below for census detail. There is no marriage record for them within the North Carolina files on Ancestry.com. It is possible that they married in another state.

49. R. Harris to Smith, December 1868, AMA Archives. Harris reported that he had hired three assistant teachers in June 1869, including Mary Green. R. Harris to Smith, June 15, 1869, AMA Archives.

50. Daniel, "Two North Carolina Families," 5.

51. Brodhead, *Journals of Charles W. Chesnutt*, 16–17.

52. Brodhead, *Journals of Charles W. Chesnutt*, May 8, 1880, 135.

53. Robert Harris, census listing, Year: *1880*; Census Place: *Fayetteville, Cumberland, North Carolina*; Roll: *960*; Tenth Census of the United States, 1880 (NARA microfilm publication T9, 1,454 rolls), Records of the Bureau of the Census, Record Group 29, National Archives, Washington, DC, Ancestry.com.

54. Deaderick and Thompson, "Amebic Dysentery."

55. Cicero Harris to Samuel Hunt, July 10, 1866, AMA Archives.

56. Theodore Sterling, recommendation letter in Cicero Harris file, July 7, 1866, AMA Archives.

57. W. Harris to Whipple, July 2, 1866, AMA Archives.

58. H. B. Knight to Executive Committee of the American Missionary Association, June 21, 1866, AMA Archives.

59. School report for Fayetteville, Robert Harris, November 1866; school report, Cicero Harris, December 1866, both in AMA Archives.

60. School report for Fayetteville, Robert Harris, C. Harris, and H. Broadfoot, January 1869, AMA Archives.

61. Daniel, "Two North Carolina Families," 5–6.

62. Worthington, *Genealogy*, 315–16. Albert Worthington and family census listing, 1860 census. Albert Worthington and his wife, Ruth, lives with three offsprings: Clarra or Claria, 23; Elizabeth, 20; and Albert, 18. Albert was a preacher with $8,000 in personal estate. Both girls were listed as teachers of music, living in Annsville, NY. This makes Elizabeth born in 1840. Year: *1860*; Census Place: *Annsville, Oneida, New York*; Roll: *M653_825*; Page: *166*; Image: *170*, Ancestry.com.

63. Albert Payson Worthington b. Milford Michigan, July 5, 1842. PBK at Harvard. D May 6, 1867. P. 129, The Delta Upsilon Quinquennial Catalog. Boston: The Fraternity, 1891. Educational Institutions. American Antiquarian Society, Worcester, Massachusetts. Ancestry.com. *U.S., School Catalogs, 1765–1935*. Ancestry.com.

64. Elizabeth Worthington to E. P. Smith, March 29, May 13, 1867, AMA Archives.

65. Elizabeth Worthington to Rev. George Whipple, June 10, 1864, AMA Archives.

66. Herman H. Sanford, Cortland Academy, Homer, unaddressed letter of recommendation for Elizabeth Worthington, June 10, 1864, AMA Archives.

67. Albert Worthington regarding Elizabeth Worthington, unaddressed letter of recommendation, June 1864, AMA Archives.

68. E. Worthington to Whipple, June 10, 1864, AMA Archives.

69. Elizabeth Worthington to W. E. Whiting, February 9, 1865, AMA Archives.

70. E. Worthington to W. E. Whiting, March 31, April 29, 1865, AMA Archives.

71. E. Worthington to Whipple, April 4, 1865 (incorrectly cataloged as April 4, 1866, but internal evidence confirms that the ambiguous final number is a 5), AMA Archives.

72. E. Worthington to Whipple, August 24, 1865, AMA Archives.

73. E. Worthington to Whipple, September 1865, AMA Archives.

74. E. Worthington to Rev. S. Hunt, September 7, 1865, AMA Archives.

75. E. Worthington to Whipple, September 1865, AMA Archives.

76. E. Worthington to Whipple, September 1865, AMA Archives.

77. H. D. Burnett et al. to W. E. Whiting, December 1864 (board bill), AMA Archives.

78. Elizabeth Worthington, Teacher's Monthly Report, Morehead and Carolina City, NC, January 1867, AMA Archives.

79. E. Worthington to W. E. Whiting, March 1867, AMA Archives.

80. E. Worthington to Smith, March 27, 1867. See also E. Worthington to Smith, March 18, 1867; to W. E. Whiting, March 1867; and to Smith, March 29, 1867, AMA Archives.

81. E. Worthington to Smith, May 13, 1867, AMA Archives.

82. E. Worthington to Smith, March 29, 1867, AMA Archives.

83. E. Worthington to Smith, October 1, 1867, AMA Archives.

84. Thomas Kennedy to Miss E. P. Worthington, February 8, 1868, Morehead City, NC, AMA Archives.

85. Wayne County, Marriage Register, 1861–1988, reproduced in *North Carolina, Marriage Records, 1741–2011*. Original data: North Carolina County Registers of Deeds. Microfilm. Record Group 048. North Carolina State Archives, Raleigh, NC. Ancestry.com.

86. E. Worthington to Smith, June 20, 1868, and Elizabeth Worthington to AMA, July 16, 1868, from Vineland, NJ (body of letter is missing), AMA Archives.

87. [Democratic National Committee], *Miscegenation*. See also Lemire, *"Miscegenation."*

88. Frederick, "'Loving'"; Anonymous, "Report of the Committee regarding the 14th Amendment," 96.

89. Mrs. Dr. Harris to W. E. Whiting, April 7, 1869, AMA Archives.

90. Mrs. Dr. Harris to E. P. Smith, July 13, 1869, AMA Archives.

CHAPTER 9

1. On the broader story of federal health care for the freed people during Reconstruction, see Foster, "Limitations of Federal Health Care for Freedmen"; and Downs, *Sick from Freedom*.

2. J. H. Franz to George F. Shepley, October 4, 1864, Maine Memory Network, MMN #76607, Maine Historical Society, Portland.

3. J. D. Harris, Personal Papers.

4. W. T. Sherman to Abraham Lincoln, December 22, 1864. Telegram available at *Pieces of History: A Blog of the US National Archives*, "The Must-Have Christmas Gift of 1864," ARC 311637, November 16, 2010, https://prologue.blogs.archives.gov/2010/11/16/the-must-have-christmas-gift-of-1864/.

5. J. D. Harris to Hon. E. M. Stanton, February 18, 1865, from Balfour US General Hospital, Portsmouth, VA, J. D. Harris, Personal Papers.

6. Service Record of Alexander Augusta ["Carded Records"], 7th US Colored Infantry, Volunteer Organizations, series 519, RG 94, NARA; Butts, "Alexander Thomas Augusta"; Baker, "American Medical Association." See also Humphreys, *Intensely Human*, 57–80; and Newmark, *Without Concealment*.

7. "The Emancipation Proclamation," National Archives, accessed December 8, 2023, www.archives.gov/exhibits/featured-documents/emancipation-proclamation. This website reproduces the Emancipation Proclamation both in manuscript and typescript forms.

8. J. B. McPherson et al. to President Abraham Lincoln, February 1864, reprinted in Berlin, Reidy, and Rowland, *Freedom*, 356–57.

9. Joel Morse to Senator John Sherman of Ohio, May 1864, in Berlin, Reidy, and Rowland, *Freedom*, 357.

10. George Luckley to W. A. Conover, March 24, 1865; J. D. Harris to Hon. E. M. Stanton, February 18, 1865, from Balfour US General Hospital, Portsmouth, VA, J. D. Harris, Personal Papers.

11. Collection in J. D. Harris, Personal Papers.

12. Humphreys, *Intensely Human*, 119–41; on Pease, see 63, 137–38.

13. BRFAL M1913.

14. J. Simons to Surgeon General Joseph Barnes, October 18, 1865, telling Barnes that he, Simons, annulled Harris's army contract on August 26, 1865, J. D. Harris, Personal Papers.

15. Contract with a private physician, October 1, 1865, made at Richmond, VA, in J. D. Harris, Personal Papers.

16. Anon., "Dedication of the New Medical College," *Cleveland Medical Gazette* 2 (1887): 175.

17. *Richmond Whig*, April 10, 1865, reported on hospital transition.

18. "Howard's Grove Hospital," Civil War Richmond, accessed December 8, 2023, www.civilwarrichmond.com/hospitals/howard-s-grove-hospital.

19. W. D. S., "A Letter from Richmond, Nov. 7," *Christian Recorder*, December 23, 1865.

20. Marcia Colton to George Whipple, October 16, 1865, AMA Archives. For a testimonial and mention of her work with the Choctaw Mission, see George Ainslie to Marcia Colton, March 4, 1864, AMA Archives. On hospital conditions, see Colton to Whipple, November 8, 1865, AMA Archives.

21. Colton to Whipple, May 29, 1866, AMA Archives.

22. Colton to Whipple, March 27, 1866, AMA Archives.

23. H. S. Merrill to O. Brown, December 18, 1865, roll 168, frame 102, BRFAL M1913.

24. Paul Lambrick to De Lamater, inspection report for quarter ending June 30, 1868, in the 3rd Sub District of Virginia, roll 168, frame 572, BRFAL M1913.

25. L. A. Edwards section on the "Medical Department" in his larger state report (October 20, 1866), part of the overall Commissioner of the Bureau of Refugees, Freedmen, and Abandoned Lands, *Report of 1867*, 17.

26. L. A. Edwards, Chief Medical Officer, BRFAL, October 8, 1866, to J. J. De Lamater, roll 168, Letters Received, Richmond, 1865–1868, BRFAL M1913.

27. L. A. Edwards section on the "Medical Department" in his larger state report, part of the overall Commissioner of the Bureau of Refugees, Freedmen, and Abandoned Lands, *Report of 1867*, 17.

28. Edwards, section on the "Medical Department," in Commissioner of the Bureau of Refugees, Freedmen, and Abandoned Lands, *Report of 1867*, 17.

29. Reyburn, *Type of Disease*, 16.

30. Downs, *Sick from Freedom*, 95–119.

31. Humphreys, *Marrow of Tragedy*, 91–94, 243–70.

32. Hicks, "Scabrous Matters," 123–50. On the varieties of vaccine viruses analyzed genomically using historical sources, see Duggan et al., "Origins and Genomic Diversity."

33. Reyburn, *Type of Disease*, 13.

34. L. A. Edwards section on the "Medical Department" in his larger state report, part of the overall Commissioner of the Bureau of Refugees, Freedmen, and Abandoned Lands, *Report of 1867*, 13.

35. See, for example, J. D. Harris, Requisition for Fuel for Freedmen's Hospital, April 1867. Here he says that the regular order is for six fireplaces times, two cords each, but now he needs only nine cords overall. Monthly Reports (cont.) covering November 1866 to October 1867, roll 87, frame 602, BRFAL M1913, Subordinate Field Offices, Fredericksburg. See also frame 437 for the February order.

36. This information is compiled from the reports of Major James Johnson, Superintendent of the 6th BRFAL district in Virginia, all in Monthly Reports (cont.) covering November 1866 to October 1867, roll 87, BRFAL M1913, Subordinate Field Offices, Fredericksburg.

37. J. D. Harris, Requisition for Straw for the month of September 1867, approved by cross signatures by J. J. De Lamater and O. Brown; bottom section indicates that Harris received the straw and confirmed it with his signature. In roll 87, frame 370, BRFAL M1913, Subordinate Field Offices, Fredericksburg.

38. For Lincoln Hospital Records, Savannah, see Family Search.org, accessed December 8, 2023, www.familysearch.org/ark:/61903/1:1:QLPP-L43C.

39. Humphreys, *Marrow of Tragedy*; Humphreys, *Yellow Fever*; Rosenberg, *Cholera Years*.

40. L. A. Edwards, Chief Medical Officer, BRFAL, Washington, DC, to J. J. De Lamater, Chief Medical Officer Virginia, January 4, 1867, Letters Sent, June 1865–August 1870, E98, RG 105, BRFAL M1913.

41. This record comes from an "endorsement" file. Such a file was a series of images from the backs of letters, wherein the recipient of the letter says whether he agrees (endorses) or disagrees. Then it goes up the chain to the proper authority. James Johnson, endorsement, August 6, 1867, to J. D. Harris request, Endorsements, roll 84, frame 12, BRFAL M1913, Subordinate Field Offices, Fredericksburg.

42. See S. C. Armstrong, Monthly Report of Fort Monroe to the Bureau of Refugees, Freedmen and Abandoned Lands, from March 1867 to December 1868, roll 125, BRFAL M1913, Subordinate Field Offices, Fort Monroe.

43. Endorsements, roll 128, frame 341, BRFAL M1913. At this point Elizabeth City County was legally separate from the town of Hampton, but for the bureau's purposes they were merged.

44. Office of the Chief Medical Officer, BRFAL, to J. J. De Lamater, Surgeon in Chief, District of Virginia, July 10, 1868, Letters Sent, June 1865–August 1870, Washington Headquarters: Chief Medical Officer, E98, RG 105, BRFAL M1913. Jim Downs describes both the original rationale and denouement of the bureau in *Sick with Freedom*.

45. Office of the Chief Medical Officer, BRFAL, Washington, DC, to J. J. De Lamater, in charge of Freedmen's Hospital, Richmond, September 29, 1869, Letters Sent, June 1865–August 1870, Washington Headquarters: Chief Medical Officer, E98, RG 105, BRFAL M1913.

46. My summary here only superficially describes this process. For detailed analysis see Lowe, *Republicans and Reconstruction*.

47. Lowe, *Republicans and Reconstruction*.

48. "The Charges against Governor Wells," *Richmond Whig*, March 10, 1869, 4. Page 1 of the online file contains the *Richmond Whig and Advertiser* for March 12, 1869. Apparently some of the March 10 columns were reprinted in the Friday edition.

49. *Daily Enquirer and Examiner* (Richmond), March 10, 1869.

50. *Daily Enquirer and Examiner*, March 10, 1869, 1.

51. "Petersburg Convention. Second Day's Proceedings," *Richmond Whig and Advertiser*, Friday, March 12, 1869, 1.

52. Philip W. Stanley, "Lewis Lindsey (1843–1908)," Encyclopedia Virginia, last updated December 22, 2021, www.Encyclopedia Virginia.org/Lindsey Lewis 1843–1908. Lowe, *Republicans and Reconstruction*, spells the last name "Lindsay," as do the contemporary newspapers cited here.

53. "Petersburg Convention. Second Day's Proceedings," 1.

54. "The Petersburg Convention. A Few Closing Notes," *Richmond Whig and Advertiser*, March 12, 1869, 2.

55. "The Petersburg Convention. A Few Closing Notes," 2.
56. "The Petersburg Convention. A Few Closing Notes," 2.
57. "The Petersburg Convention. A Few Closing Notes," 2.
58. *Daily Enquirer and Examiner*, March 15, 1869, 3.
59. *Daily Enquirer and Examiner*, March 11, 1869, 1.
60. *Daily Enquirer and Examiner*, March 15, 1869, 1.
61. *Daily Enquirer and Examiner*, March 12, 1869, 1.
62. *Daily Enquirer and Examiner*, June 1, 1869, 2.
63. *Daily Enquirer and Examiner*, April 26, 1869, 1.
64. *Daily Enquirer and Examiner*, April 26, 1869, 1.
65. "State Colored Convention," *Daily Dispatch*, May 29, 1869, 1, in *Report of the Virginia State Colored Convention held in Richmond, May 27, 1869* (Richmond, VA: Richmond Dispatch, 1869), CCP.
66. *Daily Enquirer and Examiner*, May 29, 1869, 1.
67. *Daily Enquirer and Examiner*, June 29, 1869, 2.
68. *Daily Enquire and Examiner*, June 3, 1869, 1.
69. *Daily Enquirer and Examiner*, June 25, 1869, 2.
70. *Daily Enquirer and Examiner*, June 25, 1869, 2.
71. *Daily Enquirer and Examiner*, June 25, 1869, 2.
72. Lowe, *Republicans and Reconstruction*, 164–82. On this election and politics in Reconstruction Virginia, see also Taylor, "Reconstruction through Compromise."
73. *Journal of the Senate of the Commonwealth of Virginia*, October 5, 1869 (Richmond, VA: James E. Goode, 1870), 34.
74. *Daily Enquirer and Examiner*, June 5, 1869, 2.
75. Pryor, *Colored Travelers*.
76. Butts, "Alexander Thomas Augusta."
77. Reported in the *Virginian-Pilot* (Norfolk), June 19, 1869, reprinted in the *Alexandria Gazette*, June 22, 1869, 4.
78. *Virginian-Pilot* (Norfolk), June 23, 1869.

CHAPTER 10

1. Reynolds, *Reconstruction in South Carolina*, 124.
2. Minutes of the Board of Regents, February 24, 1870, and April 2, 1870, Minutes of the Mental Health Commission 1828–1885, Microfilm ST 0833 (AD 671), Richland County, SCDAH.
3. Mrs. Dr. Harris to E. P. Smith, March 28, 1870, AMA Archives.
4. McCandless, *Moonlight*, 220.
5. McCandless, *Moonlight*, 213–34.
6. Joshua F. Ensor, "Superintendent's Report," November 15, 1870, Report of the Lunatic Asylum, November 1870, 417–63, in *Reports and Resolutions*.
7. Mrs. Dr. Harris to E. P. Smith, March 28, 1870, AMA Archives.
8. Simkins and Woody, *South Carolina*, 327. See also *Charleston (WV) Daily News*, April 23 and June 21, 1869.

9. "The Negro in Georgia," *Charleston Daily News,* June 23, 1869, 4.

10. William D. Harris to George Whipple, November 7, 1868, AMA Archives.

11. William D. Harris to E. P. Smith, February 15, 1869, AMA Archives.

12. W. Harris to Smith, March 1869, AMA Archives.

13. William D. Harris, 1870 census listing, Year: *1870;* Census Place: *Columbia, Richland, South Carolina;* Roll: *M593_1507;* Page: *168A; 1870 United States Federal Census,* Ancestry.com.

14. William D. Harris, death record, *South Carolina, Death Records, 1821–1961,* Columbia, SCDAH. On typhoid fever research in the nineteenth century, see Hardy, *Salmonella Infections.* On the American South and typhoid in the Spanish-American War, see Cirillo, *Bullets and Bacilli.* Troesken, *Water, Race, and Disease,* describes the provision of clean water in southern cities in the 1910s and 1920s and the impact of changed typhoid incidence on overall health. The rural South still relied in part on latrines that ultimately drained into creeks and lakes. I had to get typhoid shots to attend Girl Scout camp in the 1960s, which was situated on Kentucky Lake, a Tennessee River reservoir.

15. William D. Harris, Probate Administration Papers, *Richland County, South Carolina Miscellaneous Estate Records, 1799–1955.* Author: *South Carolina. County Court (Richland County);* Probate Place: *Richland, South Carolina,* Ancestry.com.

16. Minutes of the Mental Health Commission, 1828–1885 [Minutes of the Board of Regents, SCDAH], Microfilm ST 0833 (AD 671), April 9, 1870, SCDAH. Harris signed the minutes as recording secretary.

17. Reynolds, *Reconstruction in South Carolina,* 124–25; Minutes of the Mental Health Commission, 1828–1885, January 14, 1871, Microfilm ST 0833 (AD 671), Richland County, Minutes of the Board of Regents, SCDAH.

18. Thompson, *Ousting the Carpetbagger,* 67. The frontispiece says, "Dedicated to the red shirts of 1876, whose unceasing vigilance led to overthrow of republican misrule and ousting the carpet bagger from SC."

19. J. D. Harris to the editor, *Columbia Daily Phoenix,* November 23, 1870.

20. Humphreys, *Marrow of Tragedy,* 67.

21. Lemire, *"Miscegenation."*

22. Cobb, *First Negro Medical Society.*

23. Vol. I, Statistics. Table 1. Population of the United States, (by States and Territories,) in the Aggregate, and as White, Colored, Free Colored, Slave, Chinese, and Indian, at Each Census, 4, in *Ninth US Census, 1870;* "Today in History—April 16," Library of Congress, accessed December 8, 2023, www.loc.gov/item/today-in-history/april-16/.

24. Summers, *Madness in the City of Magnificent Intentions,* 15–24.

25. Daniel, "Two North Carolina Families," 3–12, 14, 23.

26. Boyd, *Boyd's Directory,* 37.

27. Both catalogs are reproduced in the Digital Howard Collection sponsored by Howard University Archives: *Catalog of the Officers and Students of Howard University, 1871–72,* 33, Howard University Catalogs, Howard University Archives, https//dh.howard.edu/hucatalogs/33; *Catalog of the Officers and Students of Howard University, 1873–74,* 32, Howard University Catalogs, Howard University Archives, https//dh.howard.edu/hucatalogs/32. There is not a catalog for 1872–73 in this collection or, to my knowledge, anywhere. Walter Dyson, an early historian of the school, said none was printed. Dyson, *Founding the School,* 27; Lamb, *Howard University Medical Department.*

28. Case Records for J. D. Harris, SEH.

29. "In the Matter of the Alleged Lunacy of Joseph D. Harris," Equity Docket No. 5780, Supreme Court of the District of Columbia, September 4, 1877, Records of the District Courts of the United States, RG 21, NARA.

30. Joseph D. Harris vs. John Brauman and Caroline Walte and minor heir of Thomas Walter, deceased, October 15, 1874, Equity Case Files, 1863–1938, Records of the District Courts of the United States, RG 21, NARA.

31. Mrs. Dr. Harris to Dr. A. H. Witmer, February 24, 1877, SEH.

32. Harris to Witmer, February 24, 1877, SEH.

33. Anonymous, *Act Regulating the Rights of Married Women*, 45.

34. Elizabeth Harris to Dr. A. H. Witmer, February 28, 1877, SEH.

35. Elizabeth Harris to Dr. Charles Nichols, March 21, 1877, SEH.

36. Elizabeth Harris to William Godding, October 9, 1884, SEH.

37. Alexander Hughes and Daniel McCarty vs. Joseph D. Harris and Elizabeth Harris, Equity Case Files #4726, box 342, entry 69, Equity Case Files, 1863–1938, Records of the District Courts of the United States, RG 21, NARA.

38. Deposition of Alexander J. Hughes, February 12, 1876; Deposition of Joseph D. Harris, March 3, 1876, both in Equity Case Files, 1863–1938, Records of the District Courts of the United States, RG 21, NARA.

39. Henry W. Garnett, Report of the Special Auditor, October 18, 1876, in Equity Case Files #4726.

40. Documents in court file regarding Kitty S. Harris, admin., v. E. W. Harris, trustee, March 25, 1880, Equity No. 7218, Docket 20, in the Supreme Court of the District of Columbia, March 25, 1880. "Equity Case Files, 1863–1938," Records of the District Courts of the United States, RG 21, NARA.

41. Holt, Smith-Parker, and Terborg-Penn, *Special Mission*, 7–11, quotation on 11.

42. Holt, Smith-Parker, and Terborg-Penn, *Special Mission*, 11.

43. Dyson, *Founding the School*, 24.

44. Holt, Smith-Parker, and Terborg-Penn, *Special Mission*.

45. Lamb, *Howard University Medical Department*, 76.

46. G. D. Palmer, surgeon-in-chief Freedmen's Hospital, to Columbus Delano, Secretary of the Interior, June 30, 1875, Records of the Freedmen's Hospital 1872–1910, Correspondence and Memoranda, 6 reels, NG 48, NARA.

47. Lamb, *Howard University Medical Department*, 107–8.

48. Mrs. Harris to Dr. Chase and Dr. Witmer, September 12, 1877, SEH.

49. Mrs. Harris to Dr. Chase, December 1876, SEH.

CHAPTER 11

1. J. D. Harris, Certificate of Death, December 25, 1884. Facsimile reproduction in G. Harris, *Harris Family History*, n.p.

2. Elizabeth Harris to J. D. H[arris], March 15, 1877, SEH.

3. I believe the historian who asked the question was Jennifer L. Morgan, professor of social and cultural analysis and history at New York University. I appreciate her useful intervention.

4. E. Harris to Dr. Chase, December 1876, SEH.

5. E. Harris to Dr. Chase, [date unknown but likely late 1876–77], SEH.

6. "In the Matter of the Alleged Lunacy of Joseph D. Harris," Equity Docket No. 5780, Supreme Court of the District of Columbia, September 4, 1877, Records of the District Courts of the United States, RG 21, NARA.

7. Affidavits from Dr. C. H. Nichols, Superintendent of the Government Hospital for the Insane, August 22, 1877, and Dr. A. H. Witmer, Assistant Physician at the Government Hospital for the Insane, August 22, 1877. The quoted sentence is identical in the two affidavits (except that Witmer excludes the "of" before the word "taking," an indication that they were repeating a set legal language that established that a person needed a guardian). Located in packet of materials relating to Equity Docket No. 5780, Supreme Court of the District of Columbia, September 4, 1877, Records of the District Courts of the United States, RG 21, NARA.

8. E. Harris to Dr. Charles Nichols, May 25, 1877, SEH.

9. Otto, *St. Elizabeths Hospital*.

10. Summers, *Madness in the City of Magnificent Intentions*.

11. Tomes, *A Generous Confidence*.

12. Otto, *St. Elizabeths Hospital*, 6–15.

13. Charles Nichols, quoted in Otto, *St. Elizabeths Hospital*, 37.

14. Summers, *Madness in the City of Magnificent Intentions*, 6–7.

15. Otto, *St. Elizabeths Hospital*, 114–15; Millikan, "Wards of the Nation," 149–50.

16. Blackburn, *Intracranial Tumors*, 94.

17. See, for example, E. Harris to W. W. Godding, April 2, September 1, and December 31, 1880, all in SEH.

18. J. D. Harris to W. W. Godding, Thanksgiving, 1879. The letter is dated 1869, but it is filed together with an 1879 letter, and Harris did not enter St. Elizabeths and begin correspondence with Godding until the mid-1870s.

19. J. Harris to Godding, January 14, 1880, SEH.

20. J. Harris to Godding, December 27, 1881, SEH.

21. E. Harris to J. Harris, March 15, 1877, SEH.

22. E. Harris to Nichols, March 30, June 9, 1877 (remarks that Dr. Harris became ill after attending chapel in a thick coat), SEH.

23. E. Harris to Nichols, July 8, 1877, SEH.

24. Register entry for Elizabeth Harris, November 26, 1871, entry no. 7253, roll 4, Register of Signatures of Depositors in Branches of the Freedman's Savings and Trust Co., 1868–1873, Freedman's Bank Records, 1865–1874, NARA. The records are freely available at Family Search, www.familysearch.org/search/catalog/133425. See also Osthaus, *Freedmen*. On Douglass's role as titular head of the bank, see Blight, *Frederick Douglass*, 546–49.

25. E. Harris to Nichols, March 26, 1879, SEH.

26. E. Harris to Nichols, October 14, 1879, SEH.

27. E. Harris to Godding, April 2, 1880, SEH.

28. Summers, *Madness in the City of Magnificent Intentions*, 68–70.

29. E. Harris to Godding, January 18, 1883, SEH.

30. Featherstonhaugh, *Instructions to Examining Surgeons of the Bureau of Pensions*.

31. E. Harris to Godding, January 18, 1883, SEH.

32. E. Harris to Godding, January 1883, SEH.

33. E. Harris to Godding, January 1883, SEH.
34. E. Harris to Godding, January 18, 1883, SEH.
35. E. Harris to Godding, January 18, 1883, SEH.
36. Joshua F. Ensor, "Superintendent's Report," November 15, 1870, Report of the Lunatic Asylum, November 1870, 417–63, in *Reports and Resolutions*.
37. Sieveking, *On Epilepsy*, 200, 201.
38. Sieveking, *On Epilepsy*, 170–71, 207, 159.
39. Sieveking, *On Epilepsy*, 160–62.
40. Sieveking, *On Epilepsy*, 204–5, italics in original.
41. Sieveking *On Epilepsy*, 216, 218–22, 226, 235, 236.
42. Hammond, *Treatise*; Blustein, *Preserve Your Love for Science*.
43. Hammond, *Treatise*, 560, 563.
44. Hammond, *Treatise*, 565. On the history of epilepsy, see Temkin, *Falling Sickness*.
45. Hammond, *Treatise*, 570, 572.
46. Hammond, *Treatise*, 572, 574–75, 582, 583.
47. Hammond, *Treatise*, 583–85.
48. J. D. Harris to The Honorable Superintendent, March 26, 1877, SEH.
49. Temkin, *Falling Sickness*, 257–58.
50. E. Harris to Nichols, June 9, 1877, SEH.
51. E. Harris to Witmer, July 16, 1878, SEH.
52. Dr. J. D. Harris, "Sympathetic Diseases, 1878," December 27, 1878, SEH.
53. Temkin discussed eighteenth-century versions of this idea in *Falling Sickness*, 216–17.
54. Barker-Benfield, *Horrors of the Half-Known Life*; Morantz-Sanchez, *Sympathy and Science*.
55. J. Harris, "Sympathetic Diseases, 1878."
56. E. Harris to Godding, February 20, 1878, SEH.
57. E. Harris to Godding, February 10, 1879, SEH.
58. J. Harris to Godding, April 13, 1879, SEH.
59. J. Harris to Godding, April 13, 1879, SEH.
60. E. Harris to Godding, April 29, 1879, SEH.
61. E. Harris to Godding, May 2, 1879, SEH.
62. E. Harris to Godding, May 14, 1879, SEH.
63. E. Harris to Godding, September 30, 1879, SEH.
64. J. Harris to Godding, January 14, 1880, SEH.
65. On the innovation and high expectations of chloral hydrate, see Warner, *Therapeutic Perspective*, 270.
66. On the rise of stimulants, and especially alcohol, in mid-nineteenth-century medicine, see Warner, *Therapeutic Perspective*, 143–61.
67. J. Harris, "Sympathetic Diseases, 1878."
68. E. Harris to Godding, October 4, 1883, SEH.
69. J. Harris to Godding, January 18, 1880, SEH.
70. E. Harris to Nichols, March 30, 1877, SEH.
71. E. Harris to Nichols, July 8, 1877, SEH.
72. E. Harris to Chase, December 1876, SEH.
73. E. Harris to Witmer, August 3, 1877, SEH.

74. E. Harris to Nichols, March 30, 1877, SEH.

75. E. Harris to Chase, December 1876, SEH.

76. E. Harris to Nichols, March 30, 1877, SEH.

77. J. Harris to Godding, Sycamore Ward, December 27, 1881, SEH.

78. E. Harris to Godding, January 3, 1882, SEH.

79. E. Harris to Godding, October 4, 1882, SEH.

80. "In the Matter of the Alleged Lunacy of Joseph D. Harris," Equity Docket No. 5780, Supreme Court of the District of Columbia, September 4, 1877, Records of the District Courts of the United States, RG 21, NARA.

81. E. Harris to Nichols, March 10, 1877, SEH.

82. E. Harris to Witmer, February 24, 1877, SEH.

83. E. Harris to Nichols, May 25, 1877, SEH.

84. E. Harris to Godding, July 10, 1882, SEH.

85. E. Harris to Godding, [n.d.], 1883, SEH.

86. E. Harris to Godding, July 2, 1883, SEH.

87. Engel and Pedley, *Epilepsy*. See especially Frank Benson and Bruce Hermann, "Personality Disorders," in Engel and Pedley, *Epilepsy*, 2065–70, 2065.

88. Sigmund Freud, quoted in Geschwind, "Personality Changes," 426. Freud's essay, "Dostoevsky and Parricide," is reproduced in *Sigmund Freud Complete Psychological Works*, 177–94.

89. Devinsky and Schacter, "Norman Geschwind's Contribution," 417–24, 423.

90. J. D. Harris, Certificate of Death, December 25, 1884. Facsimile reproduction in G. Harris, *Harris Family History*, n.p.

CONCLUSION

1. Carpio, Escobar, and Hauser, "Progress in Epilepsy Research," 1025. See also Fleury et al., "Cysticercosis."

2. "Parasites—Cysticercosis," Centers for Disease Control and Prevention, accessed October 19, 2023, www.cdc.gov/parasites/cysticercosis/index.html.

3. G. Harris, *Harris Family History*.

4. G. Harris, *Harris Family History*.

5. Newmark, *Without Concealment*.

BIBLIOGRAPHY

PRIMARY SOURCES

Manuscript and Archival Collections

Boston, Massachusetts
    Boston Public Library, Rare Book and Manuscript Department
        Hunt, Benjamin P., Papers, Catalogue of Books, Pamphlets, Maps & Charts, Manuscripts & Engravings, Relating to the West Indies

Charleston, West Virginia
    West Virginia Archives and History
        Documents Relative to the Harpers Ferry Invasion Appended to Governor Wise's Message
        "His Soul Goes Marching On," *The Life and Legacy of John Brown* online exhibit

Cleveland, Ohio
    Case Western Reserve University
        Dittrick Medical History Center

Columbia, South Carolina
    South Carolina Department of Archives and History
        Miscellaneous Estate Records, 1799–1955 (accessed through Ancestry.com)
        Records of the State Lunatic Asylum
            Minutes of the Mental Health Commission, 1828–85, Microfilm ST 0833 (AD 671), Richland County, SC, Members of the Board of Regents

New Orleans, Louisiana
    Tulane University, Amistad Research Collection
        American Missionary Association Archives

New York, New York
    Columbia University, Rare Book and Manuscript Library

John Brown Manuscripts, 1839–1943 (accessed through ProQuest)
New York Public Library, Manuscripts and Archives Division
   United States Sanitary Commission Records, 1861–79, microfilm
Portland, Maine
   Maine Memory Network, Maine Historical Society, MMN #76607,
      www.mainememory.net/search?keywords=76607
Raleigh, North Carolina
   State Archives of North Carolina
Richmond, Virginia
   Library of Virginia
      Henry A. Wise Papers
State College, Pennsylvania
   Penn State University Libraries
      Colored Conventions Project (accessed online)
Washington, DC
   Howard University, Howard University Archives
      Digital Howard Collection, 1871–74
   National Archives and Records Administration
      Records of St. Elizabeth's Hospital, Washington, DC, RG 418
         Case Records of Patients, 1855–1950
      Records of the Adjutant General's Office, US Army, RG 94
         Personal Papers of Medical Officers and Physicians
         J. D. Harris Papers, box 249
      Records of the Bureau of Refugees, Freedmen, and Abandoned Lands
         Records of the Field Offices for the State of Virginia,
            1865–72, Microfilm Collection M1913
      Records of the Bureau of the Census, RG 29
            (microfilm, accessed through Ancestry.com)
         Fifth Census of the United States, 1830, M19
         Sixth Census of the United States, 1840, M704
         Seventh Census of the United States, 1850, M432
         Eighth Census of the United States, 1860, M653
         Ninth Census of the United States, 1870, M593
         Tenth Census of the United States, 1880, T9
      Records of the District Courts of the United States, RG 21

Published Primary Sources

Aikin, John, Mrs. Barbauld, Arthur Aiken, and Miss Aikin. *Evenings at Home; or, The Juvenile Budget Opened*. 16th ed. London: Longman and Company, 1846.
Alcott, William A. *Familiar Letters to Young Men on Various Subjects, Designed as a Companion to the Young Man's Guide*. Buffalo, NY: George H. Derby and Co., 1850.
Anonymous. *An Act Regulating the Rights of Married Women in the District of Columbia*. April 10, 1869, 41st Cong., 1st Sess., ch. 23, in *The Statutes at Large and Publications of the United*

States of America, from December 1869 to March 1871, edited by George Sanger, 44–45. Boston: Little, Brown, 1871.

Anonymous. "Report of the Committee regarding the 14th Amendment." *Journal of the Senate and House of Commons of the General Assembly of North Carolina, 1866–1867*. Raleigh, NC: Wm. E. Pell, 1867.

Blair, Frank P., Jr. *The Destiny of the Races of this Continent*. Washington, DC: Buell and Blanchard Printers, 1859.

———. *Speech of Hon. Frank P. Blair, Jr. of Missouri, on the Acquisition of Territory in Central and South America, to be Colonized with Free Blacks, and Held as a Dependency by the United States*. Pamphlet. Washington, DC: Buell and Blanchard, Printers, 1858.

Boyd, William H. *Boyd's Directory of the District of Columbia*. Washington, DC: R. L. Polk and Co., 1875.

Christy, David. *A Lecture on African Civilization: Including a Brief Outline of the Social and Moral Condition of Africa; and the Relations of American Slavery* . . . Cincinnati: J. A. and U. P. James, 1849.

Coke, Thomas. *A History of the West Indies* . . . 3 vols. Liverpool: Printed by Nuttall, Fisher, and Dixon, 1808–11.

Commissioner of the Bureau of Refugees, Freedmen, and Abandoned Lands. *Report of the Commissioner of the Bureau of Refugees, Freedmen and Abandoned Lands for the Year 1865*. Washington, DC: Government Printing Office, 1865.

———. *Report of the Commissioner of the Bureau of Refugees, Freedmen, and Abandoned Lands for the Year 1867*. Washington, DC: Government Printing Office, 1867.

Courtney, W. S. *The Gold Fields of St. Domingo*. New York: A. P. Norton, 1860.

[Democratic National Committee]. *Miscegenation. Endorsed by the Republican Party*. New York, 1864.

Edwards, Bryan. *An Historical Survey of the French Colony in the Island of St. Domingo*. London: John Stockdale, 1797.

———. *The History, Civil and Commercial, of the British West Indies* . . . 5th ed. 5 vols. London: G. and W. B. Whitaker, 1818–19.

Edwards, L. A. "Medical Supplies." In *Report of the Commissioner of the Bureau of Refugees, Freedmen, and Abandoned Lands for the Year 1867*, by Commissioner of the Bureau of Refugees, Freedmen, and Abandoned Lands, 10–21. Washington, DC: Government Printing Office, 1867.

Emerson, Ralph Waldo. *Essays*. New York: FM Lupton Publishing Co., 1870.

Featherstonhaugh, Thomas. *Instructions to Examining Surgeons of the Bureau of Pensions, 1893*. Washington, DC: Government Printing Office, 1893.

Fielder, Brigette, Cassander Smith, and Derrick R. Spires, eds. Introduction to "Weekly Anglo-African and The Pine and Palm: Excerpts from 1861–1862." *Just Teach One: Early African American Print*, no. 4 (Spring 2018). https://jtoaa.americanantiquarian.org/welcome-to-just-teach-one-african-american/weekly-anglo-african-and-the-pine-and-palm/.

Hammond, William. *A Treatise on Diseases of the Nervous System*. New York: Appleton, 1871.

Harris, J. Dennis. *Love and Law, South and West: A Poem*. Chicago: Charles Scott, 1856.

———. *A Summer on the Borders of the Caribbean Sea*. Introduction by George William Curtis. New York: A. B. Burdick, 1860. Reprinted with an introduction in *Black Separatism and the Caribbean 1860*, edited by Howard H. Bell, 1–16. Ann Arbor: University of Michigan Press, 1970.

Holly, James Theodore. *A Vindication of the Capacity of the Negro Race for Self-Government, and Civilized Progress, as Demonstrated by Historical Events of the Haytian Revolution; and the Subsequent Acts of that People since Their National Independence.* New Haven, CT: Afric-American Printing Co., 1857. Reprinted with an introduction in *Black Separatism and the Caribbean 1860,* edited by Howard H. Bell, 17–66. Ann Arbor: University of Michigan Press, 1970.

Howe, Julia Ward. "Battle-Hymn of the Republic." 1861. Poetry Foundation. www.poetry foundation.org/poems/44420/battle-hymn-of-the-republic.

[Hunt, Benjamin P.]. *Remarks on Hayti as a Place of Settlement for Afric-[A]mericans; and on the Mulatto as a Race for the Tropics.* Philadelphia: T. B. Pugh, 1860.

Hunt, Benjamin P. *Report of the Committee for the Securing to Colored People the Use of the Street-cars.* Philadelphia: Merrihew & Sons, Printers, 1865.

Lamb, Daniel Smith. *Howard University Medical Department, Washington, D.C.: A Historical, Biographical and Statistical Souvenir.* 1900. Reprint, Freeport, NY: Books for Libraries Press, 1971.

Langston, John Mercer. *From the Virginia Plantation to the National Capitol: or The First and Only Negro Representative in Congress from the Old Dominion.* Hartford, CT: American Publishing Company, 1894.

———. "The Oberlin Wellington Rescue." *Anglo-African Magazine* 1 (July 1859): 210–14.

Lothrop, Charles H. *The Medical and Surgical Directory of the State of Iowa.* Lyons, IA: J. G. Hopkins Printer, 1876.

Merry, John F., ed. *History of Delaware County, Iowa, and Its People.* Vol. 1. Chicago: S. J. Clarke, 1914.

Moreau de Saint-Méry, Médéric-Louis-Élie. *A Civilization That Perished: The Last Years of White Colonial Rule in Haiti.* Philadelphia, published by the author, 1797–98. Translated, abridged, and edited by Ivor D. Spencer. Lanham, MD: University Press of America, 1985.

———. *Description topographique, physique, civile, politique, et historique de la partie française de l'isle Saint-Domingue.* Philadelphia, published by the author, 1797–98.

Morton, Samuel George. *Crania Americana.* Philadelphia: J. Dobson, 1839.

Northup, Solomon. *Twelve Years a Slave.* Auburn: Derby and Miller, 1853.

Phillips, Wendell. *The Lesson of the Hour: Lecture of Wendell Phillips Delivered at Brooklyn, N.Y., Tuesday Evening, November 1, 1859.* n.p.: n.p., 1859. Americana Collection, Library of Congress, Washington, DC.

Priest, Josiah. *Bible Defence of Slavery, and Origin Fortunes, and History of the Negro Race.* Glasgow, KY: W. S. Brown, 1852.

———. *Slavery, as It Relates to the Negro, or African Race: Examined in the Light of Circumstances, History, and the Holy Scriptures . . . with Strictures on Abolitionism.* Albany: C. Van Benthuysen and Co., 1843.

Rainsford, Marcus. *A Memoir of the Transactions That Took Place in St. Domingo, in the Spring of 1799* [. . .]. London: R. B. Scott, Printer, 1802.

Redpath, James, ed. *Echoes of Harper's Ferry.* Boston: Thayer and Eldridge, 1860.

Reports and Resolutions of the General Assembly of the State of South Carolina at the Regular Session, 1870–71. Columbia, SC: Republican Printing Co., 1871.

Reyburn, Robert. *Type of Disease among Freed People of the United States Consolidated . . . under Treatment from 1865 to June 30 1872 by Medical Officers on Duty in Bureau of Refugees*

Freedmen and Abandoned Lands. Submitted as a report to Surgeon General Joseph Barnes, 1874; printed as a separate pamphlet. Washington, DC: Gibson Bros., 1891.

Reynolds, John S. *Reconstruction in South Carolina, 1865–1877.* Columbia, SC: State Co., 1905. Reprint, New York: Negro Universities Press, 1969.

Sanger, George P., ed. *The Statutes at Large and Proclamations of the United States of America, from December 1869 to March 1871.* Boston: Little, Brown, 1871.

Sieveking, Edward Henry. *On Epilepsy and Epileptiform Seizures: Their Causes, Pathology, and Treatment.* London: John Churchill, 1858.

Stauffer, John, ed. *The Works of James McCune Smith: Black Intellectual and Abolitionist.* New York: Oxford University Press, 2006.

US Public Health Service. *Annual Report of the Supervising Surgeon General of the Marine Hospital Service of the United States for the Fiscal Year 1896.* Washington, DC: Government Printing Office, 1896.

Van Evrie, J. H. *Negroes and Negro "Slavery": The First an Inferior Race: The Latter Its Normal Condition.* New York: Van Evrie, Horton, 1863.

Wells, Samuel R. *Hand-Books for Home Improvement, Comprising How to Write. How to Talk. How to Behave. How to Do Business.* New York: Fowler and Wells, 1869.

Woodward, R. A. "Historical Sketch of the United States Marine-Hospital Service at Cleveland, Ohio." In *Annual Report of the Supervising Surgeon General of the Marine Hospital Service of the United States for the Fiscal Year 1896,* by US Public Health Service, 291–96. Washington, DC: Government Printing Office, 1896.

Worthington, George. *The Genealogy of the Worthington Family.* Cleveland: n.p., 1894.

Newspapers and Periodicals

Alexandria Gazette
Anglo-African Magazine
Annals of the Early Settlers' Association of Cuyahoga County (OH)
The Atlantic
Atlantic Monthly
Carolina Observer (Fayetteville)
Charleston (WV) Daily News
Chicago Tribune
Christian Recorder
Cleveland Medical Gazette
Cleveland Morning Leader
Cleveland Plain Dealer
Columbia Daily Phoenix
Congressional Globe
Daily Enquirer and Examiner (Richmond)
Fayetteville Observer
Iowa Medical Journal
Jamaica Journal
JAMA Network Open
Journal of the Senate of the Commonwealth of Virginia
Liberator
Norfolk Virginian Pilot
North Carolina Standard (Raleigh)
Philadelphia Inquirer
Pine and Palm
Richmond Whig
Richmond Whig and Advertiser
Virginian-Pilot (Norfolk)
Weekly Anglo-African

SECONDARY SOURCES

Books

Aptheker, Herbert. *American Negro Slave Revolts*. New York: International Publishers, 1970.
Ball, Erica L. *To Live an Antislavery Life: Personal Politics and the Antebellum Black Middle Class*. Athens: University of Georgia Press, 2012.
Barcia, Manuel. *The Yellow Demon of Fever: Fighting Disease in the Nineteenth-Century Transatlantic Slave Trade*. New Haven, CT: Yale University Press, 2020.
Barker-Benfield, G. *The Horrors of the Half-Known Life: Male Attitudes toward Women and Sexuality in Nineteenth-Century America*. New York: Harper and Row, 1977.
Beckert, Sven. *Empire of Cotton: A New History of Global Capitalism*. New York: Alfred A. Knopf, 2014.
Bell, Howard H., ed. *Black Separatism and the Caribbean, 1860*. Ann Arbor: University of Michigan Press, 1970.
Berlin, Ira. *Slaves without Masters: The Free Negro in the Antebellum South*. New York: Pantheon Books, 1974.
Berlin, Ira, ed., and Joseph P. Reidy and Leslie Rowland, assoc. eds. *Freedom: A Documentary History of Emancipation, 1861–1867. Selected from the Holdings of the National Archives of the United States. Series II: The Black Military Experience*. Cambridge: Cambridge University Press, 1982.
Bishir, Catherine W. *Crafting Lives: African American Artisans in New Bern, North Carolina, 1770–1900*. Chapel Hill: University of North Carolina Press, 2013.
Blackburn, Isaac Wright. *Intracranial Tumors among the Insane: A Study of Twenty-Nine Intracranial Tumors found in Sixteen Hundred and Forty-Two Autopsies in Cases of Mental Disease*. Washington, DC: Government Printing Office, 1908.
Blight, David. *Frederick Douglass: Prophet of Freedom*. New York: Simon and Schuster, 2018.
Blustein, Bonnie. *Preserve Your Love for Science: Life of William A. Hammond, American Neurologist*. New York: Cambridge University Press, 1991.
Bonilla-Silva, Eduardo. *Racism without Racists: Color-Blind Racism and the Persistence of Racial Inequality in America*. 5th ed. Lanham, MD: Rowman and Littlefield, 2018.
Bourdieu, Pierre. *Outline of a Theory of Practice*. Translated from the French by Richard Nice. Cambridge: Cambridge University Press, 1972 (French), 1977 (English).
Boyd, W. D. "James Redpath and American Negro Colonization in Haiti, 1860–1862." *The Americas* 12, no. 2 (1955): 169–82.
Boyer, Paul, and Stephen Nissenbaum. *Salem Possessed: The Social Origins of Witchcraft*. Cambridge, MA: Harvard University Press, 1974.
Brodhead, Richard, ed. *The Journals of Charles W. Chesnutt*. Durham, NC: Duke University Press, 1993.
Butts, Heather. *African American Medicine in Washington, D.C.: Healing the Capital during the Civil War Era*. Charleston, SC: History Press, 2014.
Campbell, Tom. *Fighting Slavery in Chicago: Abolitionists, the Law of Slavery, and Lincoln*. Chicago: Ampersand, 2009.

Cecelski, David. *The Waterman's Song: Slavery and Freedom in Maritime North Carolina*. Chapel Hill: University of North Carolina Press, 2001.

Chanoff, David, and Louis W. Sullivan. *We'll Fight It Out Here: A History of the Ongoing Struggle for Health Equity*. Baltimore: Johns Hopkins University Press, 2022.

Cheek, William, and Aimee Lee Cheek. *John Mercer Langston and the Fight for Black Freedom, 1829–1865*. Urbana: University of Illinois Press, 1989.

Childs, Frances Sergeant. *French Refugee Life in the United States, 1790–1800: An American Chapter of the French Revolution*. Baltimore: Johns Hopkins University Press, 1940.

Cirillo, Vincent. *Bullets and Bacilli: The Spanish-American War and Military Medicine*. New Brunswick, NJ: Rutgers University Press, 2004.

Cobb, W. Montague. *The First Negro Medical Society*. Washington, DC: Associated Publishers, 1939.

Cohen, Rich. *The Fish That Ate the Whale: The Life and Times of America's Banana King*. New York: Farrar, Straus and Giroux, 2012.

Delbanco, Andrew. *The War before the War: Fugitive Slaves and the Struggle for America's Soul from the Revolution to the Civil War*. New York: Penguin Press, 2018.

Demos, John. *A Little Commonwealth: Family Life in Plymouth Colony*. New York: Oxford University Press, 1970.

Dixon, Chris. *African America and Haiti: Emigration and Black Nationalism in the Nineteenth Century*. Westport, CT: Greenwood Press, 2000.

Downs, Jim. *Sick from Freedom: African-American Illness and Suffering during the Civil War and Reconstruction*. New York: Oxford University Press, 2012.

Drachman, Virginia. G. *Hospital with a Heart: Women Doctors and the Paradox of Separatism at the New England Hospital, 1862–1969*. Ithaca: Cornell University Press, 1984.

Dubois, Laurent. *Avengers of the New World*. Cambridge, MA: Harvard University Press, 2004.

———. *Haiti: The Aftershocks of History*. New York: Henry Holt, 2012.

Duffin, Jacalyn. *Langstaff: A Nineteenth-Century Medical Life*. Toronto: University of Toronto Press, 1993.

Dykstra, Robert R. *Bright Radical Star: Black Freedom and White Supremacy on the Hawkeye Frontier*. Cambridge, MA: Harvard University Press, 1993.

Dyson, Walter. *Founding the School of Medicine of Howard University, 1868–1873*. Washington, DC: Howard University Press, 1929.

Earle, Jonathan. *John Brown's Raid on Harpers Ferry: A Brief History with Documents*. New York: Bedford/St. Martin's, 2008.

Engel, Jerome, Jr., and Timothy A. Pedley, eds. *Epilepsy: A Comprehensive Textbook*. Vol. 2. Philadelphia: Lippincott-Raven, 1998.

Engs, Robert Francis. *Freedom's First Generation: Black Hampton, Virginia, 1861–1890*. New York: Fordham University Press, 1979.

Ernest, John. *Liberation Historiography: African American Writers and the Challenge of History, 1794–1861*. Chapel Hill: University of North Carolina Press, 2004.

Fehrenbacher, Don E. *The Dred Scott Case: Its Significance in American Law and Politics*. New York: Oxford University Press, 1978.

Fett, Sharla. *Working Cures: Health Healing and Power on Southern Slave Plantations*. Chapel Hill: University of North Carolina Press, 2002.

Fiske, David, Clifford W. Brown, and Rachel Seligman. *Solomon Northup: The Complete Story of the Author of "Twelve Years a Slave."* Santa Barbara, CA: Praeger, 2013.

Foner, Eric. *Gateway to Freedom: The Hidden History of America's Fugitive Slaves.* New York: Oxford University Press, 2015.

Franklin, John Hope. *The Free Negro in North Carolina, 1790–1860.* Chapel Hill: University of North Carolina Press, 1943.

Frederickson, George M. *The Black Image in the White Mind: The Debate on Afro-American Character and Destiny, 1817–1914.* New York: Harper and Row, 1971.

Ginzburg, Carlo. *The Cheese and the Worms: The Cosmos of a Sixteenth-Century Miller.* Translated by John Tedeschi and Anne Tedeschi. Baltimore: Johns Hopkins University Press, 1992.

Glass, Brent D. *The Textile Industry in North Carolina: A History.* Raleigh: Division of Archives and History, 1992.

Gobat, Michel. *Empire by Invitation: William Walker and Manifest Destiny in Central America.* Cambridge, MA: Harvard University Press, 2018.

Gordon-Reed, Annette. *The Hemingses of Monticello: An American Family.* New York: W. W. Norton, 2008.

Gregory, James N. *The Southern Diaspora: How the Great Migrations of Black and White Southerners Transformed America.* Chapel Hill: University of North Carolina Press, 2005.

Griffler, Keith P. *Front Line of Freedom: African Americans and the Forging of the Underground Railroad in the Ohio Valley.* Lexington: University of Kentucky, 2004.

Haller, John S. *Outcasts from Evolution: Scientific Attitudes of Racial Inferiority, 1859–1900.* Urbana: University of Illinois Press, 1971.

Hardy, Anne. *Salmonella Infections, Networks of Knowledge, and Public Health in Britain, 1880–1975.* Oxford: Oxford University Press, 2015.

Harris, Greg. *Harris Family History.* Berwyn, IL: n.p., ca. 2015.

Harris, Sharon M. *Dr. Mary Walker: An American Radical, 1832–1919.* New Brunswick, NJ: Rutgers University Press, 2009.

Hogarth, Rana A. *Medicalizing Blackness: Making Racial Difference in the Atlantic World, 1780–1840.* Chapel Hill: University of North Carolina Press, 2017.

Hollyday, Joyce. *On the Heels of Freedom: The American Missionary Association's Bold Campaign to Educate Minds, Open Hearts, and Heal the Soul of a Divided Nation.* New York: Crossroad Publishing, 2005.

Holt, Thomas, Cassandra Smith-Parker, and Rosalyn Terborg-Penn. *A Special Mission: The Story of Freedmen's Hospital, 1862–1962.* Washington, DC: Academic Affairs Division, Howard University, 1975.

Horton, James Oliver, and Lois E. Horton. *In Hope of Liberty: Culture, Community and Protest among Northern Free Blacks, 1700–1800.* New York: Oxford University Press, 1997.

Humphreys, Margaret. *Intensely Human: The Health of the Black Soldier in the American Civil War.* Baltimore: Johns Hopkins University Press, 2008.

———. *Malaria: Poverty, Race and Public Health in the United States.* Baltimore: Johns Hopkins University Press, 2001.

———. *Marrow of Tragedy: The Health Crisis of the American Civil War.* Baltimore: Johns Hopkins University Press, 2013.

———. *Yellow Fever and the South*. New Brunswick, NJ: Rutgers University Press, 1992.

Jackson, Debra. "'A Cultural Stronghold': The 'Anglo-African' Newspaper and the Black Community of New York." *New York History* 85, no. 4 (Fall 2004): 331–57.

Jordan, Ryan P. *Slavery and the Meetinghouse: The Quakers and the Abolitionist Dilemma, 1820–1865*. Bloomington: Indiana University Press, 2007.

Knight, Edgar W. *Public School Education in North Carolina*. Boston: Houghton Mifflin, 1916.

LaRoche, Cheryl Janifer. *Free Black Communities and the Underground Railroad: The Geography of Resistance*. Champaign: University of Illinois Press, 2012.

Lemire, Elise. *"Miscegenation": Making Race in America*. Philadelphia: University of Pennsylvania Press, 2010.

Lin, Nan, Karen Cook, and Ronald S. Burt, eds. *Social Capital: Theory and Research*. New York: Aldine de Gruyter, 2001.

Litwack, Leon F. *North of Slavery: The Negro in the Free States, 1790–1860*. Chicago: University of Chicago Press, 1961.

Logan, Shirley Wilson. *Liberating Language: Sites of Rhetorical Education in Nineteenth-Century Black America*. Carbondale: Southern Illinois University Press, 2008.

Long, Gretchen. *Doctoring Freedom: The Politics of African American Medical Care in Slavery and Emancipation*. Chapel Hill: University of North Carolina Press, 2012.

Lowe, Richard. *Republicans and Reconstruction in Virginia, 1856–70*. Charlottesville: University of Virginia Press, 1991.

Lubet, Steven. *The "Colored Hero" of Harper's Ferry: John Anthony Copeland and the War against Slavery*. New York: Cambridge University Press, 2015.

May, Robert E. *The Southern Dream of a Caribbean Empire, 1854–1861*. 1973. Reprint, Gainesville: University of Florida Press, 2002.

McCandless, Peter. *Moonlight, Magnolias and Madness: Insanity in South Carolina from the Colonial Period to the Progressive Era*. Chapel Hill: University of North Carolina Press, 1996.

McKivigan, John. *Forgotten Firebrand: James Redpath and the Making of Nineteenth-Century America*. Ithaca: Cornell University Press, 2008.

McMullan, Fitzhugh. *Plagues and Politics: The Story of the United States Public Health Service*. New York: Basic Books, 1989.

Miller, Floyd J. *The Search for a Black Nationality: Black Emigration and Colonization, 1787–1863*. Urbana: University of Illinois Press, 1975.

Morais, Herbert M. *The History of the Negro in Medicine*. International Library of Negro Life and History. New York: Publishers Company, 1967.

Morantz-Sanchez, Regina. *Sympathy and Science: Women Physicians in American Medicine*. New York: Oxford University Press, 1975.

Morris, J. Brent. *Oberlin, Hotbed of Abolitionism: College, Community, and the Fight for Freedom and Equality in Antebellum America*. Chapel Hill: University of North Carolina Press, 2014.

Newmark, Jill. *Without Concealment, without Compromise: The Courageous Lives of Black Civil War Surgeons*. Carbondale: Southern Illinois University Press, 2023.

Oates, John A. *The Story of Fayetteville and the Upper Cape Fear*. Charlotte, NC: Dowd Press, 1950.

Oates, Stephen B. *The Fires of Jubilee: Nat Turner's Fierce Rebellion*. New York: Harper and Row, 1975.

Olivarius, Kathryn. *Necropolis: Disease, Power, and Capitalism in the Cotton Kingdom*. Cambridge, MA: Harvard University Press, 2022.

Osthaus, Carl. *Freedmen, Philanthropy, and Fraud: A History of the Freedman's Savings Bank*. Champaign: University of Illinois Press, 1976.

Otto, Thomas J. *St. Elizabeths Hospital: A History*. Washington, DC: GSA, 2013.

Pons, Frank Moya. *The Dominican Republic: A National History*. New Rochelle, NY: Hispaniola Books, 1995.

Pryor, Elizabeth Stordeur. *Colored Travelers: Mobility and the Fight for Citizenship before the Civil War*. Chapel Hill: University of North Carolina Press, 2016.

Raimon, Eve Allegra. *The "Tragic Mulatta" Revisited: Race and Nationalism in Nineteenth-Century Antislavery Fiction*. New Brunswick, NJ: Rutgers University Press, 2004.

Rasmussen, Daniel. *American Uprising: The Untold Story of America's Largest Slave Revolt*. New York: HarperCollins, 2011.

Régent, Frédéric. *Les Maîtres de la Guadeloupe : propriétaires d'esclaves, 1635-1848*. Paris: Tallandier, 2019.

Richardson, Joe M. *Christian Reconstruction: The American Missionary Association and Southern Blacks, 1861–1890*. Athens: University of Georgia Press, 1986.

Robisheaux, Thomas. *The Last Witch of Langenburg: Murder in a German Village*. New York: W. W. Norton, 2009.

Rosenberg, Charles. *The Cholera Years: The United States in 1832, 1849, and 1866*. Chicago: University of Chicago Press, 1962.

Rothstein, William G. *American Physicians in the Nineteenth Century: From Sects to Science*. Baltimore: Johns Hopkins University Press, 1985.

Savitt, Todd. *Medicine and Slavery: The Diseases and Healthcare of Blacks in Antebellum Virginia*. Urbana: University of Illinois Press, 1978.

———. *Race and Medicine in Nineteenth- and Early-Twentieth-Century America*. Kent, OH: Kent State Press, 2007.

Schwalm, Leslie A. *Medicine, Science, and Making Race in Civil War America*. Chapel Hill: University of North Carolina Press, 2023.

Simkins, Francis Butler, and Robert Hilliard Woody. *South Carolina during Reconstruction*. Chapel Hill: University of North Carolina Press, 1932.

Sloan, De Villo. *The Crimsoned Hills of Onondaga: Romantic Antiquarians and the Euro-American Invention of Native American Prehistory*. Amherst, NY: Cambria Press, 2008.

Smail, Daniel Lord. *On Deep History and the Brain*. Berkeley: University of California Press, 2008.

Smedley, Brian D., Adrienne Y. Stith, and Alan R. Nelson, eds. *Unequal Treatment: Confronting Racial and Ethnic Disparities in Health Care*. Washington, DC: National Academies Press, 2003.

Sollors, Werner. *Neither Black nor White Yet Both*. New York: Oxford University Press, 1997.

Starobin, Paul. *Madness Rules the Hour: Charleston, 1860 and the Mania for War*. New York: Public Affairs, 2017.

Summers, Martin. *Madness in the City of Magnificent Intentions: A History of Race and Mental Illness in the Nation's Capital*. New York: Oxford University Press, 2019.

Taylor, Elizabeth Dowling. *The Original Black Elite: Daniel Murray and the Story of a Forgotten Era*. New York: Amistad, 2017.

Taylor, Nikki Marie. *Frontiers of Freedom: Cincinnati's Black Community, 1802–1868*. Columbus: Ohio State University Press, 2005.

Temkin, Oswei. *The Falling Sickness: A History of Epilepsy from the Greeks to the Beginning of Modern Neurology*. 2nd ed., rev. Baltimore: Johns Hopkins University Press, 1971.

Thompson, Henry T. *Ousting the Carpetbagger from South Carolina*. Columbia, SC: R. L. Bryan Co., 1926. Reprint, New York: Negro Universities Press, 1969.

Tise, Larry. *A History of the Defense of Slavery in America, 1701–1840*. Athens: University of Georgia Press, 1987.

Tomes, Nancy. *A Generous Confidence: Thomas Story Kirkbride*. Cambridge: Cambridge University Press, 1994.

Troesken, Werner. *Water, Race, and Disease*. Cambridge, MA: Massachusetts Institute of Technology Press, 2004.

Tuchman, Arleen Marcia. *Science Has No Sex: The Life of Marie Zakrzewska, M.D.* Chapel Hill: University of North Carolina Press, 2008.

Ulrich, Laurel Thatcher. *A Midwife's Tale: The Life of Martha Ballard, Based on Her Diary, 1785–1812*. New York: Knopf, 1990.

Waite, Frederick Clayton. *Western Reserve University Centennial History of the School of Medicine*. Cleveland: Western Reserve University Press, 1946.

Walls, William Jacob. *Joseph Charles Price: Educator and Race Leader*. Boston: Christopher Publishing House, 1943.

Warner, John Harley. *The Therapeutic Perspective: Medical Practice, Knowledge, and Identity in America, 1820–1885*. Cambridge, MA: Harvard University Press, 1986.

Weeks, Stephen B. *Southern Quakers and Slavery: A Study in Institutional History*. Baltimore: Johns Hopkins University Press, 1896.

Wilkerson, Isabel. *The Warmth of Other Suns: The Epic Story of America's Great Migration*. New York: Vintage, 2010.

Williamson, Joel. *A New People: Miscegenation and Mulattoes in the United States*. New York: Free Press, 1980.

Willoughby, Chris, and Sean Smith, eds. *Medicine and Healing in the Age of Slavery*. Baton Rouge: Louisiana State University Press, 2021.

Willoughby, Urmi Engineer. *Yellow Fever, Race, and Ecology in Nineteenth-Century New Orleans*. Baton Rouge: Louisiana State University Press, 2017.

Articles and Dissertations

Alexander, Philip. "John H. Rapier Jr. and the Medical Profession in Jamaica, 1861–1862." Pts. 1 and 2. *Jamaica Journal* 24 (February 1993): 37–36; 25 (October 1993): 55–62.

Baker, Robert B. "The American Medical Association and Race." *AMA Journal of Ethics* 16, no. 6 (June 2014): 479–88.

Banner, Lois W. "Biography as History." *American Historical Review* 114 (2009): 579–86.

Butts, Heather M. "Alexander Thomas Augusta—Physician, Teacher and Human Rights Activist." *Journal of the National Medical Association* 97, no. 1 (2005): 106–9.

Carpio, Arturo, Alfonso Escobar, and W. Allen Hauser. "Progress in Epilepsy Research: Cysticercosis and Epilepsy: A Critical Review." *Epilepsia* 39 (1998): 1005–40.

Daniel, Constance R. H. "Two North Carolina Families—the Harrises and the Richardsons." *Negro History Bulletin* 13 (October 1949): 3–12, 14, 23.

Deaderick, William H., and Loyd Thompson. "Amebic Dysentery." In *The Endemic Diseases of the Southern States*, 437–44. Philadelphia: W. B. Saunders Co., 1916.

De Boer, Clara M. "The Role of Afro-Americans in the Origin and Work of the American Missionary Association: 1839–1877." PhD diss., Rutgers, State University of New Jersey–New Brunswick, 1972. ProQuest (AAT 7327914).

Devinsky, Julie, and Steven Schacter. "Norman Geschwind's Contribution to the Understanding of Behavioral Changes in Temporal Lobe Epilepsy: The February 1974 Lecture." *Epilepsy and Behavior* 15, no. 4 (August 2009): 417–24.

Duggan, Ana T., Jennifer Klunk, Ashleigh F. Porter, Anna N. Dhody, Robert Hicks, Geoffrey L. Smith, Margaret Humphreys, et al. "The Origins and Genomic Diversity of American Civil War Era Smallpox Vaccine Strains." *Genome Biology* 21, no. 175 (2020): 175–85.

Fleury, Agnès, Edda Sciutto, Aline S. de Aluja, and Arturo Carpio. "Cysticercosis: A Preventable, but Embarrassing, Neglected Disease Still Prevalent in Non-developed Countries." In *Zoonoses in Food-Chain Animals with Public Health Relevance*, edited by Andreas Sing, 335–54. Dordrecht: Springer Science, 2015.

Foster, Gaines. "The Limitations of Federal Health Care for Freedmen, 1860–1868." *Journal of Southern History* 48 (1982): 349–72.

Frederick, Candace. "'Loving' and the History of Anti-miscegenation Laws in Virginia and Washington." Schomberg Center for Research in Black Culture (blog), New York Public Library. November 3, 2016. www.nypl.org/blog/2016/11/03/loving-and-history.

Freud, Sigmund. "Dostoevsky and Parricide." In *Sigmund Freud Complete Psychological Works*, edited by Norman Geschwind, 177–94. London: Hogarth Press, 1961.

Geschwind, Norman. "Personality Changes in Temporal Lobe Epilepsy (1974)." Reprinted in *Epilepsy Behavior* 15, no. 4 (August 2009): 425–33.

Hicks, Robert. "Scabrous Matters: Spurious Vaccinations in the Confederacy." In *War Matters: Material Culture in the Civil War Era*, edited by Joan Cashin, 123–50. Chapel Hill: University of North Carolina Press, 2018.

Kessler-Harris, Alice. "Why Biography?" *American Historical Review* 114 (2009): 625–30.

Kibre, Pearl. "The Faculty of Medicine at Paris, Charlatanism, and Unlicensed Medical Practices in the Later Middle Ages." *Bulletin of the History of Medicine* 27, no. 1 (January–February 1953): 1–20.

Lawlor, Andrew. "Fort Monroe's Lasting Place in History." *Smithsonian Magazine*, July 24, 2011. www.smithsonianmag.com/history/fort-monroes-lasting-place-in-history-25923793/.

Lawrence, Susan. "Iowa Physicians: Legitimacy, Institutions, and the Practice of Medicine. Part One: Establishing a Professional Identity, 1833–1886." *Annals of Iowa* 62 (Spring 2003): 151–200.

Lett, Elle, H. Moses Murdock, Whitney U. Orji, Jaya Aysola, and Ronnie Sebro. "Trends in Racial/Ethnic Representation among US Medical Students." *JAMA Network Open* 2, no. 9 (September 2019): e1910490.

McClintock, John T. "Medical Education in Iowa." In *One Hundred Years of Iowa Medicine: Commemorating the Centenary of the Iowa State Medical Society, 1850–1950*, [by Iowa State Medical Society], 224–309. Iowa City, IA: Athens Press, 1950.

McKay, Richard A. "Why Do We Do What We Do? The Values of the Social History of Medicine." *Social History of Medicine* 33, no. 1 (February 2020): 13–17.

Millikan, Frank Rives. "Wards of the Nation: The Making of St. Elizabeth's Hospital, 1852–1920." PhD diss., George Washington University, 1990.

Morris, Charles Edward. "Panic and Reprisal: Reaction in North Carolina to the Nat Turner Insurrection, 1831." *North Carolina Historical Review* 62, no. 1 (January 1985): 29–52.

Nasaw, David. Introduction to "AHR Roundtable: Historians and Biography." *American Historical Review* 114, no. 3 (June 2009): 573–78.

Perry, Matthew Leary. "The Negro in Fayetteville." In *The Story of Fayetteville and the Upper Cape Fear*, by John A. Oates, 695–715. Charlotte, NC: Dowd Press, 1950. Reprint with index, 1972.

Pettigrew, T. F., and J. Martin. "Shaping the Organizational Context for Black American Inclusion." *Journal of Social Issues* 43, no. 1 (1987): 41–78.

Reverby, Susan, and David Rosner. "Beyond 'the Great Doctors.'" In *Health Care in America: Essays in Social History*, edited by Susan Reverby and David Rosner, 3–16. Philadelphia: Temple University Press, 1979.

Richmond, Stephanie J. "Microhistories of Slavery and Racism in Antebellum America." *Reviews in American History* 46, no. 3 (2018): 385–90.

Taylor, A. A. "Reconstruction through Compromise." *Journal of Negro History* 11, no. 3 (July 1926): 494–512.

Vinovskis, Maris A. "Have Social Historians Lost the Civil War? Some Preliminary Demographic Speculations." In *Toward a Social History of the American Civil War: Exploratory Essays*, edited by Maris A. Vinovskis, 1–29. Cambridge: Cambridge University Press, 1990.

Wagstaff, Henry McGilbert, ed. Prefatory note to *The Harris Letters*, vol. 14, no. 1, edited by J. G. de Roulhac Hamilton and Henry McGilbert Wagstaff, 5–7. Durham, NC: James Sprunt Historical Publications, 1916.

West, Earle H. "The Harris Brothers: Black Northern Teachers in the Reconstruction South." *Journal of Negro Education* 48, no. 2 (Spring 1979): 126–38.

———. "The Peabody Education Fund and Negro Education, 1867–1880." *History of Education Quarterly* 6, no. 2 (Summer 1966): 3–21.

Wilkinson, Doris Y. "The 1850 Harvard Medical School Dispute and the Admission of African American Students." *Harvard Library Bulletin* 3, no. 3 (Fall 1992): 13–27.

INDEX

Page numbers in italics refer to illustrations.

abolitionist movement, 88; AMA's work in, 152–53; Black congresses and, 32, 47; on John Brown, 87; in Cleveland, 80–81, 137; college admittance and, 6; detractors of, 41; leaders of, 75, 86, 88–89, 112, 138, 205–6; newspapers of, 52; at Oberlin College, 75, 80–81, 101; in Philadelphia, 135; supporters of, 49, 139. *See also* slave revolts; *and names of specific leaders*
Adams, John, 93, 120
African Methodist Episcopal (AME) Church, 39, 156, 164
African Methodist Episcopal Zion (AMEZ) Church, 164
African Protestant Church, 39
agricultural utopia, 11
Alcott, W. A., 52
AMA (American Missionary Association), 17, 28, 30, 151–53, 154, 158–62, 168–69, 188
AME (African Methodist Episcopal Church), 39, 156, 164
American Civil War, 1, 3, 6, 7, 71, 134–35, 182, 244, 245
American Colonization Society, 6, 41
American Medical Association, 4, 51
American Missionary Association (AMA), 17, 28, 30, 151–53, 154, 158–62, 168–69, 188
American Neurological Society, 229
American Revolution, 32, 43
AMEZ (African Methodist Episcopal Zion Church), 164
Amistad (ship), 152
Anglo-African empire, 11, 89–90, 94, 95, 111
Anglo-African Magazine, 97
antislavery movement. *See* abolitionist movement
Appeal (Walker), 33
apprenticeships: of J. D. Harris, 28, 138, 139; of Harris family, 22–23, 24, 25–26, 27, 158, 243; legislation on, 32
Aptheker, Herbert, 65–66
Artibonite River valley (Haiti), 11, 124, 125, 126, 126, 127, 128. *See also* Haiti
Artis, Owen Clinton, 22, 26
Augusta, Alexander, 174–75, 177, 185, 205
autopsies, 219–20

295

Ball, Erica L., 32
Ballard, Martha, 9
Banks, Nathaniel P., 116–17
Barnum, P. T., 117
Barrett, P. G., 176
Bell, Howard H., 14, 100; *Black Separatism and the Caribbean*, 14, 262n43
Bell, W. S., 155
"Beyond 'the Great Doctors'" (Reverby and Rosner), 2, 3
Bible Defence of Slavery (Priest), 62–63
Bishir, Catherine, 19, 20
Blackburn, Isaac W., 219
Black Codes, 49, 54, 61, 64, 70
Black conventions, 8, 40–44, 47, 52, 64, 72, 95–96
Black lives matter, as concept, 3
Black people: conventions of, 8, 40–44, 47, 52, 64, 72, 95–96, 245; educated community of, in Washington, DC, 12; on emigration, 41, 81–87, 96–99, 121–28; as health professionals, 6–7; literacy and, 7, 14, 20, 31, 243; as medical patients, 218–19; as physicians, 5–7, 10, 14, 134–36; population statistics on, 7. *See also* free Black people; mixed-race people; mulatto, as legally recognized category; *and names of specific Black people*
Black physicians, 5–7, 10, 14, 134–36. *See also* Harris, J. D. (Joseph Dennis)
Black Separatism and the Caribbean (Bell), 14, 262n43
Blair, Francis Preston, Jr., 81–83, 111; *The Destiny of the Races of this Continent*, 82
bonds of apprenticeships, 22–23
Boyer, Paul, 9
brain tumors, 247–48
Brigham, Amariah, 218
Brimage, Thomas, 24, 26
Brodhead, Richard, 160, 163
Brooks, Martin Luther, 137, 138
Brown, John, 7, 11, 70, 71, 78–81, 87, 101, 194, 244
Brown, John, Jr., 77–78, 98, 122

Brown, William Wells, 123
Buchanan, James, 74, 111
Bureau of Refugees, Freedmen, and Abandoned Lands. *See* Freedmen's Bureau
Burnett, William, 22, 26
business and social structure, 30–31
Butler, Benjamin, 152

California, 42
Canada, 122
cancer, 249
Cartwright, Samuel, 8
Cass, Lewis, 74
caste system, 13
Central American Land Company, 84, 85
Chesnutt, Charles, 31, 35, 160, 163, 164
Chesnutt, Mary, 202
Chillicothe, OH, 38–39, 40, 46
cholera, 157, 180–81, 185
Christian Recorder (publication), 123, 146, 147, 173
chronic alcoholism, 247
citizenship, 43, 44, 45, 177. *See also* Freedmen's Bureau
Civil War. *See* American Civil War
Clark, Alexander, 48, 49
Cleveland, OH, 46, 137–41
Cleveland Anti-Slavery Society, 78
Cleveland Morning Leader (publication), 86–87
colonization, 14, 110–11, 121–28, 245
Colored Conventions, 8, 40–44, 47, 52, 64, 72, 95–96, 245
colorism, 13
Colton, Marcia, 179–80
Columbia, SC, 201. *See also* South Carolina Lunatic Asylum
Compromise of 1850, 49
Conservative Republicans, 188–89, 200
constitutional convention, 41–42
conventions, 40–44, 52, 64, 72, 95–96, 192, 245
Cope, Peregrine (pseudonym). *See* Harris, J. D. (Joseph Dennis)

Copeland, John, 75, 80
Copeland, John, Jr., 79
cotton gin, 20
cotton plantations, 20–21
Courtney, W. S., 113; *Gold Fields of St. Domingo*, 120
Crania Americana (Morton), 124
Cuba, 120
Curtis, George William, 112
Cuyahoga County Anti-Slavery Society, 78
cysticercosis, 248–49

Daily Enquirer and Examiner (*E&E*; publication), 192–93, 194–95
Daniel, Constance, 39
Day, Thomas, 26
Day, William Howard, 40, 43
death of Harris, 12, 215, 239–41. *See also* Harris, J. D. (Joseph Dennis)
De Lamater, John J., 139, 185, 187
Delany, Martin, 6, 40, 86
Delaware, OH, 46
Delbanco, Andrew, 72; *The War before the War*, 72
dementia, 12
Democratic Party, 71, 188
Demos, John, 27, 28, 29, 30
Dennis, Joseph, 24
Dessalines, Jean-Jacques, 105
Destiny of the Races of this Continent, The (Blair), 82
diseases: cholera, 157, 180–81, 185; dysentery, 158, 163, 203, 246; insanity from infectious, 246–47; meningitis, 247; neurocysticercosis, 248–49; smallpox, 130, 146, 181–83, 184–86, 213, 216, 250, 269n12; syphilis, 247; tuberculosis, 149, 165, 169, 247
Dismukes, Alexander Hamilton, 19
Dismukes, Charlotte, 18–19, 20. *See also* Harris, Charlotte Dismukes
Dismukes, George, 18–19, 26
Dismukes, William, 19
District of Columbia Freedmen's Hospital, 211–14

Dixon, Chris, 109
Doctoring Freedom (Long), 10
Dominican Republic, 11, 86, 105, 111–21
Douglas, Stephen, 52
Douglas, W. W. C., 189
Douglass, Frederick, 8–9, 40, 74, 86, 222, 239
Douglass, H. F., 43, 84
Downs, Jim, 181; *Sick from Freedom*, 181–82
drapetomania, 8
Dred Scott case (1857), 8, 12, 71, 73–74, 77, 92, 136, 250
Dubois, Laurent, 87, 98, 120
Du Bois, W. E. B., 152
Duffin, Jacalyn, 9; *Langstaff*, 9
dysentery, 158, 163, 203, 246

economic recession, 142, 207, 222
Edwards, Bryan, 103, 104
Edwards, L. A., 181
election of 1869, 188–97
Élie, Auguste, 126
Emancipation Proclamation, 8, 12, 14, 140, 175
emigration, 81–87, 96–99, 121–28. *See also* migration stories
Ensor, Joshua, 200, 203
epilepsy, 12, 209, 216, 220, 225, 226, 247, 248–49; association with insanity of, 227, 230, 240–41; treatment of, 229–31, 233, 236–37
Erikson, Erik, 27
Ernest, John, 59
escaped enslaved people, 8, 15, 38, 39, 42, 57, 72, 75, 107, 113, 122–23. *See also* Fugitive Slave Act (1850); *and names of specific persons*

family culture of Harris, 27–33. *See also* Harris, J. D. (Joseph Dennis)
Fanz, J. H., 173
farming techniques, 11
Fayetteville, NC, 21–27, 55, 59
Fehrenbacher, Don, 73

Fett, Sharla, 10; *Working Cures*, 10–11
financial mismanagement of Harrises, 206–11, 222–23. *See also* Harris, J. D. (Joseph Dennis)
fire (1831), 21, 22
Flight (ship), 124–26
Flight I colony, 129, 131–32, 246
Fore, James, 26
Fourteenth Amendment, 16
Franklin, John Hope, 3, 16, 24, 26, 32, 250
Fredericksburg Freedmen's Bureau hospital, 183–87, *184*
free Black people: Blair on, 82; on emigration, 41; kidnappings of, 12, 42, 67, 72, 109, 190, 237; literacy of, 7, 14, 20; migration stories of, 36–40; of New Bern, NC, 18–21, 23; political activism by, 32; as slave owners, 26; trades of, 19–20, 22–23, 28, 30–31. *See also* Black people
Freedmen's Bureau, 12, 14, 36, 39, 146, 152, 182
Freedmen's Bureau hospital system: conditions of, 178–83; in District of Columbia, 211–14; in Fredericksburg, 183–87; in Hampton, 170, 171, 173–74, 186, 197, 198; indigent patients and, 200
Freedmen's Savings and Trust Co., 222–23
freedom, as theme, 45
Free-Soil Party, 71
Free West (publication), 52
Frémont, John C., 117
French language, 29
French medical professionalism, 4–5
Freud, Sigmund, 240
Fugitive Slave Act (1850), 15, 42, 43–44, 47, 49, 64, 71, 72, 95. *See also* escaped enslaved people; slavery

Garrison, William Lloyd, 137
Geffrard, Fabre, 86, 87, 89, 99, 105–6, 124, 132
George III (king), 93
Geschwind, Norman, 240–41

Ginzburg, Carlo, 9
Godding, William Whitney, 219, 220
Gold Fields of St. Domingo (Courtney), 120
Goldsboro Patriot (publication), 33
Gordon-Reed, Annette, 19
Government Hospital for the Insane. *See* St. Elizabeths Hospital
Grand Turks and Caicos islands, 111
Grant, Ulysses S., 196
Griffler, Keith P., 38
Gross, Samuel D., 146; *Manual of Military Surgery*, 146
Guide to Hayti (Redpath), 99

Hahnemann, Samuel, 5
Haiti, 109, *125*, *126*; caste system in, 13; colonization scheme in, 11, 14, 86–87, 110–11, 121–28, 245; Harris's language skills in, 29, 60; political sovereignty of, 110–11
Haitian Revolution, 8, 29, 59, 88–89, 96, 99–109, 120. *See also* Haiti
Hamilton, Thomas, 97, 111
Hammond, William A., 145, 227, 229–31; *On Epilepsy and Epileptiform Seizures*, 227; *Treatise on Diseases of the Nervous System*, 227
Hampton Freedmen's Bureau hospital, 170, 171, 173–74, 186, 197, 198
Hampton Institute, 170
Hand-Books for Home Improvement (Wells), 31
Harper, R. A., 84
Harris, Agnes Hart, 249
Harris, Catherine Webber, 22, 24, 29–30, 34–35
Harris, Charlotte Dismukes, 17–21, 28, 38–39, 243
Harris, Cicero Richardson, 17, 22, 31, 35, 39, 151, 158, 163–65, 244
Harris, Elizabeth Worthington, 165–69; declaration of J. D. Harris's insanity by, 209, 215, 216–17; financial management and, 208–11, 217, 222–23; on J. D. Harris's position at South

Carolina asylum, 198, 199; Robert Harris and, 159; meeting J. D. Harris and marriage of, 168, 170–71, 202, 245; work of, 198, 201
Harris, George, 24
Harris, Greg, 249
Harris, Hannah Brimage, 24
Harris, Jacob, 17, 18, 19, 21, 27–28, 34–35, 38–39
Harris, J. D. (Joseph Dennis), xvi, 1–3, 7–8, 11, 243–50; abolitionism of, 88–92; apprenticeships of, 28, 138, 139; as army surgeon, 133, 172–77, 224–26; as assistant superintendent of South Carolina Lunatic Asylum, 198–204, 246; at Colored Conventions, 76–77; death of, 12, 215, 239–41; as doctor-in-charge at Fredericksburg Freedmen's Bureau hospital, 133, 183–87; on Dominican Republic, 111–21; early life of, 3, 17–18, 24; early work of, 28, 50; election of 1869 and, 188–97; Elizabeth and financial management by, 206–11; Elizabeth's declaration of J. D. Harris's insanity, 209, 215, 216–17; emigration of, 81–87, 98–99; on emigration, 83–87, 96–97; epilepsy and insanity of, 12, 209, 216, 220, 225, 226–31, 233, 236–37, 240–41, 248; family culture of, 27–33; Fayetteville household of, 21–27; as Freedmen's Bureau surgeon, 177–83; on Fugitive Slave Act, 95–96; on Haiti, 99–109; Haiti colonization and, 14, 41, 110–11, 121–33, 245; Hunt's publication and, 92–95; insanity of, 153, 187, 200, 209, 215, 218–19, 230, 232, 233, 239; language skills of, 29, 111; *Love and Law, South and West*, 40, 45–48, 50–70, 244; medical career of, 244–45; medical training of, 12, 50–51, 133, 134, 136–44, 245–46; meeting Elizabeth and marriage of, 168, 170–71, 202, 217, 245; migration stories of, 34–40, 44, 46; parents of, 18–21; as patient, 2, 13, 16, 25, 205, 217–26, 231–39, 247; poem on temperance by, 42–43; property of, 79; pseudonym of, 123; *A Summer on the Borders of the Caribbean Sea*, 11, 14, 93, 99–109, 110–11

Harris, Kitty Stanley, 210–11, 249
Harris, Mary, 21, 249
Harris, Robert W., 24, 25, 26, 31, 35, 39, 151, 158–63, 238, 244
Harris, Sarah, 18, 21, 26, 28, 30, 39
Harris, Thoro, 13, 249–50
Harris, William D., 153–58; AMA and, 151; birth of, 21, 25–26; in Charleston, 198; at conventions, 40, 44; farm and family life of, 39, 244; naming of, 19; work of, 29; Elizabeth Worthington on, 167
Harris, Worthie, 13, 202, 249
Harvard Medical School, 6
Hauger, Jessica, 10
"Have Social Historians Lost the Civil War?" (Vinovskis), 3
Health Care in America (publication), 2
heatstroke, 216
Helper, Hinton R., 91
Hemings, Sally, 19
herbal remedies, 5
Holden, William B., 249
Holly, James Theodore, 86, 124
homeopathy, 5, 51, 143, 145
Honduras, 107, 111
Howard, O. O., 202, 212
Howard Hospital, 205, 211–13, 245–47
Howard Medical School, 12, 205, 212, 246
Howard School, 160–61, 162. *See also* State Colored Normal School of Fayetteville
Howard's Grove Hospital, 1, 14, 147, 153, 156, 183, 185, 198–99, 226; J. D. Harris in charge of, 153, 146–47, 148, 150, 178–79
Howard University, 7, 12, 165
Howe, Julia Ward, 106
Hughes, Langston, 36
Huilliad, Mariette Scholastique "French Mary," 29

INDEX   299

Humphreys, Margaret: *Intensely Human*, 4, 10; *Malaria*, 3; *Marrow of Tragedy*, 4, 147; *Yellow Fever and the South*, 3, 8
Hunt, Benjamin S., 92–95
Hunter, William H., 210
Huntington, Charlotte, 23, 26

infectious diseases. *See* diseases
insanity, 153, 187, 200, 209, 215, 218–19, 226–31, 232, 233, 239. *See also* South Carolina Lunatic Asylum; St. Elizabeths Hospital
insurrection of John Brown, 7, 11
Intensely Human (Humphreys), 4, 10
Iowa, 44, 48–50
Iowa Constitution, 49–50
Iowa State University, 141

Jackson, Andrew, 43
Jackson, Calvin, 26
Jamaica, 59–60, 92, 136, 192
Jefferson, Thomas, 19
Johnson, Matthew, 80
Johnson, William Henry, 117
Jordan, Ryan P., 37, 38

Kagi, J. Henrie, 78, 79
Keokuk medical school, 51, 141–42
kidnappings of free Black people, 12, 42, 67, 72–73, 109, 190, 237
Kirtland, Jared Potter, 139–40

Ladies Anti-slavery Society of Delaware, 44
Lamater, J. J. De, 178
Lancet, The (publication), 144
Langstaff (Duffin), 9
Langston, Charles: case against, 75–76, 115; at conventions, 40, 76; dentistry work of, 50; on *Dred Scott* case, 77; emigration of, 36–39; Wellington rescue and, 90
Langston, John Mercer, 36; on abolishing Fugitive Slave Law, 95; charges against, 75; at conventions, 40, 41–43; emigration of, 37; as family friend and advisor, 222; J. D. Harris and, 47; on J. D. Harris's insanity, 239–40; legal work of, 50, 135, 205–6
Langston, Lucy, 36
LaRoche, Cheryl, 38
Laud, William, 93
Lawrence, George, 122
Lawrence, Susan, 142
Leary, Lewis Sheridan, 75, 78, 80, 90
Leary, Matthew, 23, 24, 26–27, 29
Leary family, 29
Lee, Robert E., 174
Lessons of the Hour, The (Phillips), 88
Liberator (publication), 57, 66
Liberia, 33, 41, 83
Lincoln, Abraham, 71, 137, 175, 244, 245
Lindsay, Lewis, 189
literacy, 7, 14, 20, 31, 243
Long, Gretchen, 10; *Doctoring Freedom*, 10
L'Ouverture, Toussaint, 105
Love and Law, South and West (Harris), 40, 45–48, 50–70, 244
Loving v. State of Virginia, 170
Luckley, George, 176

malaria, 8
Malaria (Humphreys), 3
mania. *See* insanity
Manual of Military Surgery (Gross), 146
manumission, 26–27
Marrow of Tragedy (Humphreys), 4, 147
Martin, James M., 148
Marvin, John A., 48
McCandless, Peter, 200
McCaskill, John, 27
McPherson, Aimee Semple, 250
McSimpson, Joshua, 57
medical career of J. D. Harris, 12, 133, 134, 172–87, 244–45. *See also* Harris, J. D. (Joseph Dennis)
medical licensing and professionalism, 4–5
medical training of J. D. Harris, 12, 50–51, 133, 136–44, 245–46. *See also* Harris, J. D. (Joseph Dennis)

Medicine and Healing in the Age of Slavery (Willoughby and Smith), 10–11
Medicine and Slavery (Savitt), 10–11
Melrose, Henry, 129–33
meningitis, 247
mental asylum (Columbia, SC). *See* South Carolina Lunatic Asylum
mental asylum (Washington, DC). *See* St. Elizabeths Hospital
mental illness. *See* insanity
Mercer, Charles, 40
Mercer, John, 36, 40
microhistory, as strategy, 9–10, 17
Midwife's Tale, A (Ulrich), 9
migration stories, 36–40. *See also* emigration
military service, 43, 175, 224–25
Miller, Floyd, 86
Minor, Lawrence, 40–41
miscegenation, 84, 170–71, 175, 192, 202
Mitchell, I., 78–79
mixed-race couples, 84, 170–71, 175, 192, 202
mixed-race people: alleged superiority of, 89, 92, 94–97, 113, 133, 149, 192; and amalgamationism, 94–96, 175; as passing for white people, 51, 141; and J. D. Harris's identity, 11, 13, 18, 51, 149–50; in J. D. Harris's poetry, 45–46, 53; rights of, in the United States, 41, 47, 49, 97–98, 114, 150, 170–71; violence against, 29, 98, 100–104. *See also* mulatto, as legally recognized category
modern farming, 11
Montford, Donum, 21, 22
Morais, Herbert, 134
Moreau de Saint-Méry, Médéric-Louis-Élie, 94, 98
Morehouse School of Medicine, 6
Morris, C. E., 66
Morton, Samuel, 124; *Crania Americana*, 124
mulatto, as legally recognized category, 13, 94, 100–104

National Emigration Convention of Colored People, 43
National Library of Medicine, 4
neurocysticercosis, 248–49
neurosyphilis, 247
New Bern, NC, 18–21, 153
New England Hospital, 5
Newmark, Jill, 2, 4, 45, 250
Nicaragua, 81, 107–8
Nichols, Charles, 218–19, 220, 223–24
Nissenbaum, Stephen, 9
North Carolina. *See* Fayetteville, NC; New Bern, NC
Northup, Solomon, 8, 12, 42, 72; *Twelve Years a Slave*, 8, 12, 42

Oberlin College, 75, 80–81, 101
octaroons, 45, 97. *See also* mixed-race people
Ohio, 38–44, 46
Ohio Anti-Slavery Society, 47, 77–78
Ohio Colored American League, 41–42
Olivarius, Kathryn, 8
On Epilepsy and Epileptiform Seizures (Sieveking and Hammond), 227
Otto, Thomas, 218

Panic of 1857, 142, 207, 222, 245
parasitic diseases, 248–49
Parker, John W., 199
Pastorisa Place, 115–16
Patterson, John E., 23
Payne, Daniel, 156, 157
Peabody Education Fund, 161
Peake, Mary, 153
Pease, E. M., 177
pellagra, 247
pensions, 225–26
Perry, Matthew, 55
Phillips, Wendell, 88; *The Lessons of the Hour*, 88
Pine and Palm (publication), 123, 125, 127, 132
plantations, 20–21, 120–21
Plumb, Ralph, 75

Plymouth colony, 27–28, 166
politics of respectability, 31–32, 40. *See also* literacy
population statistics, 7
pork tapeworm, 248–49
Port-au-Prince, Haiti, 87, 100, 123, *126*, 127, 130
poverty, 3
Price, John, 75, 77
Priest, Josiah, 62; *Bible Defence of Slavery*, 62
public education, 72
public market, 59
Purvis, Charles, 134, 135, 139–41, 143, 205

quadroons, 53, 97, 114. *See also* mixed-race people
Quakers, 37–38
Quarles, Ralph, 36
Quinn, William Paul, 38

racism: Chesnutt on, 35; *Dred Scott* case and, 8, 12; Haiti caste system, 13; J. D. Harris's medical career and, 203–4; of human exhibit, 117; by medical providers, 218–19
Radical Republicans, 12, 14, 188–89, 193–94, 198, 199
Ragland, George W., 23–24
Rainsford, Marcus, 100
Rapier, John, 134–36, 142
Reconstruction: impact of, on J. D. Harris, 195, 216, 246; and interracial marriage, 170; opposition to, 161, 171, 245; Radical Reconstruction, 188; in South Carolina, 199–200; in Virigina, 12, 151, 187, 188
Redpath, James, 86, 99, 100, 110–11, 121, 132–33; *Guide to Hayti*, 99
Reed, M. S., 186
religious beliefs of Harris family, 29–30; of J. D. Harris, 95, 113
Remarks on Hayti as a Place of Settlement for Afric-[A]mericans (Hunt), 92

Republican Party, 71, 188–90, *191*, 195, 246
respectability, 31–32, 40. *See also* literacy
Reverby, Susan, 2; "Beyond 'the Great Doctors,'" 2, 3
Reyburn, Robert, 183, 213
Rice, Valerie Montgomery, 6
Richardson, Alexander, 39
Richardson, Cicero, 22, 23, 26, 30–31, 78, 170
Richardson, Jacob, 39
Richardson, Joseph, 36
Richardson, Sarah Harris, 18, 21, 26, 28, 30, 39
Richmond Whig (publication), 190
Robinson, Benjamin, 24
Robinson, Hiram, 23
Robinson, Moses, 48
Robisheaux, Thomas, 9
Rosner, David, 2; "Beyond 'the Great Doctors,'" 2, 3
Ruatan, 107–8
Russell, Ira, 1–2, 148–50

Salem witchcraft trials, 9
Sanborn, John, 142
Santana, Pedro, 121
Santo Domingo (present-day Dominican Republic), 89, 111, 112, 120, 132
Santo Domingo (Hispaniola Island), 32, 90, 93, 94, 100, 112
Savitt, Todd, 10; *Medicine and Slavery*, 10–11
Saxton, Rufus, 175
Schwalm, Leslie, 149
Scott, Charles, 52
Scott, Dred, 73
Scott, Robert K., 203–4
segregation, 16
seizures, 215, 222, 228, 229, 231–32. *See also* epilepsy
Shepley, George F., 173
Sherman, W. T., 174, 200
Sick from Freedom (Downs), 181–82

Sieveking, Edward, 227–29; *On Epilepsy and Epileptiform Seizures*, 227
slave revolts, 7, 11, 22, 32, 46, 65–66, 72, 78–81, 103. *See also* abolitionist movement; Haitian Revolution
slavery, 20–21, 26, 37–38; Christianity in justification of, 62–63, 95. *See also* American Civil War; escaped enslaved people; Fugitive Slave Act (1850)
Smail, Daniel Lord, 15
smallpox, 130, 146, 181–83, 184–86, 213, 216, 250, 269n12
Smith, James McCune, 8, 113
Smith, Parker T., 123
social history of medicine, 2–4, 15
social history of war, 4
Society for Social Medicine, 2
South Carolina Lunatic Asylum, 12, 14, 198–204, 201, 246. *See also* insanity
Spelman, Asa, 20
Stanley, Kate "Kitty," 153
Stanley, S., 78
Sta[n]ley, Sara G., 44
Stanly, John C., 22, 153
Stanton, E. M., 174
State Colored Normal School of Fayetteville, 162–63
St. Elizabeths Hospital, 2, 13, 16, 25, 205, 217–26, 221, 224, 247. *See also* insanity
Stone, Andrew, 48
Stowe, Harriet Beecher, 46; *Uncle Tom's Cabin*, 46
Sturtevant, Mary, 80
suffrage, 50, 72
sugar, 121
Summer on the Borders of the Caribbean Sea, A (Harris), 11, 14, 93, 99, 110–11
Summers, Martin, 219
syphilis, 247

Taney, Roger B., 73, 92
Taylor, E. C., 48, 50, 51, 189
temperance, 42–43, 243
Texas, 42
therapeutics, 235–36

Thirteenth Amendment, 16
Thompson, Alfred V., 83
Thompson, Henry, 203
tobacco, 121
trades, 19–20, 22–23, 28, 30–31, 153
translation skills, 29
Treatise on Diseases of the Nervous System (Hammond), 227
True Republicans, 188, 193, 194, 195
tuberculosis, 149, 165, 169, 247
Turner, Nat, 22, 66
Twelve Years a Slave (Northup), 8, 12, 42

Ulrich, Laurel Thatcher, 9; *A Midwife's Tale*, 9
Uncle Tom's Cabin (Stowe), 46
Underground Railroad, 38, 122, 137, 245
University of Iowa, 51, 141–42
US Army hospital, 172
US Army surgeon, 133, 172–77, 224–26
US Colored Infantry, 175
US Colored Troops, 6, 135, 143, 173
US Constitution, 16
US Marine Hospital in Cleveland, 138, *138*
US National Archives, 3
US Sanitary Commission, 1, 148

vaccines, 182, 183, 184. *See also* diseases
Van Evrie, J. H., 73–74
Vinovskis, Maris A., 3, 4; "Have Social Historians Lost the Civil War?," 3
Virginia, 182
voting rights, 50, 72

Waite, Frederick, 140, 141
Walker, E. P., 77, 96
Walker, Gilbert C., 189
Walker, Mary, 5–6
Walker, William, 81, 108
Walter, Thomas, 207
War before the War, The (Delbanco), 72
War of 1812, 43
Washington, DC, 12, 211–14
Watkins, William H., 95
Webber, Catharine "Caty," 22

INDEX   303

Weekly Anglo-African (publication), 86, 99, 111, 122
Wellington rescue, 72, 76, 80, 90, 114, 244
Wells, Horace, 188–89
Wesleyan Methodist Convention, 156
West, Earle, 161
Western Citizen (publication), 52
Western Female Seminary, 165
Western Reserve Medical School, 140, 141, 143–44
"What Is It?" exhibit, 117
Whiting, W. E., 166
Whitney, Eli, 20
Williams, David, 26
Williams, George, 26, 41
Williams, James, 34

Windsor, ON, 122
Wise, Henry A., 88
women physicians, 5
work crew, 224
Working Cures (Fett), 10–11
Worthington, Albert, 222, 249
Worthington, Clara, 165, 167
Worthington, Elizabeth. *See* Harris, Elizabeth Worthington
Worthington family, 165

yellow fever, 3, 8, 180, 181, 185
Yellow Fever and the South (Humphreys), 3, 8

Zakrzewska, Marie, 139
Zouave people, 96